Principles of Immunology

Principles of Immunology

Joffrey Butler

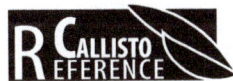

www.callistoreference.com

Callisto Reference,
118-35 Queens Blvd., Suite 400,
Forest Hills, NY 11375, USA

Visit us on the World Wide Web at:
www.callistoreference.com

ISBN: 978-1-64116-551-8 (Hardback)

Cataloging-in-Publication Data

Principles of immunology / Joffrey Butler.
    p. cm.
Includes bibliographical references and index.
ISBN 978-1-64116-551-8
1. Immunology. 2. Serology. 3. Molecular immunology. I. Butler, Joffrey.
QR181 .P75 2022
571.96--dc23

Table of Contents

Preface

Immunology is a domain of biology that is concerned with the study of immune systems in different organisms. It is involved in measuring and contextualizing the physiological functioning of the immune system in both healthy and diseased state. It also studies the malfunctions of the immune system during immunological disorders as well as the chemical, physical and physiological characteristics of the constituents of immune system. There are various fields of immunology such as classical immunology, clinical immunology, developmental immunology, diagnostic immunology, reproductive immunology and theoretical immunology. It plays a vital role in diverse fields of medicine such as organ transplantation, oncology, rheumatology, bacteriology, parasitology, virology, psychiatry and dermatology. This textbook provides comprehensive insights into the field of immunology. Some of the diverse topics covered herein address the varied branches that fall under this category. Those in search of information to further their knowledge will be greatly assisted by this book.

A foreword of all Chapters of the book is provided below:

Chapter 1 - The defense system of organisms which is responsible for providing protection against diseases is termed as the immune system. Its two major sub-types are innate immune system and adaptive immune system. This chapter provides a brief introduction to these types of immune systems.; **Chapter 2** - The protein which is used by the immune system for neutralizing various pathogens is known as an antibody. The structures which are bound by antibodies are known as antigens. The set of genes which are integral for the recognition of foreign molecules by the acquired immune system is termed as major histocompatibility complex. This chapter discusses in detail the concepts related to antigens, antibodies and major histocompatibility complex.; **Chapter 3** - The lymphocytes which develop in the thymus gland and are vital for the immune response in organisms are known as T cells. B cells refer to a type of white blood cells which belong to the subtype lymphocyte. This chapter closely examines the key concepts of B cells and T cells such as their development and activation to provide an extensive understanding of the subject.; **Chapter 4** - The body's response when antigens activate the immune system is known as the immune response. The process of fortifying an individual's immune system with respect to a particular agent is termed as the immunization. This chapter has been carefully written to provide an easy understanding of the varied facets of immune responses and immunization as well as the immunology of vaccination.; **Chapter 5** - The state where the ability of the immune system to fight infectious diseases or cancer is reduced or completely absent is called immunodeficiency. Immunosuppression refers to the reduction of the activation of the immune system. The network of immune responses of an organism against its own healthy tissues and cells is termed as autoimmunity. The diverse aspects of immunodeficiency, immunosuppression and autoimmunity have been thoroughly discussed in this chapter;

I would like to thank the entire editorial team who made sincere efforts for this book and my family who supported me in my efforts of working on this book. I take this opportunity to thank all those who have been a guiding force throughout my life.

Joffrey Butler

Chapter 1

Understanding the Immune System

The defense system of organisms which is responsible for providing protection against diseases is termed as the immune system. Its two major sub-types are innate immune system and adaptive immune system. This chapter provides a brief introduction to these types of immune systems.

The immune system, which is made up of special cells, proteins, tissues, and organs, defends people against germs and microorganisms every day. In most cases, the immune system does a great job of keeping people healthy and preventing infections. But sometimes problems with the immune system can lead to illness and infection. The immune system is the body's defence against infectious organisms and other invaders. Through a series of steps called the immune response, the immune system attacks organisms and substances that invade body systems and cause disease.

The immune system is made up of a network of cells, tissues, and organs that work together to protect the body. One of the important cells involved are white blood cells, also called leukocytes, which come in two basic types that combine to seek out and destroy disease-causing organisms or substances.

Leukocytes are produced or stored in many locations in the body, including the thymus, spleen, and bone marrow. For this reason, they're called the lymphoid organs. There are also clumps of lymphoid tissue throughout the body, primarily as lymph nodes, that house the leukocytes. The leukocytes circulate through the body between the organs and nodes via lymphatic vessels and blood vessels. In this way, the immune system works in a coordinated manner to monitor the body for germs or substances that might cause problems.

The two basic types of leukocytes are:

1. Phagocytes, cells that chew up invading organisms.

2. Lymphocytes, cells that allow the body to remember and recognize previous invaders and help the body destroy them.

A number of different cells are considered phagocytes. The most common type is the neutrophil, which primarily fights bacteria. If doctors are worried about a bacterial infection, they might order a blood test to see if a patient has an increased number of neutrophils triggered by the infection. Other types of phagocytes have their own jobs to make sure that the body responds appropriately to a specific type of invader.

The two kinds of lymphocytes are B lymphocytes and T lymphocytes. Lymphocytes start out in the bone marrow and either stays there and mature into B cells, or they leave for the thymus gland, where they mature into T cells. B lymphocytes and T lymphocytes have separate functions: B lymphocytes are like the body's military intelligence system, seeking out their targets and sending defenses to lock onto them. T cells are like the soldiers, destroying the invaders that the intelligence system has identified.

When antigens (foreign substances that invade the body) are detected, several types of cells work together to recognize them and respond. These cells trigger the B lymphocytes to produce antibodies, which are specialized proteins that lock onto specific antigens.

Once produced, these antibodies stay in a person's body, so that if his or her immune system encounters that antigen again, the antibodies are already there to do their job. So if someone gets sick with a certain disease, like chickenpox, that person usually won't get sick from it again.

This is also how immunizations prevent certain diseases. An immunization introduces the body to an antigen in a way that doesn't make someone sick, but does allow the body to produce antibodies that will then protect the person from future attack by the germ or substance that produces that particular disease.

Although antibodies can recognize an antigen and lock onto it, they are not capable of destroying it without help. That's the job of the T cells, which are part of the system that destroys antigens that have been tagged by antibodies or cells that have been infected or somehow changed. (Some T cells are actually called "killer cells.") T cells also are involved in helping signal other cells (like phagocytes) to do their jobs.

Antibodies also can neutralize toxins (poisonous or damaging substances) produced by different organisms. Lastly, antibodies can activate a group of proteins called complement that are also part of the immune system. Complement assists in killing bacteria, viruses, or infected cells. All of these specialized cells and parts of the immune system offer the body protection against disease. This protection is called immunity.

Immunity

Humans have three types of immunity — innate, adaptive and passive:

Innate Immunity

Everyone is born with innate (or natural) immunity, a type of general protection. Many of the germs that affect other species don't harm us. For example, the viruses that cause leukemia in cats or distemper in dogs don't affect humans. Innate immunity works both ways because some viruses that make humans ill — such as the virus that causes HIV/AIDS — don't make cats or dogs sick.

Innate immunity also includes the external barriers of the body, like the skin and mucous membranes (like those that line the nose, throat, and gastrointestinal tract), which are the first line of defense in preventing diseases from entering the body. If this outer defensive wall is broken (as through a cut), the skin attempts to heal the break quickly and special immune cells on the skin attack invading germs.

Adaptive Immunity

The second kind of protection is adaptive (or active) immunity, which develops throughout our lives. Adaptive immunity involves the lymphocytes and develops as people are exposed to diseases or immunized against diseases through vaccination.

Passive Immunity

Passive immunity is "borrowed" from another source and it lasts for a short time. For example, antibodies in a mother's breast milk give a baby temporary immunity to diseases the mother has been exposed to. This can help protect the baby against infection during the early years of childhood.

Everyone's immune system is different. Some people never seem to get infections, whereas others seem to be sick all the time. As people get older, they usually become immune to more germs as the immune system comes into contact with more and more of them. That's why adults and teens tend to get fewer colds than kids — their bodies have learned to recognize and immediately attack many of the viruses that cause colds.

Problems of the Immune System

Disorders of the immune system fall into four main categories:

- Immunodeficiency disorders (primary or acquired).

- Autoimmune disorders (in which the body's own immune system attacks its own tissue as foreign matter).

- Allergic disorders (in which the immune system overreacts in response to an antigen).

- Cancers of the immune system.

Immunodeficiency Disorders

Immunodeficiencies happen when a part of the immune system is missing or not working properly. Some people are born with an immunodeficiency (known as primary immunodeficiencies), although symptoms of the disorder might not appear until later in life. Immunodeficiencies also can be acquired through infection or produced by drugs (these are sometimes called secondary immunodeficiencies).

Immunodeficiencies can affect B lymphocytes, T lymphocytes, or phagocytes. Examples of primary immunodeficiencies that can affect kids and teens are:

- IgA deficiency is the most common immunodeficiency disorder. IgA is an immunoglobulin that is found primarily in the saliva and other body fluids that help guard the entrances to the body. IgA deficiency is a disorder in which the body doesn't produce enough of the antibody IgA. People with IgA deficiency tend to have allergies or get more colds and other respiratory infections, but the condition is usually not severe.

- Severe combined immunodeficiency (SCID) is also known as the "bubble boy disease" after a Texas boy with SCID who lived in a germ-free plastic bubble. SCID is a serious immune system disorder that occurs because of a lack of both B and T lymphocytes, which makes it almost impossible to fight infections.

- DiGeorge syndrome (thymic dysplasia), a birth defect in which kids are born without a thymus gland, is an example of a primary T-lymphocyte disease. The thymus gland is where T lymphocytes normally mature.

- Chediak-Higashi syndrome and chronic granulomatous disease (CGD) both involve the inability of the neutrophils to function normally as phagocytes.

Acquired (or secondary) immunodeficiencies usually develop after someone has a disease, although they can also be the result of malnutrition, burns, or other medical problems. Certain medicines also can cause problems with the functioning of the immune system.

Acquired (secondary) immunodeficiencies include:

- HIV (human immunodeficiency virus) infection/AIDS (acquired immunodeficiency syndrome) is a disease that slowly and steadily destroys the immune system. It is caused by HIV, a virus that wipes out certain types of lymphocytes called T-helper cells. Without T-helper cells, the immune system is unable to defend the body against normally harmless organisms, which can cause life-threatening infections in people who have AIDS. Newborns can get HIV infection from their mothers while in the uterus, during the birth process, or during breastfeeding. People can get HIV infection by having unprotected sexual intercourse with an infected person or from sharing contaminated needles for drugs, steroids, or tattoos.

- Immunodeficiencies caused by medications: Some medicines suppress the immune system. One of the drawbacks of chemotherapy treatment for cancer, for example, is that it not only attacks cancer cells, but other fast-growing, healthy cells, including those found in the bone marrow and other parts of the immune system. In addition, people with autoimmune disorders or who have had organ transplants may need to take immunosuppressant medications, which also can reduce the immune system's ability to fight infections and can cause secondary immunodeficiency.

Autoimmune Disorders

In autoimmune disorders, the immune system mistakenly attacks the body's healthy organs and tissues as though they were foreign invaders. Autoimmune diseases include:

- Lupus: A chronic disease marked by muscle and joint pain and inflammation (the abnormal immune response also may involve attacks on the kidneys and other organs).

- Juvenile idiopathic arthritis: A disease in which the body's immune system acts as though certain body parts (such as the joints of the knee, hand, and foot) are foreign tissue and attacks them.

- Scleroderma: A chronic autoimmune disease that can lead to inflammation and damage of the skin, joints, and internal organs.

- Ankylosing spondylitis: A disease that involves inflammation of the spine and joints, causing stiffness and pain.

- Juvenile dermatomyositis: A disorder marked by inflammation and damage of the skin and muscles.

Allergic Disorders

Allergic disorders happen when the immune system overreacts to exposure to antigens in the environment. The substances that provoke such attacks are called allergens. The immune response can cause symptoms such as swelling, watery eyes, and sneezing, and even a life-threatening reaction called anaphylaxis. Medicines called antihistamines can relieve most symptoms.

Allergic disorders include:

- Asthma, a respiratory disorder that can cause breathing problems, often involves an allergic response by the lungs. If the lungs are oversensitive to certain allergens (like pollen, molds, animal dander, or dust mites), breathing tubes can become narrowed and swollen, making it hard for a person to breathe.

- Eczema is an itchy rash also known as atopic dermatitis. Although not necessarily caused by an allergic reaction, eczema most often happens in kids and teens who have allergies, hay fever, or asthma or who have a family history of these conditions.

- Allergies of several types can affect kids and teens. Environmental allergies (to dust mites, for example), seasonal allergies (such as hay fever), drug allergies (reactions to specific medications or drugs), food allergies (such as to nuts), and allergies to toxins (bee stings, for example) are the common conditions people usually refer to as allergies.

Cancers of the Immune System

Cancer happens when cells grow out of control. This can include cells of the immune system. Leukemia, which involves abnormal overgrowth of leukocytes, is the most common childhood cancer. Lymphoma involves the lymphoid tissues and is also one of the more common childhood cancers. With current treatments, most cases of both types of cancer in kids and teens are curable.

Cells and Organs of the Immune System

Specific as well as non-specific immunity is maintained in the body the lymphoreticular system that is a complex organization of cells of diverse morphology and distributed widely in different parts of the body. Lymphoreticular cells include reticuloendothelial cells and lymphoid cells.

Reticuloendothelial System

The reticuloendothelial system mainly comprise of phagocytic cells whose function is to engulf microbes, immune complex from blood and tissues and participate in inflammation. This way they contribute to non-specific immunity. These cells also participate in specific immunity by way of antigen presentation and cytokine secretions. The role of phagocytes was highlighted by Elie Metchnikoff. The deficiency of phagocytic system can lead to disorders such as Chronic Granulomatous

Disease.

The major phagocytic cells are:

- Polymorphonuclear leucocytes (PMNLs), also called neutrophils, microphages.

- Blood and tissue monocytes.

They both are derived from the bone marrow during hematopoiesis.

Neutrophils have short life span - They circulate in the blood for 6-7 hours, then migrate through the endothelial cell junctions and reside in tissue spaces where they live only for few days and do not multiply. Neutrophils are the most abundant of the leukocytes, normally accounting for 54-75% of the WBCs. An adult typically has 3,000-7,500 neutrophils/mm^3 of blood but the number may increase two- to three-fold during active infections. Adult body usually produces 10^{11} neutrophils per day. Some neutrophils may remain attached to endothelial lining of large veins and can be mobilised during inflammation. The nucleus of a neutrophil is segmented into 3-5 connected lobes, hence the name polymorphonuclear leukocyte. They are called neutrophils because their granules stain poorly with the mixture of dyes used in staining leukocytes. Because of the granules, they are considered as one of the granulocytes. There are two types of granules, the specific granules and azurophilic granules. Specific granules are present in abundance and contain proteolytic enzymes such as lysozyme, collagenase and elastase. They stain neither with acidic nor basic dyes. The azurophilic granules are actually lysosomes.

Monocytes have rounded or kidney-shaped nuclei with finely granular cytoplasm measure 12-15 µm and have half-life of 3 days in circulation. Monocytes normally make up 2-8% of the WBCs (100-500/mm^3 of blood). Once monocytes leave circulation and enter tissue, they are called macrophages. There are two types of macrophages, one that wander in the tissue spaces and the other that are fixed to vascular endothelium of liver, spleen, lymph node and other tissue. Tissue macrophages survive for months and can multiply. Macrophages present in different organs have been given different names. They are Histiocytes (in tissue), Kupffer cells (in liver), Alveolar macrophages (in lungs), Peritoneal macrophages (in peritoneum), Microglial cells (in brain), Mesangial cells (in kidneys) and Osteoclasts (in bone). Some macrophages develop abundant cytoplasm and are called epitheloid cells. Macrophages can fuse to form multi-nucleated giant cells. Some mononuclear cells differentiate into dendritic cells. Functions of macrophage include killing of microbes, infected cells, and tumor cells, secretion of immunomodulatory cytokines, antigen processing and presentation to T cells. Macrophages respond to infections as quickly as neutrophils but persist much longer; hence they are dominant effector cells in the later stage of infection.

Microbial Killing by Phagocytes

Phagocytosis involves two steps namely attachment and ingestion. Following attachment of the organism, invagination of the phagocyte results in the formation of a phagosome. Some capsulated bacteria don't attach to the phagocyte, but they can still be phagocytosed if they are coated with opsonins such as IgG and complement component (C3b). The engulfed bacteria are held inside a vacuole called phagosome. The formation of phagosome triggers respiratory bursts and fusion of lysosome with phagosome to form phagolysosome.

The phagocytes appear to kill engulfed bacteria by two pathways, oxygen independent pathway and oxygen dependent pathway. The microbicidal mechanisms of the respiratory burst are termed oxygen dependent and phagolysosome formations are termed oxygen independent.

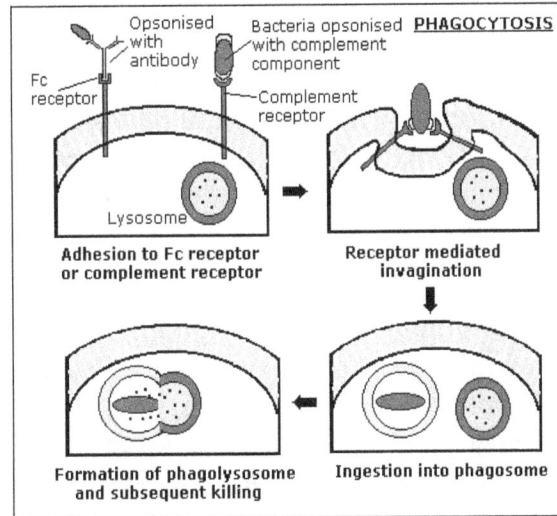

Phagocytosis

Oxygen dependent mechanism involves catalytic conversion of molecular oxygen to oxyhalide free radicals, which are highly reactive oxidizing agents. The phagocyte oxidase present in the plasma membrane and phagolysosome reduce oxygen into reactive oxygen intermediates such as superoxide radicals. Superoxide is converted to H_2O_2, which is used by enzyme myeloperoxidase to convert unreactive halide ions to reactive hypohalous acids that are toxic to bacteria.

Oxygen independent mechanism involves release of lysosomal contents into phagolysosomes. The content of lysosome includes lactoferrin, cathepsin G, lysozyme and defensins etc.

In addition to the phagocyte oxidase system, macrophages have free-radical generating system, namely inducible nitric oxide synthase. This cytosolic enzyme is absent in resting macrophages but can be induced in response to bacterial lipopolysaccharides and IFN-γ. This enzyme catalyses the conversion of arginine to citrulline, and in the process releases nitric oxide gas. Nitric oxide may then combine with H_2O_2 or superoxide to form highly reactive peroxynitrite radicals that kill the microbes.

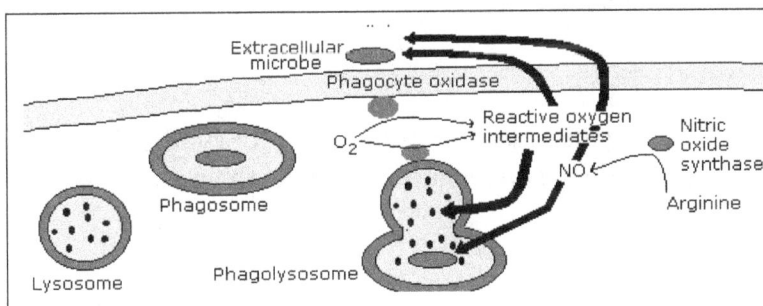

Dendritic Cells

These cells are derived from myeloid progenitor in the bone marrow and are morphologically identified by spiny membranous projection on their surfaces. Immature dendritic cells are located in epithelia of skin, gastrointestinal tract and respiratory tract and are called langerhan cells. They express low levels of MHC proteins on their surface and their main function is to capture and transport protein antigen to the draining lymph node. During their migration to the lymph node, dendritic cells mature into excellent antigen presenting cells (APC). Mature dendritic cells reside in the T cell area (paracortex) of the lymph node. Here, they are referred as interdigitating dendritic cells. These cells are distinct from the dendritic cells that occur in the germinal centers of lymphoid follicles (follicular dendritic cells) in lymph node, spleen and MALT. The follicular dendritic cells are not derived from the bone marrow and their role is to present antigen-antibody complex and complement products to B cell.

Lymphoid System

Lymphoid organs are stationed throughout the body and are concerned with the growth, development and deployment of lymphocytes. These structurally and functionally diverse lymphoid organs and tissues are interconnected by the blood vessels and lymphatic vessels through which lymphocytes circulate. The organs involved in specific as well as non-specific immunity are classified as primary (central) lymphoid organs and secondary (peripheral) lymphoid organs. The blood and lymphatic vessels that carry lymphocytes to and from the other structures can also be considered lymphoid organs. Recently, it has become accepted that the liver is also a hematopoietic organ, giving rise to all leukocyte lineages.

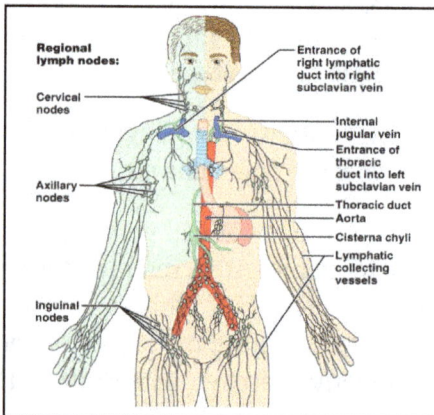

Overview of Lymphatic System.

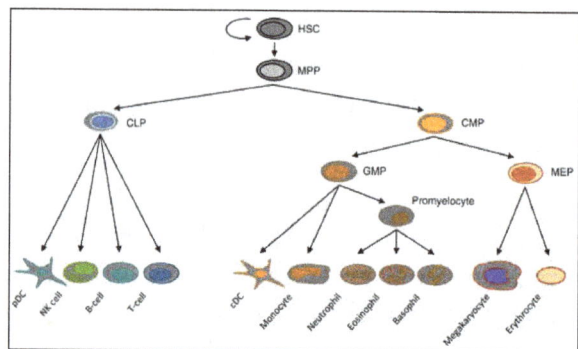

Overview of Hematopoiesis

Primary Lymphoid Organs

Also called central lymphoid organs, these are responsible for synthesis and maturation of immunocompetant cells. These include the bone marrow and the thymus.

Bone Marrow

All the cells of the immune system are initially derived from the bone marrow through a process called hematopoiesis. During foetal development hematopoiesis occurs initially in yolk sac and para-aortic mesenchyme and later in the liver and spleen. This function is taken over gradually by the bone marrow. During hematopoiesis, bone marrow-derived stem cells differentiate into either mature cells or into precursors of cells that migrate out of the bone marrow to continue their maturation in thymus.

The bone marrow produces B cells, natural killer cells, granulocytes and immature thymocytes, in addition to red blood cells and platelets. It is both a primary and secondary lymphoid organ. The proliferation and maturation of precursor cells in the bone marrow are stimulated by cytokines, many of which are called colony stimulating factors (CSFs). The bone marrow also contains antibody secreting plasma cells, which have migrated from the peripheral lymphoid tissue.

Thymus

The thymus is a gland located in the anterior mediastinum just above the heart, which reaches its greatest size just prior to birth, then atrophies with age. This lymphoepithelial organ develops from ectoderm derived from the third branchial cleft and endoderm of the third branchial pouch.

Immature lymphocytes begin to accumulate in the thymus of human embryos at about 90-100 days after fertilization. Initially most of these immature lymphocytes have come from the yolk sac and fetal liver rather than the bone marrow. Cells from the bone marrow later migrate to the thymus as precursors and develop into mature peripheral T cells. Once the immature lymphocytes have passed the blood-thymus barrier they are called thymocytes. Mature T cells migrate from the thymus to secondary lymphoid organs such as lymph node, Peyer's patches and spleen.

Ultimately the thymus becomes an encapsulated and consists of many lobes, each divided into an outer cortical region and an inner medulla. The cortex contains mostly immature thymocytes, some of which mature and migrate to the medulla, where they learn to discriminate between self and non-self during foetal development and for a short time after birth. T cells leave the medulla to enter the peripheral blood circulation, through which they are transported to the secondary lymphoid organs. About 98% of all T cells die in the thymus.

The greatest rate of T cell production occurs before puberty. After puberty, the thymus shrinks and the production of new T cells in the adult thymus drops away. Children with no development of thymus suffer from DiGeorge syndrome that is characterized by deficiency in T cell development but normal numbers of B cells.

Peripheral Lymphoid Organs

While primary lymphoid organs are concerned with production and maturation of lymphoid cells, the secondary or peripheral lymphoid organs are sites where the lymphocytes localise, recognise foreign antigen and mount response against it. These include the lymph nodes, spleen, tonsils, adenoids, appendix, and clumps of lymphoid tissue in the small intestine known as Peyer's patches. They trap and concentrate foreign substances, and they are the main sites of production of antibodies.

Some lymphoid organs are capsulated such as lymph node and spleen while others are non-capsulated, which include mostly mucosa-associated lymphoid tissue (MALT).

Lymph Node

Clusters of lymph nodes are strategically placed in the neck, axillae, groin, mediastinum and abdominal cavity, where they filter antigens from the interstitial tissue fluid and the lymph during its passage from the periphery to the thoracic duct. The key lymph nodes are the axillary lymph nodes, the inguinal lymph nodes, the mesenteric lymph nodes and the cervical lymph nodes. Lymph nodes that protect the skin are termed somatic nodes, while deep lymph nodes protecting the respiratory, digestive and genitourinary tracts are termed visceral nodes. Each lymph node is surrounded by a fibrous capsule that is pierced by numerous afferent lymphatics that drain lymph into marginal sinus. The lymph flows through the medullary sinus and leaves through efferent lymphatics. Each lymph node is divided into an outer cortex, inner medulla and intervening paracortical region. The cortex is also referred as B cell area, which mainly consists of B cells. The cortex is a high traffic zone where recirculating T- and B lymphocytes enter from the blood. Aggregates of cells called follicles are present in the cortex, which in turn may have central areas called germinal centers. Follicles without germinal centers are called primary follicles and those with germinal centers are called secondary follicles. Primary follicles are rich in mature but resting B cells. Germinal centers develop in response to antigenic stimulation and consist of follicular dendritic cells and reactive B cells. The medulla contains a mixture of B cells, T cells, plasma cells and macrophages. The medulla consists of medullary cords that lead to the medullary sinus. The cords are populated by plasma cells and macrophages. Between these two zones, lie the paracotex (T cell area) that contains T lymphocytes, dendritic cells and mononuclear phagocytes. Most of the T cells (70%) located there are CD4+ helper cells.

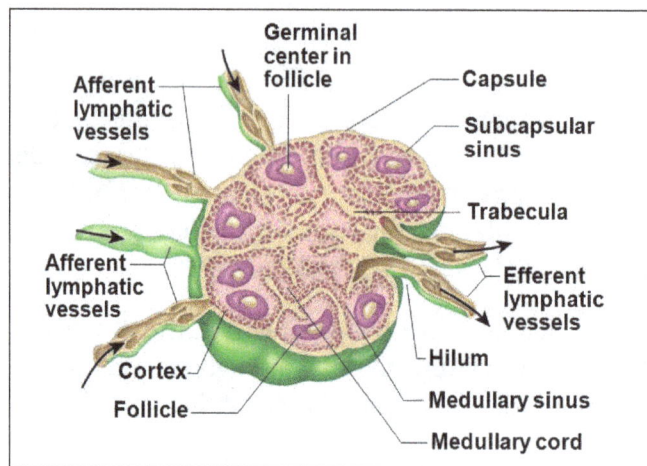

Structure of a Lymph Node.

Spleen

Situated in the left upper quadrant of the abdomen and weighing about 150 grams, spleen is the largest single lymphoid organ in the body. It has a dense fibrous capsule with muscular trabeculae extending inward to subdivide the spleen into lobules. It filters blood and is the major organ in which antibodies are synthesized and released into circulation. In addition to capturing foreign antigens from the blood that passes through the spleen, migratory macrophages and dendritic cells also bring antigens to the spleen via the bloodstream. Persons lacking spleen (e.g. splenectomy) are highly susceptible to infections with capsulated bacteria such as pneumococci and meningococci.

Spleen is the major site for phagocytosis of antibody coated bacteria and destruction of aged RBCs.

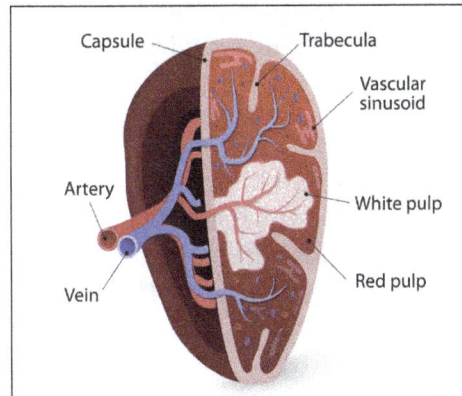

Spleen

It is supplied by splenic artery, which pierces the capsule at hilum and divides into smaller branches that are surrounded by fibrous trabeculae. The spleen is composed of two types of tissue, the red pulp and the white pulp. The red pulp contains vascular sinusoids, large number of erythrocytes, resident macrophages, dendritic cells, granulocytes, few plasma cells and lymphocytes. It is the site where aged platelets and erythrocytes are destroyed. The white pulp contains the lymphoid tissue clustered around small arterioles and is known as a periarteriolar lymphoid sheath (PALS). PALS contain mainly T lymphocytes, about 75% of which are CD4+ helper T cells. Attached to this are lymphoid follicles, some of which contain germinal centers. Follicles and germinal center predominantly contain B cells. The PALS and follicles are surrounded by rim of lymphocytes and macrophages, called marginal zone. Marginal zone is composed of macrophages, B cells, and CD4+ helper T cells. The arterioles end in vascular sinusoids in the red pulp, which in turn end in venules that drain into splenic vein. Antigens and lymphocytes enter the spleen through vascular sinusoids. Activation of B cells occurs at the juncton between follicle and PALS. Activated B cells then migrate to the germinal centers or into the red pulp.

Mucosa associated Lymphoid Tissue (Malt)

Approximately >50% of lymphoid tissue in the body is found associated with the mucosal system. MALT is composed of gut-associated lymphoid tissues (GALT) lining the intestinal tract, bronchus-associated lymphoid tissue (BALT) lining the respiratory tract, and lymphoid tissue lining the genitourinary tract. The respiratory, alimentary and genitourinary tracts are guarded by subepithelial accumulations of lymphoid tissue that are not covered by connective tissue capsule. They may occur as diffuse collections of lymphocytes, plasma cells and phagocytes throughout the lung and lamina propria of intestine or as clearly organised tissue with well-formed lymphoid follicles. The well-formed follicles include the tonsils (lingual, palatine and pharyngeal), Peyer's patches in the intestine and appendix. The major function of these organs is to provide local immunity by way of sIgA (also IgE) production. Diffuse accumulations of lymphoid tissue are seen in the lamina propria of the intestinal wall. The intestinal epithelium overlying the Peyer's patches is specialized to allow the transport of antigens into the lymphoid tissue. This function is carried out by cuboidal absorptive epithelial cells termed "M" cells, so called because they have numerous microfolds on their luminal surface. M cells endocytose, transport and present antigens to subepithelial lymphoid cells.

Majority of intra-epithelial lymphocytes are T cells, and most often CD8+ lymphocytes. The intestinal lamina propria contains CD4+ lymphocytes, large number of B cells, plasma cells, macrophages, dendritic cells, eosinophils and mast cells. Peyer's patches contain both B cells and CD4+ T cells.

Lymphocytes

Lymphocytes are stem cells derived cells that mature either in the bone marrow or thymus. Together, the thymus and marrow bone marrow produce approximately 10^9 mature lymphocytes each day and the adult human body contains approximately 10^{12} lymphocytes. Lymphocytes comprise 20-40% (1000 - 4000 cells/μl) of all leukocytes. The lymphocytes are distributed to blood, lymph and lymphoid organs.

Typically, lymphocyte is small, round, cell with diameter of 5-10μm, spherical nucleus, densely compacted nuclear chromatin and scanty cytoplasm. Though the cytoplasm contains mitochondria and ribosomes, other organelles are not detectable. Such mature but resting lymphocytes are known as naïve cells. They are mitotically inactive but when stimulated can undergo cell division. Naïve lymphocytes have a short life span and die in few days after leaving bone marrow or thymus unless they are stimulated. Once the lymphocyte is activated (stimulated), they become large (10-12μm), have more cytoplasm and more organelles. Activated lymphocytes may undergo several successive rounds of cell division over a period of several days. Some of the progeny cells revert to the resting stage and become memory cells, but can survive for several years in the absence of any antigenic stimulus.

There are three major types of lymphocyte, B lymphocyte, T lymphocyte and NK cells. Different lymphocytes are identified by certain protein markers on their surface called "cluster of differentiation" or "CD" system. One marker that all leukocytes have in common is CD45. The presence of the markers can be detected using specific monoclonal antibodies.

Distribution of Lymphocytes

	Approximate %		
Tissue	T-Cells	B-Cells	NK Cells
Peripheral blood	70-80	10-15	10-15
Bone marrow	5-10	80-90	5-10
Thymus	99	<1	<1
Lymph node	70-80	20-30	<1
Spleen	30-40	50-60	1-5

B Lymphocyte

Also called B-cells, they are so called because in birds they were found to mature in bursa of fabricius. Humans don't have an anatomical equivalent to bursa, but the development and maturation of these cells occur in bone marrow.

Ontogeny

In mammals, the early stages of B cell maturation occur in the fetal liver and bone marrow. B cell development begins in the fetal liver and continues in the bone marrow throughout life.

The stages in B cell development in the bone marrow are:

Stem cell > pro-B cell > pre-B cell > small pre-B cell > immature B cell > mature B cell.

Distribution

They account for 5-15% of lymphocytes (250 cells/µl) in circulation and 80-90% in bone marrow, 20-30% in lymph node and 50-60% in spleen.

Surface Markers

The most important surface marker on the surface of mature B cell is the surface immunoglobulin. The surface immunoglobulins are of IgM and IgD type. A B cell will have approximately 10^9 immunoglubulins of single specificity on its surface. Markers/Receptors on B cells are Surface Immunoglobulin (IgM and IgD), CD40, B7, ICAM-1, LFA-1, MHC II, CD32 (Ig Fc receptor), CD35 (Receptor for complement component) and additional markers that distinguish B cells such as CD19, CD20, CD21 and CD22.

Demonstration of B Cells

EAC (Erythrocyte Amboceptor Complement) Rosettes: When sheep RBCs coated with antibody and treated with complement and B cells, a rosette is formed due to the presence of complement receptor on B cells. B cells can be demonstrated by immunofluorescence with fluorescent-labelled monoclonal antibodies against surface markers such as surface immunoglobulin.

On stimulation by pokeweed mitogen, they undergo blast transformation.

Functions of B-cells

Direct antigen recognition and Antigen presentation B cells may differentiate into plasma cells (which secrete large amounts of antibodies) or into memory B cells. Memory cells can survive 20 years or more.

Plasma Cells

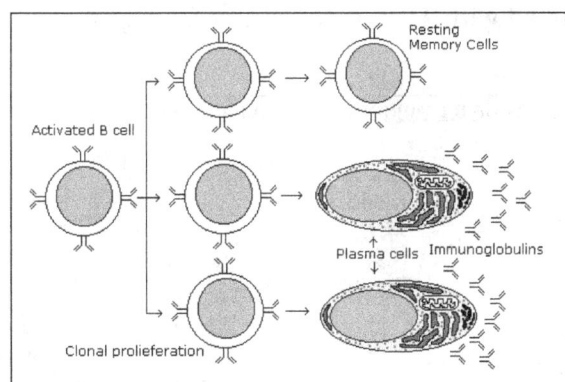

These are the effector cells of the B-cell lineage and are specialised in secreting immunoglobulins. When activated B cells divide, some of its progeny become memory cells and the reminder become immunoglobulin-secreting plasma cells. Plasma cells are oval or egg shaped, have eccentrically placed nuclei, have abundant cytoplasm containing dense rough endoplasmic reticulum (the site of antibody production), perinuclear Golgi body (where immunoglobulins are converted to final form and packaged). Unlike B cells, immunoglobulins are not present on the surface of plasma cells. They have a short life span of few days to few weeks.

T Lymphocyte

Ontogeny

The name "T-cell" is an abbreviation of "thymus dependent lymphocyte". T lymphocytes arise in the bone marrow as T-cell precursors, then migrate to and mature in the thymus. After entry into the thymus T-cell precursors are also referred to as "thymocytes".

In the thymus there are rearrangements at gene segments coding for the variable part of the TCR (T Cell Receptor) resulting in generation of diversity. T Cell Receptors are then expressed on the surface, which is followed by expression of either CD8 or CD4 surface molecules. Those cells expressing receptors that can interact with self MHC molecules are positively selected while those cells that express receptors that recognize peptides derived from self-protein in association with self MHC are negatively selected. Such cells undergo clonal deletion or anergy.

Distribution

T cell accounts for 70-80% (1500 cells/µl) lymphocytes in peripheral blood, 5-10% in bone marrow, 70-80% in lymph node and 30-40% in spleen.

Surface Markers

The most important surface receptor is TCR. TCR are polypeptides that belong to the immuno-globulin superfamily. There are two kinds of TCR, one composed of a α-β heterodimer (TCR2) and the other composed of a γ-δ heterodimer (TCR1). An individual T cell can express either α-β or γ-δ as its receptor but never both. 95% of T cells express the α-β heterodimer. The other markers/receptors present on the surface are IL-2R, IL-1R, CD2, CD3, CD4/CD8, CD28, ICAM-1 and LFA-1. Nearly all the mature T lymphocytes express both CD2 and CD3 on their surface. CD3, which is always found closely associated with TCR, is necessary for signal transduction following antigen recognition by the TCR.

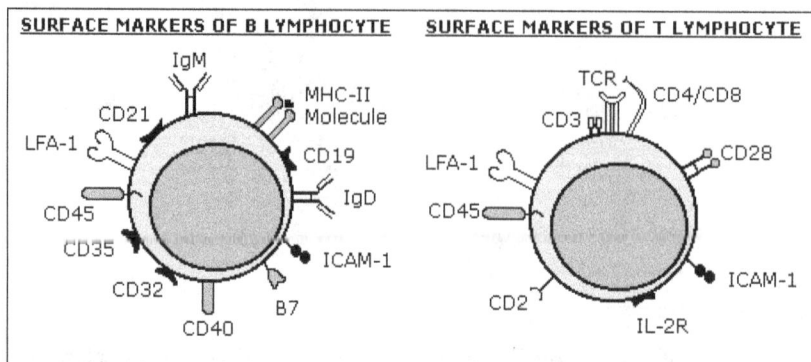

Surface markers of B Lymphocyte (Left) and Surface markers of T Lymphocyte (Right).

Subsets of T Cells

There are two major types of T cells, Helper (CD4) and Cytotoxic/Suppressor (CD8) T cells. CD4 cells account for 45% (900/µl) of lymphocytes while CD8 cells account for 30% (600/µl).

- Helper T cells (T_H) secrete cytokines that promote the proliferation and differentiation of cytotoxic T cells, B cells and macrophages and activation of inflammatory leukocytes. T_H cells are identified by the presence of the CD4 marker. They recognize antigen when presented along with Class II MHC molecules. T_H cells are further subdivided into the T_{H1} and T_{H2} subsets on the basis of the kinds of cytokines they produce. T_{H1} cells produce interleukin-2 (IL-2), interferon-gamma (IFNγ), and tumour necrosis factor-beta (TNF-β) while T_{H2} cells produce IL-4, IL-5, IL-6, IL-10 and TGF-β.

- Cytotoxic T cells (T_C) lyse cells with foreign antigens, e.g. tumour cells, virus-infected cells, and foreign tissue grafts. T_C cells are identified by the presence of the CD8 marker. They recognize antigen presented when presented along with Class I MHC molecules. The suppressor T cells have a role in downregulation of immune response.

Demonstration of T Cells

- T cells can be demonstrated by immunofluorescence using fluorescent-labelled monoclonal antibodies against TCR or other surface markers.

- E-Rosette/SRBC rosette: T cells bind to sheep RBCs at 37 °C forming rosettes.

- They undergo blast transformation on treatment with mitogens such as phytohemagglutinin (PHA) or Concanavalin A.

Functions of Helper T-cells (TH)

- Promotes differentiation of B-cells and cytotoxic T-cells.

- Activates macrophages.

Functions of Cytotoxic/Suppressor T-cells (CTL)

- Kills cells expressing appropriate antigen.

- Down regulates the activities of other cells.

NK Cells (Large Granular Lymphocytes)

Also called Large Granular Lymphocytes (LGLs), these are large lymphocytes containing azurophilic granules in the cytoplasm. NK cells derive form bone marrow but don't require thymus for development. NK cells are so called because they kill variety of target cells (such as tumour cells, virus-infected cells, and transplanted cells) without the participation of MHC molecules. They can kill target cell without a need for activation unlike cytotoxic T lymphocytes. Hence they mediate a form of natural (innate) immunity.

Distribution

They account for 10-15% of blood lymphocytes. They are rare in lymph nodes and don't circulate through lymph.

Surface Markers

NK cells lack any surface immunoglobulins, TCR or CD4 makers; instead they have CD16 (Immunoglobulin Fc receptor) and CD56. Approximately 50% of human NK cells express only one form of CD8. Other receptors include IL-2R, CD2, ICAM-1 and LFA-1.

Functions

NK cells are activated by recognition of antibody-coated cells, virus infected cell, cell infected with intracellular bacteria and cells lacking MHC I proteins. Activation of NK cell results in cytolysis of target and cytokine secretion but no clonal expansion. Interestingly, NK cells are inhibited on contact with MHC I proteins. NK cells can kill antibody-coated target cells, which is mediated through Fc receptor present on its surface. This is called antibody-dependent cell cytotoxicity (ADCC).

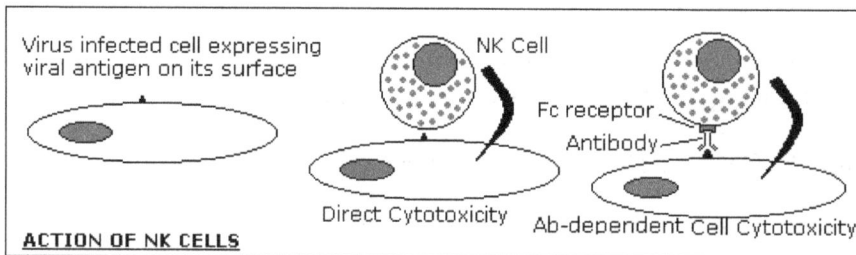

Active of NK Cells.

NK cells also participate in Graft vs. Host reaction in recipient of bone marrow transplants. NK cells can be activated by IL-2 so that their cytotoxic capacity is enhanced. Such cells are called Lymphokine Activated Killer cells (LAK) and have been used clinically to treat tumours. LAK cells have enhanced cytolytic activity and are effective against wide range of tumour cells. Activated NK cells produce cytokines such as IFN-γ, TNFα, GM-CSF and CSF-1 all of which are immunomodulators.

Lymphocte Recirculation

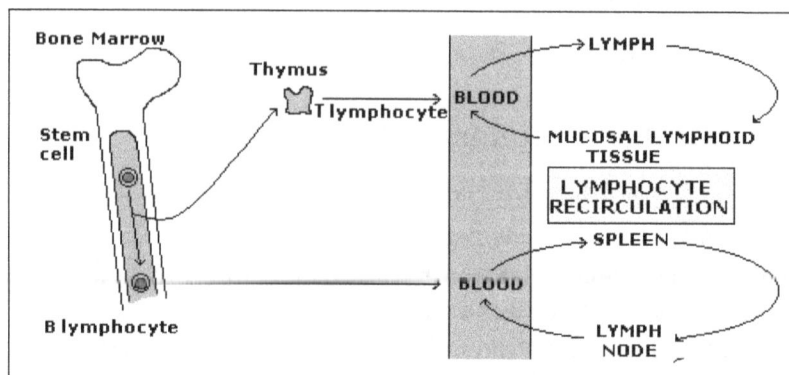

The movement of lymphocytes via the blood stream and lymphatics from peripheral tissue to another is called lymphocyte recirculation. Lymphocytes are migratory cells; mature lymphocytes continually migrate in and out of all peripheral lymphoid tissue. At an average each cell changes location once or twice each day. At any given point of time 1-2% of lymphocytes will be in transit. In most lymphoid organs, they enter through blood and exit through lymphatics, but in spleen they enter and leave directly through blood. As lymphocytes migrate, they can survey the body for foci of infection or presence of foreign antigens. Such a movement also helps to maintain a balance in distribution of lymphocytes in the body.

Innate Immune System

The innate immune system is made of defenses against infection that can be activated immediately once a pathogen attacks. The innate immune system is essentially made up of barriers that aim to keep viruses, bacteria, parasites, and other foreign particles out of your body or limit their ability to spread and move throughout the body. The innate immune system includes:

- Physical Barriers: Such as skin, the gastrointestinal tract, the respiratory tract, the naso-pharynx, cilia, eyelashes and other body hair.

- Defense Mechanisms: Such as secretions, mucous, bile, gastric acid, saliva, tears, and sweat.

- General Immune Responses: Such as inflammation, complement, and non-specific cellular responses. The inflammatory response actively brings immune cells to the site of an infection by increasing blood flow to the area. Complement is an immune response that marks pathogens for destruction and makes holes in the cell membrane of the pathogen.

The innate immune system is always general, or nonspecific, meaning anything that is identified as foreign or non-self is a target for the innate immune response. The innate immune system is activated by the presence of antigens and their chemical properties.

Cells of the Innate Immune System

There are many types of white blood cells or leukocytes that work to defend and protect the human body. In order to patrol the entire body, leukocytes travel by way of the circulatory system.

The following cells are leukocytes of the innate immune system:

- Phagocytes or Phagocytic cells: Phagocyte means "eating cell", which describes what role phagocytes play in the immune response. Phagocytes circulate throughout the body, looking for potential threats, like bacteria and viruses, to engulf and destroy. You can think of phagocytes as security guards on patrol.

- Macrophages: Macrophages, commonly abbreviated as "Mφ", are efficient phagocytic cells that can leave the circulatory system by moving across the walls of capillary vessels. The ability to roam outside of the circulatory system is important, because it allows macrophages to hunt pathogens with fewer limits. Macrophages can also release cytokines in order to signal and recruit other cells to an area with pathogens.

- Mast cells: Mast cells are found in mucous membranes and connective tissues, and are important for wound healing and defense against pathogens via the inflammatory response. When mast cells are activated, they release cytokines and granules that contain chemical molecules to create an inflammatory cascade. Mediators, such as histamine, cause blood vessels to dilate, increasing blood flow and cell trafficking to the area of infection. The cytokines released during this process act as a messenger service, alerting other immune cells, like neutrophils and macrophages, to make their way to the area of infection, or to be on alert for circulating threats.

- Neutrophils: Neutrophils are phagocytic cells that are also classified as granulocytes because they contain granules in their cytoplasm. These granules are very toxic to bacteria and fungi, and cause them to stop proliferating or die on contact.

  The bone marrow of an average healthy adult makes approximately 100 billion new neutrophils per day. Neutrophils are typically the first cells to arrive at the site of an infection because there are so many of them in circulation at any given time.

- Eosinophils: Eosinophils are granulocytes target multicellular parasites. Eosinophils secrete a range of highly toxic proteins and free radicals that kill bacteria and parasites. The use of toxic proteins and free radicals also causes tissue damage during allergic reactions, so activation and toxin release by eosinophils is highly regulated to prevent any unnecessary tissue damage.

  While eosinophils only make up 1-6% of the white blood cells, they are found in many locations, including the thymus, lower gastrointestinal tract, ovaries, uterus, spleen, and lymph nodes.

- Basophils: Basophils are also granulocytes that attack multicellular parasites. Basophils release histamine, much like mast cells. The use of histamine makes basophils and mast cells key players in mounting an allergic response.

- Natural Killer cells: Natural Killer cells (NK cells), do not attack pathogens directly. Instead, natural killer cells destroy infected host cells in order to stop the spread of an infection. Infected or compromised host cells can signal natural kill cells for destruction through the expression of specific receptors and antigen presentation.

- Dendritic cells: Dendritic cells are antigen-presenting cells that are located in tissues, and can contact external environments through the skin, the inner mucosal lining of the nose, lungs, stomach, and intestines. Since dendritic cells are located in tissues that are common points for initial infection, they can identify threats and act as messengers for the rest of the immune system by antigen presentation. Dendritic cells also act as bridge between the innate immune system and the adaptive immune system.

Inflammation

Inflammation happens in everyone, whether you're aware of it or not. Your immune system creates inflammation to protect the body from infection, injury, or disease. There are many things you wouldn't be able to heal from without inflammation.

Sometimes with autoimmune diseases, like certain types of arthritis and inflammatory bowel disease, your immune system attacks healthy cells.

Inflammation is classified into two main types:

- Acute inflammation usually occurs for a short (yet often severe) duration. It often resolves in two weeks or less. Symptoms appear quickly. This type restores your body to its state before injury or illness.

- Chronic inflammation is as lower and generally less severe form of inflammation. It typically lasts longer than six weeks. It can occur even when there's no injury, and it doesn't always end when the illness or injury is healed. Chronic inflammation has been linked to autoimmune disorders and even prolonged stress.

5 Signs of Inflammation

- Heat;
- Pain;
- Redness;
- Swelling;
- Loss of function.

The specific symptoms you have depend on where in your body the inflammation is and what's causing it. Long-term inflammation can lead to a number of symptoms and affect your body in many ways. Common symptoms of chronic inflammation can include:

- Body pain;
- Constant fatigue and insomnia;
- Depression, anxiety, and other mood disorders;
- Gastrointestinal issues, like constipation, diarrhea, and acid reflux;
- Weight gain;
- Frequent infections.

Symptoms of Common Inflammatory Conditions

Symptoms can also vary depending on the condition that has an inflammatory component.

For example, in some autoimmune conditions, your immune system affects your skin, leading to rashes. In other types, it attacks specific glands, which affect hormone levels in the body. In rheumatoid arthritis, your immune system attacks your joints. You may experience:

- Joint pain, swelling, stiffness, or loss of joint function;
- Fatigue;

- Numbness and tingling;

- Limited range of motion.

In inflammatory bowel disease, inflammation occurs in the digestive tract. Some common symptoms include:

- Diarrhea;

- Stomach pain, cramping, or bloating;

- Weight loss and anemia;

- Bleeding ulcers.

In multiple sclerosis, your body attacks the myelin sheath. This is the protective covering of nerve cells. You may experience:

- Numbness and tingling of the arms, legs, or one side of the face;

- Balance problems;

- Double vision, blurry vision, or partial vision loss;

- Fatigue;

- Cognitive problems, like brain fog.

Causes of Inflammation

Many factors can lead to inflammation, such as:

- Chronic and acute conditions;

- Certain medications;

- Exposure to irritants or foreign materials your body can't easily eliminate.

Recurrent episodes of acute inflammation can also lead to a chronic inflammatory response.

There are also certain types of foods that can cause or worsen inflammation in people with autoimmune disorders

These foods include:

- Sugar;

- Refined carbohydrates;

- Alcohol;

- Processed meats;

- Trans fats.

How is Inflammation Diagnosed?

There's no single test that can diagnose inflammation or conditions that cause it. Instead, based on your symptoms, your doctor may give you any of the tests below to make a diagnosis.

Blood Tests

There are a few so-called markers that help diagnose inflammation in the body. However, these markers are nonspecific, meaning that abnormal levels can show that something is wrong, but not *what* is wrong.

Serum Protein Electrophoresis (SPE)

SPE is considered the best way Trusted Source to confirm chronic inflammation. It measures certain proteins in the liquid part of the blood to identify any issues. Too much or too little of these proteins can point to inflammation and markers for other conditions.

C-reactive Protein (CRP)

CRP is naturally produced in the liver in response to inflammation. A high level of CRP in your blood can occur due to several inflammatory conditions. While this test is very sensitive for inflammation, it doesn't help differentiate between acute and chronic inflammation, since CRP will be elevated during both. High levels combined with certain symptoms can help your doctor make a diagnosis.

Erythrocyte Sedimentation Rate (ESR)

The ESR test is sometimes called a sedimentation rate test. This test indirectly measures inflammation by measuring the rate at which red blood cells sink in a tube of blood. The quicker they sink, the more likely you're experiencing inflammation.

The ESR test is rarely performed alone, as it doesn't help pinpoint specific causes of inflammation. Instead, it can help your doctor identify that inflammation is occurring. It can also help them monitor your condition.

Plasma Viscosity

This test measures the thickness of blood. Inflammation or infection can thicken plasma.

Other Blood Tests

If your doctor believes the inflammation is due to viruses or bacteria, they may perform other specific tests. In this case, your doctor can discuss what to expect with you.

Other Diagnostic Tests

If you have certain symptoms — for instance, chronic diarrhea or numbness on one side of your face — your doctor may request an imaging test to check certain parts of the body or brain. MRIs and X-rays are commonly used.

To diagnose inflammatory gastrointestinal conditions, your doctor may perform a procedure to see inside parts of the digestive tract. These tests can include:

- Colonoscopy

- Sigmoidoscopy

- Upper endoscopy

Complement System

The complement system is an integral part of the innate immune response and acts as a bridge between innate and acquired immunity. It consists of a series of proteins that are mostly (although not exclusively) synthesised in the liver, and exist in the plasma and on cell surfaces as inactive precursors (zymogens). Complement mediates responses to inflammatory triggers through a co-ordinated sequential enzyme cascade leading to clearance of foreign cells through pathogen recognition, opsonisation and lysis. Complement also possesses anti-inflammatory functions: it binds to immune complexes and apoptotic cells, and assists in their removal from the circulation and damaged tissues. The complement proteins are activated by, and work with IgG and IgM antibodies, hence the name 'complement'. Many complement proteins exist in a 'precursor' form and are activated at the site of inflammation. The complement system is more complex than many enzymatic cascades as it requires the formation of sequential non-covalently associated activated protein fragments. These in turn become convertases and cleave components for the next enzymatic complex in the cascade, and the rapid dissociation of these complexes (and loss of enzymatic activity) forms an integral part of the elegant regulation of complement activity.

Pathways of Activation

There are three known pathways for complement activation: Classical, Alternative and Lectin pathway.

Classical Pathway

The classical pathway is initiated by IgM or IgG antigen/antibody complexes binding to C1q (first protein of the cascade) leading to activation of C1r, which in turn cleaves C1s. This in turn activates the serine proteases that lead to cleaving of C4 and C2, leading to formation of C4b2a (C3 convertase), which in turn cleaves C3 into C3a and C3b. While C3a acts as a recruiter of inflammatory cells (anaphylatoxin), C3b binds to the C4b2a complex to form C5 convertase (C4b2a3b). The C5 convertase initiates the formation of the Membrane Attack Complex (MAC), that inserts into membrane creating functional pores in bacterial membranes leading to its lysis. The classical pathway can also be activated by other danger signals like C-reactive protein, viral proteins, polyanions, apoptotic cells and amyloid, thus providing evidence that classical pathway could be activated independent of antibodies.

Alternative Pathway

Fifty years after the discovery of the classical activation pathway, Pillemer et al. proposed a highly controversial alternative activation pathway. Initially, this was rejected by the scientific community and only substantiated and accepted more than a decade later. Pillemer's hypothesis was based on observations that the complement system could be activated by direct binding of bacteria and yeast independent of antibody interaction. It was originally named the 'properdin pathway' and is now known as the alternative pathway. The alternative pathway is not so much an activation pathway, as it is a failure to regulate the low level continuous formation of a soluble C3 convertase. The internal thioester bond of C3 is highly reactive and undergoes spontaneous hydrolysis resulting in a molecule known as C3 (H_2O) which resembles C3b. This can then bind to factor B, and be processed into a short lived soluble C3 convertase that can generate more C3b. If this C3b binds to a nearby surface that is incapable of inactivating it (such as bacteria/yeast cells or damaged host tissues), this then leads to amplification of the alternative pathway. The presence of complement regulators in healthy cells ensures the spontaneous hydrolysis of C3 is kept in check. C3 activation takes place when C3b binds to factor B and is then cleaved by factor D (a process which is stabilised by magnesium ions and properdin). The enzymatic action of factor D acts as the rate limiting step of the alternative pathway and cleaves factor B, the larger fragment of which remains bound to C3b to form the alternative pathway C3 convertase—C3bBb. C3b is able to create new C3 convertase in the presence of Factors B and D, thus acting as an 'amplification loop' for other pathways, as well as the alternative pathway. The alternative pathway omits the components C1, C2 and C4.

Lectin Pathway

Forty years after the proposal of the alternative pathway, the MBL (mannose-binding lectin)/ MASP (MBL-associated serine protease) pathway was discovered. This pathway was characterised by using proteins isolated from rabbit liver and serum, but its function remained unclear initially. Two forms of MBL (MBL-A and -C) are present in rodents compared to a single form in the humans. Studies linking the deficiency of MBL protein to immunodeficiencies in children led to its recognition as an important activator of the complement system. The initiating molecules for this pathway are collectins (MBL and ficolin), which are multimeric lectin complexes. These bind to specific carbohydrate patterns uncommon in the host, leading to activation of the pathway through enzymatic activity of MASP. There are structural similarities shared between MBL and C1 complexes (MBL- with C1q-associated serine proteases, MASP-1 and MASP-2 with C1r and C1s, respectively), leading to the belief that complement activation by MBL and C1 complexes are similar. MASP-2 cleaves C4 and C2 to form C3 convertase, while MASP-1 may cleave C3 directly bypassing the C4b2a complex, albeit at a very slow rate. Another serine protease, MASP-3 was shown to down-regulate the C4 and C2 cleaving activity of MASP-2. Following the initial characterisation of MBL, 3 other lectins (known as ficolins) have been shown to interact with MASP: ficolin-1 (or M-ficolin), ficolin-2 (or L-ficolin) and ficolin-3 (or H-ficolin or Hakata antigen). The ficolins activate the lectin pathway by forming active complexes with MASP. More recently, a new C-type lectin (CL-11) was shown to interact with MASP-1 and/or MASP-3 and could activate the lectin pathway.

Other Activators of the Complement System

Various serine proteases belonging to the coagulation system have also been shown to activate the complement cascade independent of the established pathways. *In vitro* findings suggested that the coagulation factors FXa, FXIa and plasmin can cleave both C5 and C3, leading to generation of anaphylatoxins C5a and C3a. Studies have documented FVIII and von Willebrand factor to possess lectin activity. Vice versa, complement factors are also known to interact with the coagulation system. C1 inhibitor was shown to block the endogenous coagulation pathway, while C5a was shown to induce tissue factor (membrane glycoprotein that serves as a cofactor for blood coagulation factor VIIa) activity on endothelial cells. Individual cells have also been implicated in activating certain elements of complement pathway. Huber-Lang et al. showed that phagocytic cells, especially lung macrophages could generate C5a from C5 independent of the plasma complement system using cell bound serine proteases. C-reactive protein is an acute phase reactant that can activate the classical pathway of the complement system, and its role in the complement led ischemia–reperfusion injury (IRI) has been shown in intestinal and myocardial animal IRI models. Similarly, cross-talk between complement and toll-like receptors has shown to be possible due to mitogen activated protein kinases in renal IRI setting. Cross-talk between complement system and other systems will exist, and future research will be aimed at evaluating these 'communicators' between systems.

Complement Cascade

The principal function of the complement system is protection of the host from infection/inflammation by recruiting (chemotaxis) and enhancing phagocytosis by innate immune cells (opsonisation), leading to lysis of the target cells. All three pathways lead to the generation of C3 convertase that cleaves the C3 protein into C3a and C3b. While C3a acts as an anaphylatoxin, C3b covalently binds to the activating surface and participates in the self-activation loop of complement activation via the alternate pathway. C3b also associates with C3 convertases (C4b2a or C3bBb) to form the C5 convertase, which cleaves C5 complement into C5a and C5b. Interaction of C5b with C6, C7, C8 and C9 leads to formation of C5b–9/MAC, a multimolecular structure that inserts into the membrane creating a functional pore leading to cell lysis. MAC can cause lysis of some cells (e.g. erythrocytes) with a single hit, but some nucleated cells required multiple hits, or rather, multiple channel formation to cause cell lysis. However, studies have shown that when the number of channels assembled on the cells is limited, sublytic C5b–9 can activate transcription factors and signal transduction, leading to inhibition of apoptosis and cell homeostasis. The complement cascade with the inherent inhibitors is shown in figure.

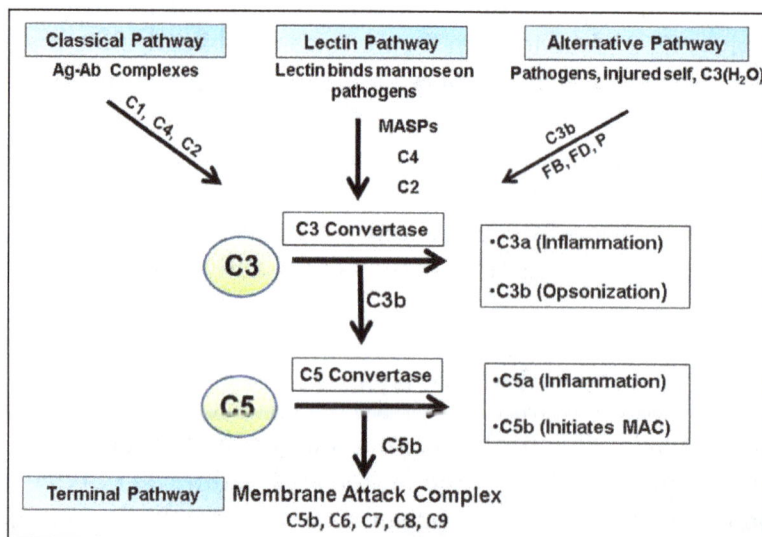

Pathways of complement activation: classical, alternative and lectin pathway.

In figure, IgM or IgG antigen/antibody complexes binding to C1q, the first protein of the cascade, initiates the classical pathway. The alternative pathway is not so much an activation pathway, as it is a failure to regulate the low level continuous formation of a soluble C3 convertase. The third pathway is known as MBL (Mannose-binding lectin)/MASP (MBL associated Serine Protease) pathway. The initiating molecules for the MBL pathway are multimeric lectin complexes that bind to specific carbohydrate patterns uncommon in the host, leading to activation of the pathway through enzymatic activity of MASP. The sites of action of the membrane bound complement regulators–CD35, CD46, CD55 & CD59 (green boxes) and the fluid phase regulators – C1-INH, Factor H, Factor I and C4bp (violet boxes) are represented with arrows. *Insert:* Membrane Attack Complex (MAC). The interaction of C5b with C6, C7, C8 and C9 leads to formation of C5b–9 or Membrane Attack Complex (MAC), a multimolecular structure that inserts into the membrane creating a functional pore leading to cell lysis

The anaphylatoxins (C3a and C5a) are key players in the recruitment of inflammatory cells and release of mediators that amplify the inflammatory response. C5a is probably the principal anaphylatoxin mediating inflammation. C5a binds to C5a receptor (C5aR or CD88) that is widely present on inflammatory and non-inflammatory cells. Apart from recruiting the neutrophils, C5a also increases neutrophil adhesiveness and aggregation. C5a causes secretion of pro-inflammatory cytokines and lysosomal enzymes from the macrophages and monocytes, thus leading to chemotaxis. C5a also up-regulates adhesion molecules such as α-integrin and β 2-integrin; in particular, Mac-1, in polymorphonuclear leukocytes. C5a was shown to be an important inflammatory mediator for the early adhesive interactions between neutrophils and endothelial cells in the acute inflammatory response. It is responsible for up-regulation of vascular adhesion molecules such as P-selectin, E-selectin, intercellular adhesion molecule-1 (ICAM-1) and vascular cell adhesion molecule-1 (VCAM-1).

C3a does not act as a chemoattractant for neutrophils, but aids migration of eosinophils and mast cells. C3a and C5a also act on their receptors expressed on innate immune cells such as dendritic cells, thus playing a role in initiating and regulating T cell responses. In the IRI setting, MAC has been shown to mediate IR injury, and its inhibition was shown to attenuate the IRI effect.

Inherent Regulation of Pathways

To prevent inadvertent injury by activated complement, the host tissues have developed intricate and elaborate mechanisms in the form of soluble and membrane bound complement regulators that inhibit complement activation. The two main regulation mechanisms are: decay-acceleration activity (DAA) which increases the rate of dissociation of (C4b2a and C3bBb) C3 convertases, and factor I cofactor activity (CA), which results in the factor I-mediated cleavage of covalently bound C3b and C4b into inactive fragments incapable of reforming the C3 convertases. The pathways are regulated by both membrane-bound and fluid phase complement regulators that keep the complement system in check.

Membrane Bound Complement Regulators

The membrane bound regulators–DAF, CR1 and MCP belong to a gene super family called as 'regulators of complement activation' (RCA)/Complement control proteins (CCP) and share a common structural motif called short consensus repeat (SCR). The SCR structure consists of around

60 amino acids held together by two disulfide bridges formed by cysteine residues. The structural moiety of the membrane bound complement regulators are depicted in figure.

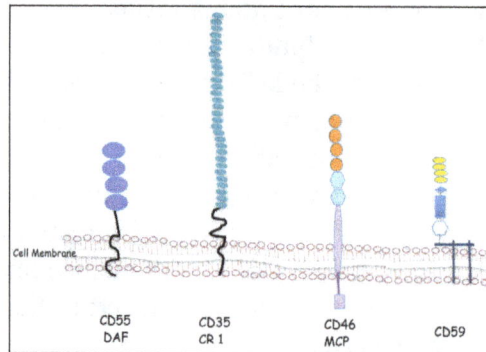

Membrane Bound Complement Regulators.

In figure, DAF, CR1 and MCP belong to a gene super family called as 'regulators of complement activation' (RCA)/complement control proteins (CCP) and share a common structural motif called short consensus repeat (SCR). The SCR structure (circles) consists of around 60 amino acids held together by two disulfide bridges formed by cysteine residues. CD59 is a GPI-anchored membrane complement that is expressed on almost all cells in the body. CD59 is the only well-characterised membrane inhibitor acting at the terminal step and prevents the assembly of the MAC.

CD35: Classical, Lectin and alternative Pathway

CD35 is a transmembrane glycoprotein that facilitates the decay of C3/C5 convertase in both the classical and alternate pathways and acts as a co-factor for factor I in the degradation of C3b and C4b. Human CR1 is found on B cells, follicular dendritic cells, erythrocytes, polymorphonuclear cells, phagocytic macrophages and on podocytes in the glomerular of the kidney. Expression of CD35 on erythrocytes is believed to be crucial in handling circulating immune complexes and abating the development of autoimmunity.

CD46: Classical, Lectin and alternative Pathway

CD46 acts as a cofactor for factor I mediated cleavage of C3b and C4b. It is widely expressed in humans apart from the erythrocytes, while in the rodents; it is expressed only in the testis. By regulating the production of interferon (IFN)-γ and interleukin (IL)-10 in the T helper cells, it is involved in the down-modulation of adaptive T helper type 1 immune responses. Deficiency of CD46 is a predisposing factor for numerous disease conditions arising from complement-mediated 'self-attack'.

CD55: Classical and alternative Pathway

CD55 is a glycosyl-phosphatidyl-inositol (GPI) anchored membrane protein that is widely expressed on vascular and non-vascular tissue cells. The main role of CD55 is the inhibition and acceleration of the decay of classical and alternative pathways C3 convertase. Apart from complement regulation, human DAF is known to act as a receptor for infection by certain viruses (echovirus and coxsackie B virus) and serves as a ligand for activation-associated leukocyte antigen CD97. Like rodent CD46, rodent CD55 is limited in its tissue expression.

CD59: Membrane Attack Complex

CD59 is a GPI-anchored membrane protein that is expressed on almost all cells in the body. CD59 is the only well-characterised membrane inhibitor acting at the terminal step, and prevents the assembly of the MAC by inhibiting the C5b-8 catalysed insertion of C9 into the lipid bilayer.

CrrY: Complement Receptor 1-related Gene/Protein Y

CrrY is a transmembrane protein specific to rodents and is widely expressed on rat and mouse cells to compensate for the lack of rodent CD55 and CD46 expression. CrrY possesses both DAA and CA properties and mimics the activities of the human DAF and MCP which regulate C3 deposition on host cells.

Fluid Phase or 'Soluble' Regulators: C1-Inhibitor: Classical and Lectin Pathway

In the fluid phase, the best-known regulatory protein is C1-Inhibitor (C1-INH), which is synthesised in the liver and by monocytes. It forms an irreversible complex with the serine proteases C1r and C1s, typical of serpin regulation, and inactivates them. This leads to the disassociation of C1r and C1s from C1q in the complex. C1-INH can also bind to MASP-1 and MASP-2 and inactivate them leading to disruption of the lectin pathway. Under physiologic conditions, activated C1 has a half-life of only 13 seconds in the presence of C1-INH (regulates nonspecific complement activation).

C1-INH inhibits other serine proteases, like kallikrein, along with coagulation factors (XIa, XIIa and plasmin), thus playing a role in coagulation regulation. Absence or low levels of C1-INH results in conditions like hereditary angioneurotic oedema where spontaneous activation of C1 and kallikrein leads to the manifestation of symptoms. Various animal IRI models have shown that C1-INH can protect liver, intestine, heart and brain tissue from ischemia–reperfusion damage.

Factor I: Classical, Lectin and alternative Pathway

Factor I cleaves C3b and C4b to form C3 and C4 fragments (iC3b, C3c, C3dg and C4c and C4d, respectively), thus blocking the formation of C3 and C5 convertase enzymes. The cofactors supporting factor I cleavage are factor H, CD35, CD46 and C4b-binding protein. Factor I is secreted by cells such as hepatocytes, macrophages, lymphocytes, endothelial cells and fibroblasts. The outcome after renal transplantation is poor in patients known to have either a complement factor H or complement factor I mutation, with approximately 80% of patients losing the graft to recurrent disease within 2 years. Mutations in factor I are linked with occurrence of atypical hemolytic uremic syndrome (HUS) in human and increases the susceptibility to pyogenic infections like meningitis and upper respiratory tract infections.

Factor H: Alternative and Classical Pathway

Factor H possesses multiple binding sites for C3b and accelerates the decay of the alternative C3 convertase through 'competitive binding' for factor B. It also facilitates the cleavage of C3b by supporting factor I activity. It plays an essential role in controlling the alternative pathway in blood and on cell surfaces. Impaired recognition of factor H by host cell surfaces due to mutations and polymorphisms can lead to complement-mediated tissue damage and disease. It is mainly synthesised in the liver, with minimal contributions from fibroblasts and endothelial cells. Genetic changes in factor H are linked to clinical conditions like HUS, membranoproliferative glomerulonephritis (dense deposit disease) and age-related macular degeneration.

C4bp: Classical and Lectin Pathway

C4bp is a regulator of the classical and lectin complement pathways. It binds to C4b and accelerates the decay of the C3 convertase []. It also acts as a cofactor for the cleavage of C4b by factor I. It is predominantly synthesised in the liver and to a lesser extent by activated monocytes. C4bp has a complex structure, mainly composed of alpha-chains with a single copy of a beta-chain. C4bp possesses binding sites for heparin and C-reactive protein as well. C4bp is up regulated in certain autoimmune diseases like lupus, but true deficiency state associated clinical conditions are yet to be reported.

Carboxypeptidase N: Anaphylatoxin Inactivator

Carboxypeptidase N was found to abolish the activity of the anaphylatoxins C3a and C5a and also those derived from bradykinin. It is synthesised in the liver and cleaves carboxy-terminal arginines and lysines from peptides (such as complement anaphylatoxins, kinins and creatine kinase MM-skeletal muscle) found in the bloodstream. Removal of the terminal arginine from C3a and C5a results in formation of C3a (desArg) and C5a (desArg), both of which have markedly lower ability to signal through receptor binding. Carboxypeptidase N plays an important role in protecting the body from excessive build-up of potentially deleterious peptides that can act as local autocrine or paracrine hormones.

Innate Immunity

In vertebrates, the skin and other epithelial surfaces, including those lining the lung and gut figure, provide a physical barrier between the inside of the body and the outside world. Tight junctions between neighboring cells prevent easy entry by potential pathogens. The interior epithelial surfaces are also covered with a mucus layer that protects these surfaces against microbial, mechanical, and chemical insults; many amphibians and fish also have a mucus layer covering their skin. The slimy mucus coating is made primarily of secreted mucin and other glycoproteins, and it physically helps prevent pathogens from adhering to the epithelium. It also facilitates their clearance by beating cilia on the epithelial cells.

The mucus layer also contains substances that kill pathogens or inhibit their growth. Among the most abundant of these are antimicrobial peptides, called defensins, which are found in all animals and plants. They are generally short (12–50 amino acids), positively charged, and have hydrophobic or amphipathic domains in their folded structure. They constitute a diverse family with a broad spectrum of antimicrobial activity, including the ability to kill or inactivate Gram-negative and Gram-positive bacteria, fungi (including yeasts), parasites (including protozoa and nematodes), and even enveloped viruses like HIV. Defensins are also the most abundant protein type in neutrophils, which use them to kill phagocytosed pathogens.

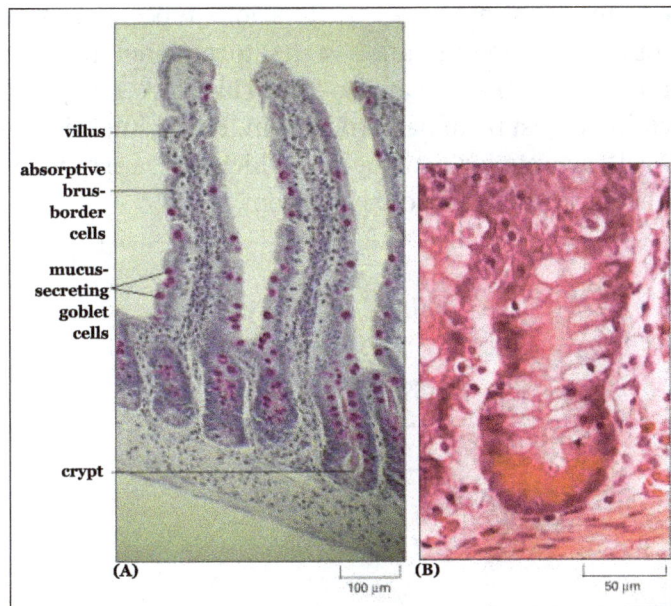

Epithelial defenses against microbial invasion.

In figure, (A) Cross section through the wall of the human small intestine, showing three villi. Goblet cells secreting mucus are stained magenta. The protective mucus layer covers the exposed surfaces of the villi. At the base of the villi lie the crypts where the epithelial cells proliferate. (B) Close-up view of a crypt stained using a method that renders the granules in the Paneth cells scarlet. These cells secrete large quantities of antimicrobial peptides and defensins into the intestinal lumen.

It is still uncertain how defensins kill pathogens. One possibility is that they use their hydrophobic or amphipathic domains to insert into the membrane of their victims, thereby disrupting membrane integrity. Some of their selectivity for pathogens over host cells may come from their preference for membranes that do not contain cholesterol. After disrupting the membrane of the pathogen, the positively-charged peptides may also interact with various negatively-charged targets within the microbe, including DNA. Because of the relatively nonspecific nature of the interaction between defensins and the microbes they kill, it is difficult for the microbes to acquire resistance to the defensins. Thus, in principle, defensins might be useful therapeutic agents to combat infection, either alone or in combination with more traditional drugs.

Human Cells Recognize Conserved Features of Pathogens

Microorganisms do occasionally breach the epithelial barricades. It is then up to the innate and adaptive immune systems to recognize and destroy them, without harming the host. Consequently, the immune systems must be able to distinguish self from non-self. The innate immune system relies on the recognition of particular types of molecules that are common to many pathogens but are absent in the host. These pathogen-associated molecules (called pathogen-associated immunostimulants) stimulate two types of innate immune responses—inflammatory responses and phagocytosis by cells such as neutrophils and macrophages. Both of these responses can occur quickly, even if the host has never been previously exposed to a particular pathogen.

The pathogen-associated immunostimulants are of various types. Procaryotic translation initiation differs from eucaryotic translation initiation in that formylated methionine, rather than regular methionine, is generally used as the first amino acid. Therefore, any peptide containing formylmethionine at the N-terminus must be of bacterial origin. Formylmethionine-containing peptides act as very potent chemoattractants for neutrophils, which migrate quickly to the source of such peptides and engulf the bacteria that are producing them.

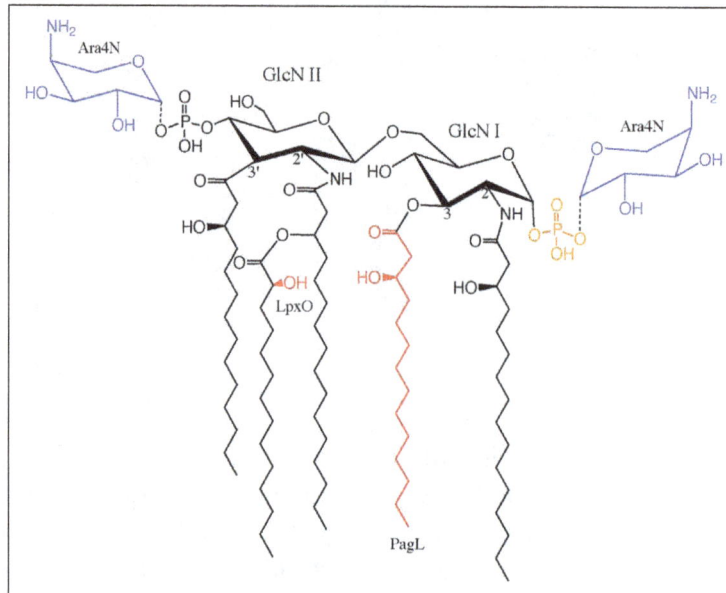

Structure of lipopolysaccharide (LPS).

In addition, the outer surface of many microorganisms is composed of molecules that do not occur in their multicellular hosts, and these molecules also act as immunostimulants. They include the peptidoglycan cell wall and flagella of bacteria, as well as lipopolysaccharide (LPS) on Gram-negative bacteria and teichoic acids on Gram-positive bacteria. They also include molecules in the cell walls of fungi such as zymosan, glucan, and chitin. Many parasites also contain unique membrane components that act as immunostimulants, including glycosylphosphatidylinositol in Plasmodium.

In figure, on the left is the 3-dimensional structure of a molecule of LPS with the fatty acids shown in yellow and the sugars in blue. The molecular structure of the base of LPS is shown on the right. The hydrophobic membrane anchor is made up of two linked glucosamine sugars attached to three phosphates and six fatty acid tails. This basic structure is elaborated by attachment of a long, usually highly branched, chain of sugars. This drawing shows the simplest type of LPS that will allow E. coli to live; it has just two sugar molecules in the chain, both 3-deoxy-D-manno-octulosonic acids. At the position marked by the arrow, wild-type Gram-negative bacteria also attach a core saccharide made up of eight to twelve linked sugars and a long O antigen, which is made up of an oligosaccharide unit that is repeated many (up to 40) times. The sugars making up the core saccharide and O antigen vary from one bacterial species to another and even among different strains of the same species. All forms of LPS are highly immunogenic.

Short sequences in bacterial DNA can also act as immunostimulants. The culprit is a "CpG motif", which consists of the unmethylated dinucleotide CpG flanked by two 5′ purine residues and two 3′

pyrimidines. This short sequence is at least twenty times less common in vertebrate DNA than in bacterial DNA, and it can activate macrophages, stimulate an inflammatory response, and increase antibody production by B cells.

The various classes of pathogen-associated immunostimulants often occur on the pathogen surface in repeating patterns. They are recognized by several types of dedicated receptors in the host that are collectively called pattern recognition receptors. These receptors include soluble receptors in the blood (components of the complement system) and membrane-bound receptors on the surface of host cells (members of the Toll-like receptor family). The cell-surface receptors have two functions: they initiate the phagocytosis of the pathogen, and they stimulate a program of gene expression in the host cell for stimulating innate immune responses. The soluble receptors also aid in the phagocytosis and, in some cases, the direct killing of the pathogen.

Complement Activation Targets Pathogens for Phagocytosis or Lysis

The complement system consists of about 20 interacting soluble proteins that are made mainly by the liver and circulate in the blood and extracellular fluid. Most are inactive until they are triggered by an infection. They were originally identified by their ability to amplify and "complement" the action of antibodies, but some components of complement are also pattern recognition receptors that can be activated directly by pathogen-associated immunostimulants.

The early complement components are activated first. There are three sets of these, belonging to three distinct pathways of complement activation—the classical pathway, the lectin *pathway*, and the alternative pathway. The early components of all three pathways act locally to activate C3, which is the pivotal component of complement. Individuals with a deficiency in C3 are subject to repeated bacterial infections. The early components and C3 are all proenzymes, which are activated sequentially by proteolytic cleavage. The cleavage of each proenzyme in the series activates the next component to generate a serine protease, which cleaves the next proenzyme in the series, and so on. Since each activated enzyme cleaves many molecules of the next proenzyme in the chain, the activation of the early components consists of an amplifying, proteolytic cascade.

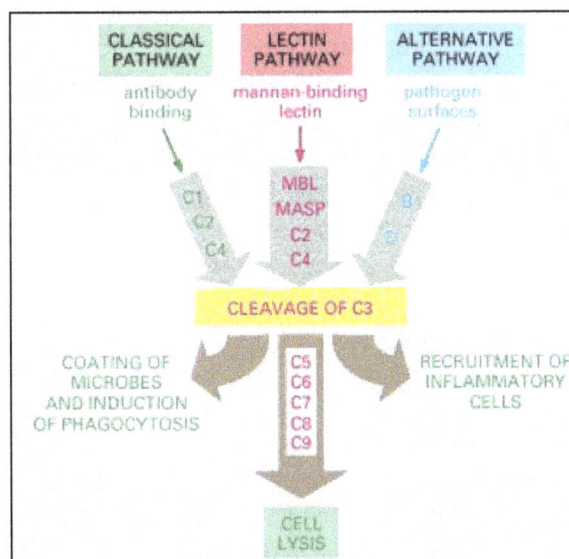

The principal stages in complement activation by the classical, lectin, and alternative pathways.

In figure, in all three pathways, the reactions of complement activation usually take place on the surface of an invading microbe, such as a bacterium. C1–C9 and factors B and D are the reacting components of the complement system; various other components regulate the system. The early components are shown within gray arrows, while the late components are shown within a brown arrow.

Many of these cleavages liberate a biologically active small peptide fragment and a membrane-binding larger fragment. The binding of the large fragment to a cell membrane, usually the surface of a pathogen, helps to carry out the next reaction in the sequence. In this way, complement activation is confined largely to the particular cell surface where it began. The larger fragment of C3, called C3b, binds covalently to the surface of the pathogen. Once in place, it not only acts as a protease to catalyze the subsequent steps in the complement cascade, but it also is recognized by specific receptors on phagocytic cells that enhance the ability of these cells to phagocytose the pathogen. The smaller fragment of C3 (called C3a), as well as fragments of C4 and C5, act independently as diffusible signals to promote an inflammatory response by recruiting phagocytes and lymphocytes to the site of infection.

The classical pathway is activated by IgG or IgM antibody molecules bound to the surface of a microbe. Mannan-binding lectin, the protein that initiates the second pathway of complement activation, is a serum protein that forms clusters of six carbohydrate-binding heads around a central collagen-like stalk. This assembly binds specifically to mannose and fucose residues in bacterial cell walls that have the correct spacing and orientation to match up perfectly with the six carbohydrate-binding sites, providing a good example of a pattern recognition receptor. These initial binding events in the classical and lectin pathways cause the recruitment and activation of the early complement components. In the alternative pathway, C3 is spontaneously activated at low levels, and the resulting C3b covalently attaches to both host cells and pathogens. Host cells produce a series of proteins that prevent the complement reaction from proceeding on their cell surfaces. Because pathogens lack these proteins, they are singled out for destruction. Activation of the classical or lectin pathways also activates the alternative pathway through a positive feedback loop, amplifying their effects.

Membrane-immobilized C3b, produced by any of the three pathways, triggers a further cascade of reactions that leads to the assembly of the late components to form membrane *attack complexes*. These complexes assemble in the pathogen membrane near the site of C3 activation and have a characteristic appearance in negatively stained electron micrographs, where they are seen to form aqueous pores through the membrane. For this reason, and because they perturb the structure of the bilayer in their vicinity, they make the membrane leaky and can, in some cases, cause the microbial cell to lyse, much like the defensins mentioned earlier.

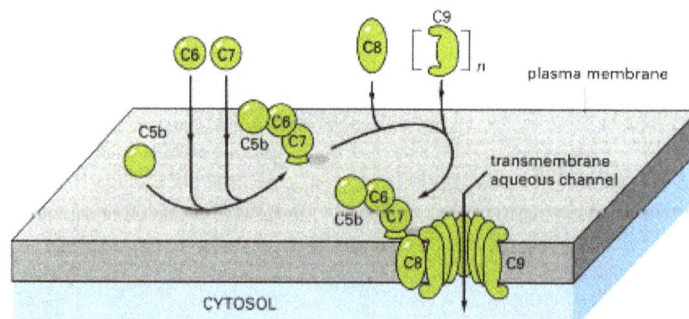

Assembly of the late complement components to form a membrane attack complex.

In figure, When C3b is produced by any of the three activation pathways, it is immobilized on a membrane, where it causes the cleavage of the first of the late components, C5, to produce C5a (not shown) and C5b. C5b remains loosely bound to C3b (not shown) and rapidly assembles with C6 and C7 to form C567, which then binds firmly via C7 to the membrane, as illustrated. To this complex is added one molecule of C8 to form C5678. The binding of a molecule of C9 to C5678 induces a conformational change in C9 that exposes a hydrophobic region and causes C9 to insert into the lipid bilayer of the target cell. This starts a chain reaction in which the altered C9 binds a second molecule of C9, where it can bind another molecule of C9, and so on. In this way, a large transmembrane channel is formed by a chain of C9 molecules.

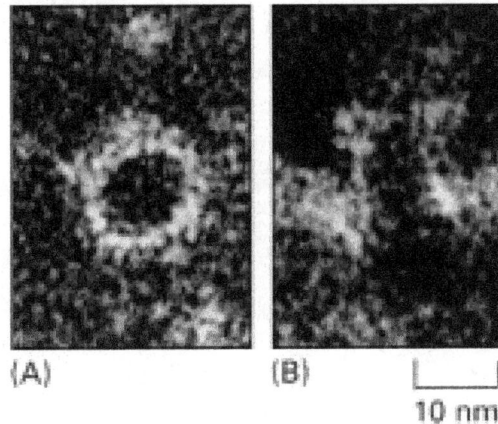

(A)   (B)

10 nm

Electron micrographs of negatively stained complement lesions in the plasma membrane of a red blood cell. The lesion in (A) is seen en face, while that in (B) is seen from the side as an apparent transmembrane channel. The negative stain fills the channels, which therefore look black.

The self-amplifying, inflammatory, and destructive properties of the complement cascade make it essential that key activated components be rapidly inactivated after they are generated to ensure that the attack does not spread to nearby host cells. Deactivation is achieved in at least two ways. First, specific inhibitor proteins in the blood or on the surface of host cells terminate the cascade, by either binding or cleaving certain components once they have been activated by proteolytic cleavage. Second, many of the activated components in the cascade are unstable; unless they bind immediately to either an appropriate component in the cascade or to a nearby membrane, they rapidly become inactive.

Toll-like Proteins are an Ancient Family of Pattern Recognition Receptors

Many of the mammalian cell-surface pattern recognition receptors responsible for triggering host cell gene expression in response to pathogens are members of the Toll-like receptor (TLR) family. Drosophila Toll is a transmembrane protein with a large extracellular domain consisting of a series of leucine-rich repeats . It was originally identified as a protein involved in the establishment of dorso-ventral polarity in developing fly embryos. It is also involved, however, in the adult fly's resistance to fungal infections. The intracellular signal transduction pathway activated downstream of Toll when a fly is exposed to a pathogenic fungus leads to the translocation of the NF-κB protein into the nucleus, where it activates the transcription of various genes, including those encoding antifungal defensins. Another member of the Toll family in Drosophila is activated by exposure to pathogenic bacteria, leading to the production of an antibacterial defensin.

Humans have at least ten TLRs, several of which have been shown to play important parts in innate immune recognition of pathogen-associated immunostimulants, including lipopolysaccharide, peptidoglycan, zymosan, bacterial flagella, and CpG DNA. As with Drosophila Toll family members, the different human TLRs are activated in response to different ligands, although many of them use the NF-κB signaling pathway. In mammals, TLR activation stimulates the expression of molecules that both initiate an inflammatory response and help induce adaptive immune responses. TLRs are abundant on the surface of macrophages and neutrophils, as well as on the epithelial cells lining the lung and gut. They act as an alarm system to alert both the innate and adaptive immune systems that an infection is brewing.

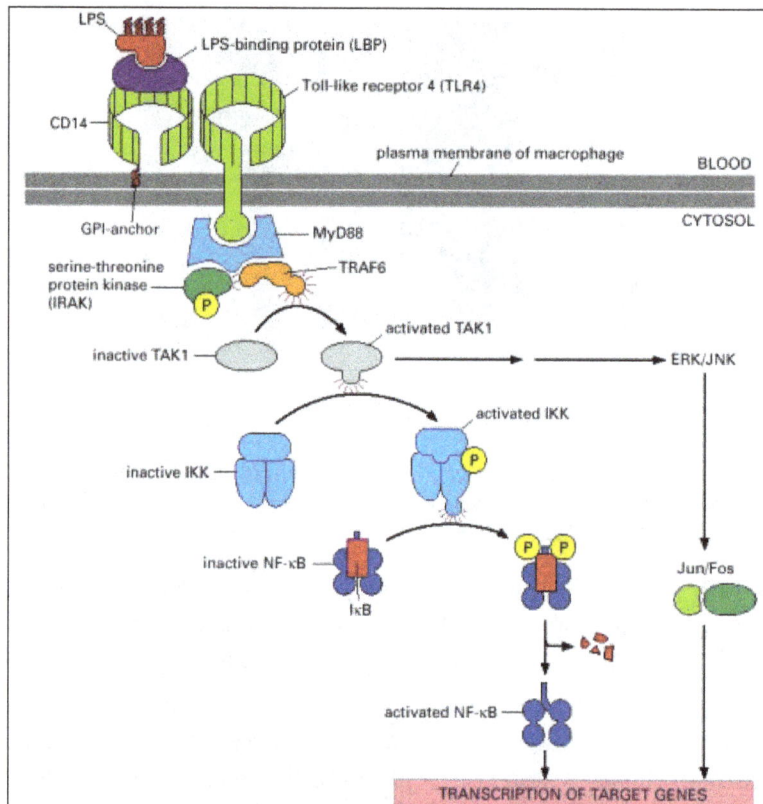

Figure shows LPS is bound by LPS-binding protein (LBP) in the blood, and the complex binds to the GPI-anchored receptor CD14 on the macrophage surface. The ternary complex then activates Toll-like receptor 4 (TLR4). Activated TLR4 recruits the adaptor protein MyD88, which interacts with the serine-threonine protein kinase IRAK. Recruitment of IRAK to the activated receptor complex results in its autophosphorylation and association with another adaptor protein, TRAF6. TRAF6, in turn, associates with and activates a MAP kinase kinase kinase, TAK1. Via several intermediate steps, TAK1 activation leads to the phosphorylation and activation of the IκB kinase (IKK). IKK phosphorylates the NF-κB inhibitor, IκB, inducing its degradation and releasing NF-κB. By way of additional MAP kinases (ERK and JNK), TAK1 also activates the AP-1 transcription family members Jun and Fos, which, together with NF-κB, activate the transcription of genes that promote immune and inflammatory responses.

Molecules related to Toll and TLRs are apparently involved in innate immunity in all multicellular organisms. In plants, proteins with leucine-rich repeats and with domains homologous to the cytosolic portion of the TLRs are required for resistance to fungal, bacterial, and viral pathogens. Thus, at least two parts of the innate immune system—the defensins and the TLRs—seem to be evolutionarily very ancient, perhaps predating the split between animals and plants over a billion years ago. Their conservation during evolution indicates the importance of these innate responses in the defense against microbial pathogens.

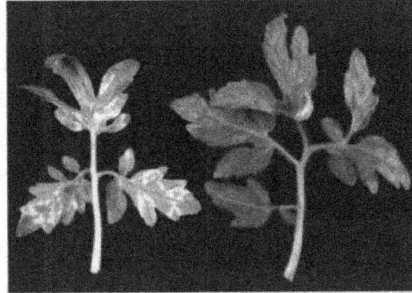

Microbial disease in a plant. These tomato leaves are infected with the leaf mold fungus Cladosporium fulvum. Resistance to this type of infection depends on recognition of a fungal protein by a host receptor that is structurally related to the TLRs.

Phagocytic Cells Seek, Engulf and Destroy Pathogens

In all animals, invertebrate as well as vertebrate, the recognition of a microbial invader is usually quickly followed by its engulfment by a phagocytic cell. Plants, however, lack this type of innate immune response. In vertebrates, macrophages reside in tissues throughout the body and are especially abundant in areas where infections are likely to arise, including the lungs and gut. They are also present in large numbers in connective tissues, the liver, and the spleen. These long-lived cells patrol the tissues of the body and are among the first cells to encounter invading microbes. The second major family of phagocytic cells in vertebrates, the neutrophils, are short-lived cells, which are abundant in blood but are not present in normal, healthy tissues. They are rapidly recruited to sites of infection both by activated macrophages and by molecules such as formylmethionine-containing peptides released by the microbes themselves.

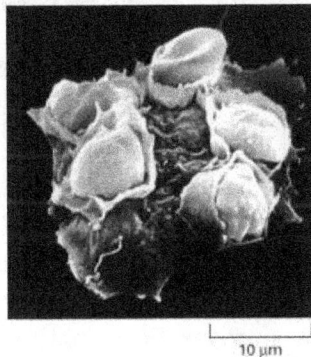

10 μm

Phagocytosis: This scanning electron micrograph shows a macrophage in the midst of consuming five red blood cells that have been coated with an antibody against a surface glycoprotein.

Macrophages and neutrophils display a variety of cell-surface receptors that enable them to recognize and engulf pathogens. These include pattern recognition receptors such as TLRs. In addition, they have cell-surface receptors for the Fc portion of antibodies produced by the adaptive immune system, as well as for the C3b component of complement. Ligand binding to any of these receptors induces actin polymerization at the site of pathogen attachment, causing the phagocyte's plasma membrane to surround the pathogen and engulf it in a large membrane-enclosed phagosome.

Once the pathogen has been phagocytosed, the macrophage or neutrophil unleashes an impressive armory of weapons to kill it. The phagosome is acidified and fuses with lysosomes, which contain lysozyme and acid hydrolases that can degrade bacterial cell walls and proteins. The lysosomes also contain defensins, which make up about 15% of the total protein in neutrophils. In addition, the phagocytes assemble an NADPH oxidase complex on the phagosomal membrane that catalyzes the production of a series of highly toxic oxygen-derived compounds, including superoxide (O_2^-), hypochlorite (HOCl, the active ingredient in bleach), hydrogen peroxide, hydroxyl radicals, and nitric oxide (NO). The production of these toxic compounds is accompanied by a transient increase in oxygen consumption by the cells, called the respiratory burst. Whereas macrophages will generally survive this killing frenzy and continue to patrol tissues for other pathogens, neutrophils usually die. Dead and dying neutrophils are a major component of the pus that forms in acutely infected wounds. The distinctive greenish tint of pus is due to the abundance in neutrophils of the copper-containing enzyme myeloperoxidase, which is one of the components active in the respiratory burst.

If a pathogen is too large to be successfully phagocytosed (if it is a large parasite such as a nematode, for example), a group of macrophages, neutrophils, or eosinophils will gather around the invader. They will secrete their defensins and other lysosomal products by exocytosis and will also release the toxic products of the respiratory burst. This barrage is generally sufficient to destroy the pathogen.

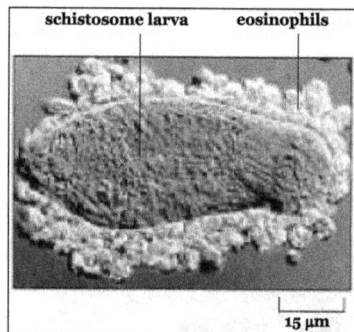

Eosinophils attacking a schistosome larva. Large parasites, such as worms, cannot be ingested by phagocytes. When the worm is coated with antibody or complement, however, eosinophils and other white blood cells can recognize and attack it.

Many pathogens have developed strategies that allow them to avoid being ingested by phagocytes. Some Gram-positive bacteria coat themselves with a very thick, slimy polysaccharide coat, or capsule, that is not recognized by complement or any phagocyte receptor. Other pathogens are phagocytosed but avoid being killed; as we saw earlier, Mycobacterium tuberculosis prevents the maturation of the phagosome and thereby survives. Some pathogens escape the phagosome entirely, and yet others secrete enzymes that detoxify the products of the respiratory burst. For such wily pathogens, these first lines of defense are insufficient to clear the infection, and adaptive immune responses are required to contain them.

Activated Macrophages Recruit additional Phagocytic Cells to Sites of Infection

When a pathogen invades a tissue, it almost always elicits an inflammatory response. This response is characterized by pain, redness, heat, and swelling at the site of infection, all caused by changes in local blood vessels. The blood vessels dilate and become permeable to fluid and proteins, leading to local swelling and an accumulation of blood proteins that aid in defense, including the components of the complement cascade. At the same time, the endothelial cells lining the local blood vessels are stimulated to express cell adhesion proteins that facilitate the attachment and extravasion of white blood cells, including neutrophils, lymphocytes, and monocytes (the precursors of macrophages).

The inflammatory response is mediated by a variety of signaling molecules. Activation of TLRs results in the production of both lipid signaling molecules such as prostaglandins and protein (or peptide) signaling molecules such as cytokines, all of which contribute to the inflammatory response. The proteolytic release of complement fragments also contribute. Some of the cytokines produced by activated macrophages are chemoattractants (known as chemokines). Some of these attract neutrophils, which are the first cells recruited in large numbers to the site of the new infection. Others later attract monocytes and dendritic cells. The dendritic cells pick up antigens from the invading pathogens and carry them to nearby lymph nodes, where they present the antigens to lymphocytes to marshal the forces of the adaptive immune system. Other cytokines trigger fever, a rise in body temperature. On balance, fever helps the immune system in the fight against infection, since most bacterial and viral pathogens grow better at lower temperatures, whereas adaptive immune responses are more potent at higher temperatures.

Some proinflammatory signaling molecules stimulate endothelial cells to express proteins that trigger blood clotting in local small vessels. By occluding the vessels and cutting off blood flow, this response can help prevent the pathogen from entering the bloodstream and spreading the infection to other parts of the body.

The same inflammatory responses, however, which are so effective at controlling local infections, can have disastrous consequences when they occur in a disseminated infection in the bloodstream, a condition called sepsis. The systemic release of proinflammatory signaling molecules into the blood causes dilation of blood vessels, loss of plasma volume, and widespread blood clotting, which an often fatal condition is known as septic shock. Inappropriate or overzealous inflammatory responses are also associated with some chronic conditions, such as asthma.

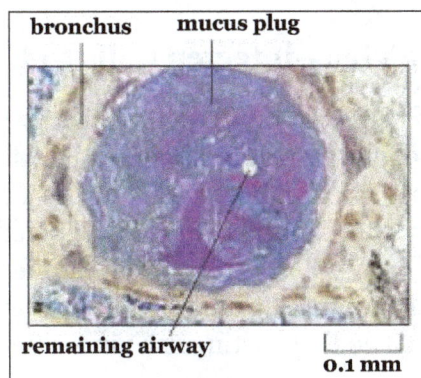

Inflammation of the airways in chronic asthma restricts breathing. Light micrograph of a section through the bronchus of a patient who died of asthma. There is almost total occlusion of the airway by a mucus plug. The mucus plug is a dense inflammatory infiltrate that includes eosinophils, neutrophils, and lymphocytes.

Just as with phagocytosis, some pathogens have developed mechanisms to either prevent the inflammatory response or, in some cases, take advantage of it to spread the infection. Many viruses, for example, encode potent cytokine antagonists that block aspects of the inflammatory response. Some of these are simply modified forms of cytokine receptors, encoded by genes acquired by the viral genome from the host. They bind the cytokines with high affinity and block their activity. Some bacteria, such as Salmonella, induce an inflammatory response in the gut at the initial site of infection, thereby recruiting macrophages and neutrophils that they then invade. In this way, the bacteria hitch a ride to other tissues in the body.

Virus-infected Cells take Drastic Measures to Prevent Viral Replication

The pathogen-associated immunostimulants on the surface of bacteria and parasites that are so important in eliciting innate immune responses are generally not present on the surface of viruses. Viral proteins are constructed by the host cell ribosomes, and the membranes of enveloped viruses are composed of host cell lipids. The only unusual molecule associated with viruses is the double-stranded RNA (dsRNA) that is an intermediate in the life cycle of many viruses. Host cells can detect the presence of dsRNA and initiate a program of drastic responses in attempt to eliminate it.

The program occurs in two steps. First, the cells degrade the dsRNA into small fragments (about 21–25 nucleotide pairs in length). These fragments bind to any single-stranded RNA (ssRNA) in the host cell with the same sequence as either strand of the dsRNA fragment, leading to the destruction of the ssRNA. This dsRNA-directed ssRNA destruction is the basis of the technique of RNA interference (RNAi) that is used by researchers to block specific gene expression. Second, the dsRNA induces the host cell to produce and secrete two cytokines—interferon α (IFN-α) and interferon β (IFN-β), which act in both an autocrine fashion on the infected cell and a paracrine fashion on uninfected neighbors. The binding of the interferons to their cell-surface receptors stimulates specific gene transcription by the Jak/STAT intracellular signaling pathway, leading to the activation of a latent ribonuclease, which nonspecifically degrades ssRNA. It also leads to the activation of a protein kinase that phosphorylates and inactivates the protein synthesis initiation factor eIF-2, shutting down most protein synthesis in the embattled host cell. Apparently, by destroying most of the RNA it contains and transiently halting most protein synthesis, the cell inhibits viral replication without killing itself. In some cases, however, a cell infected with a virus is persuaded by white blood cells to destroy itself to prevent the virus from replicating.

Natural Killer Cells Induce Virus-infected Cells to Kill themselves

Another way that the interferons help vertebrates defend themselves against viruses is by stimulating both innate and adaptive cellular immune responses. interferons enhance the expression of class I MHC proteins, which present viral antigens to cytotoxic T lymphocytes. Here, we consider how interferons enhance the activity of natural killer cells (NK cells), which are part of the innate immune system. Like cytotoxic T cells, NK cells destroy virus-infected cells by inducing the infected cell to kill itself by undergoing apoptosis. Unlike T cells, however, NK cells do not express antigen-specific receptors. How, then, do they distinguish virus-infected cells from uninfected cells.

NK cells monitor the level of class I MHC proteins, which are expressed on the surface of most vertebrate cells. The presence of high levels of these proteins inhibits the killing activity of NK cells, so that the NK cells selectively kill cells expressing low levels, including both virally-infected cells and some cancer cells. Many viruses have developed mechanisms to inhibit the expression of class I MHC molecules on the surface of the cells they infect, in order to avoid detection by cytotoxic

T lymphocytes. Adenovirus and HIV, for example, encode proteins that block class I MHC gene transcription. Herpes simplex virus and cytomegalovirus block the peptide translocators in the ER membrane that transport proteasome-derived peptides from the cytosol into the lumen of the ER; such peptides are required for newly-made class I MHC proteins to assemble in the ER membrane and be transported through the Golgi apparatus to the cell surface. Cytomegalovirus causes the retro translocation of class I MHC proteins from the ER membrane into the cytosol, where they are rapidly degraded by proteasomes. Proteins encoded by still other viruses prevent the delivery of assembled class I MHC proteins from the ER to the Golgi apparatus or from the Golgi apparatus to the plasma membrane. By evading recognition by cytotoxic T cells in these ways, however, a virus incurs the wrath of NK cells. The local production of IFN-α and IFN-β activates the killing activity of NK cells and also increases the expression of class I MHC proteins in uninfected cells. The cells infected with a virus that blocks class I MHC expression are thereby exposed and become the victims of the activated NK cells. Thus, it is difficult or impossible for viruses to hide from both the innate and adaptive immune systems simultaneously.

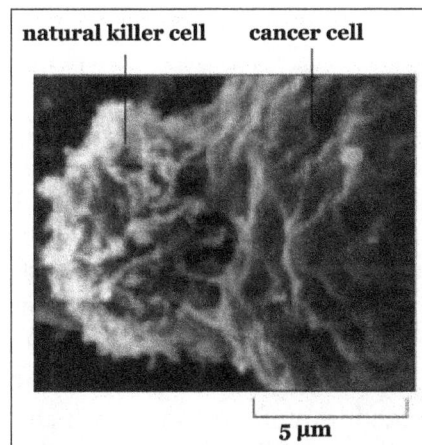

A natural killer (NK) cell attacking a cancer cell. The NK cell is the smaller cell on the left. This scanning electron micrograph was taken shortly after the NK cell attached, but before it induced the cancer cell to kill itself.

Both NK cells and cytotoxic T lymphocytes kill infected target cells by inducing them to undergo apoptosis before the virus has had a chance to replicate. It is not surprising, then, that many viruses have acquired mechanisms to inhibit apoptosis, particularly early in infection, apoptosis depends on an intracellular proteolytic cascade, which the cytotoxic cell can trigger either through the activation of cell-surface death receptors or by injecting a proteolytic enzyme into the target cell. Viral proteins can interfere with nearly every step in these pathways. In some cases, however, viruses encode proteins that act late in their replication cycle to induce apoptosis in the host cell, thereby releasing progeny virus that can infect neighboring cells.

The battle between pathogens and host defenses is remarkably balanced. At present, humans seem to be gaining a slight advantage, using public sanitation measures, vaccines, and drugs to aid the efforts of our innate and adaptive immune systems. However, infectious and parasitic diseases are still the leading cause of death worldwide, and new epidemics such as AIDS continue to emerge. The rapid evolution of pathogens and the almost infinite variety of ways that they can invade the human body and elude immune responses will prevent us from ever winning the battle completely.

In conclusion, the innate immune responses are the first line of defense against invading pathogens.

They are also required to initiate specific adaptive immune responses. Innate immune responses rely on the body's ability to recognize conserved features of pathogens that are not present in the uninfected host. These include many types of molecules on microbial surfaces and the double-stranded RNA of some viruses. Many of these pathogen-specific molecules are recognized by Toll-like receptor proteins, which are found in plants and in invertebrate and vertebrate animals. In vertebrates, microbial surface molecules also activate complement, a group of blood proteins that act together to disrupt the membrane of the microorganism, to target microorganisms for phagocytosis by macrophages and neutrophils, and to produce an inflammatory response. The phagocytic cells use a combination of degradative enzymes, antimicrobial peptides, and reactive oxygen species to kill the invading microorganisms. In addition, they release signaling molecules that trigger an inflammatory response and begin to marshal the forces of the adaptive immune system. Cells infected with viruses produce interferons, which induce a series of cell responses to inhibit viral replication and activate the killing activities of natural killer cells and cytotoxic T lymphocytes.

Adaptive Immune System

The adaptive, or acquired, immune response takes days or even weeks to become established—much longer than the innate response; however, adaptive immunity is more specific to pathogens and has memory. Adaptive immunity is an immunity that occurs after exposure to an antigen either from a pathogen or a vaccination. This part of the immune system is activated when the innate immune response is insufficient to control an infection. In fact, without information from the innate immune system, the adaptive response could not be mobilized. There are two types of adaptive responses: the cell-mediated immune response, which is carried out by T cells, and the humoral immune response, which is controlled by activated B cells and antibodies. Activated T cells and B cells that are specific to molecular structures on the pathogen proliferate and attack the invading pathogen. Their attack can kill pathogens directly or secrete antibodies that enhance the phagocytosis of pathogens and disrupt the infection. Adaptive immunity also involves a memory to provide the host with long-term protection from reinfection with the same type of pathogen; on re-exposure, this memory will facilitate an efficient and quick response.

Antigen-presenting Cells

Unlike NK cells of the innate immune system, B cells (B lymphocytes) are a type of white blood cell that gives rise to antibodies, whereas T cells (T lymphocytes) are a type of white blood cell that plays an important role in the immune response. T cells are a key component in the cell-mediated response—the specific immune response that utilizes T cells to neutralize cells that have been infected with viruses and certain bacteria. There are three types of T cells: cytotoxic, helper, and suppressor T cells. Cytotoxic T cells destroy virus-infected cells in the cell-mediated immune response, and helper T cells play a part in activating both the antibody and the cell-mediated immune responses. Suppressor T cells deactivate T cells and B cells when needed, and thus prevent the immune response from becoming too intense.

An antigen is a foreign or "non-self" macromolecule that reacts with cells of the immune system.

Not all antigens will provoke a response. For instance, individuals produce innumerable "self" antigens and are constantly exposed to harmless foreign antigens, such as food proteins, pollen, or dust components. The suppression of immune responses to harmless macromolecules is highly regulated and typically prevents processes that could be damaging to the host, known as tolerance.

The innate immune system contains cells that detect potentially harmful antigens, and then inform the adaptive immune response about the presence of these antigens. An antigen-presenting cell (APC) is an immune cell that detects, engulfs, and informs the adaptive immune response about an infection. When a pathogen is detected, these APCs will phagocytose the pathogen and digest it to form many different fragments of the antigen. Antigen fragments will then be transported to the surface of the APC, where they will serve as an indicator to other immune cells. Dendritic cells are immune cells that process antigen material; they are present in the skin (Langerhans cells) and the lining of the nose, lungs, stomach, and intestines. Sometimes a dendritic cell presents on the surface of other cells to induce an immune response, thus functioning as an antigen-presenting cell. Macrophages also function as APCs. Before activation and differentiation, B cells can also function as APCs.

After phagocytosis by APCs, the phagocytic vesicle fuses with an intracellular lysosome forming phagolysosome. Within the phagolysosome, the components are broken down into fragments; the fragments are then loaded onto MHC class I or MHC class II molecules and are transported to the cell surface for antigen presentation, as illustrated in figure. Note that T lymphocytes cannot properly respond to the antigen unless it is processed and embedded in an MHC II molecule. APCs express MHC on their surfaces, and when combined with a foreign antigen, these complexes signal a "non-self" invader. Once the fragment of antigen is embedded in the MHC II molecule, the immune cell can respond. Helper T- cells are one of the main lymphocytes that respond to antigen-presenting cells. Recall that all other nucleated cells of the body expressed MHC I molecules, which signal "healthy" or "normal."

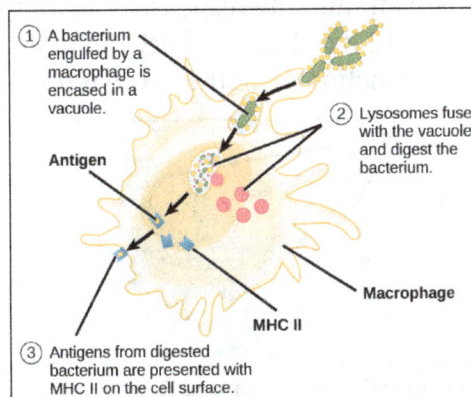

An APC, such as a macrophage, engulfs and digests a foreign bacterium. An antigen from the bacterium is presented on the cell surface in conjunction with an MHC II molecule Lymphocytes of the adaptive immune response interact with antigen-embedded MHC II molecules to mature into functional immune cells.

T and B Lymphocytes

Lymphocytes in human circulating blood are approximately 80 to 90 percent T cells, shown in figure, and 10 to 20 percent B cells. Recall that the T cells are involved in the cell-mediated immune response, whereas B cells are part of the humoral immune response.

T cells encompass a heterogeneous population of cells with extremely diverse functions. Some T cells respond to APCs of the innate immune system, and indirectly induce immune responses by releasing cytokines. Other T cells stimulate B cells to prepare their own response. Another population of T cells detects APC signals and directly kills the infected cells. Other T cells are involved in suppressing inappropriate immune reactions to harmless or "self" antigens.

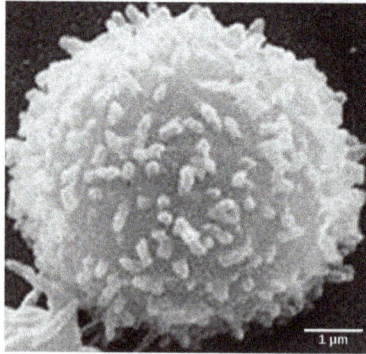

This scanning electron micrograph shows a T lymphocyte, which is responsible for the cell-mediated immune response. T cells are able to recognize antigens.

T and B cells exhibit a common theme of recognition/binding of specific antigens via a complementary receptor, followed by activation and self-amplification/maturation to specifically bind to the particular antigen of the infecting pathogen. T and B lymphocytes are also similar in that each cell only expresses one type of antigen receptor. Any individual may possess a population of T and B cells that together express a near limitless variety of antigen receptors that are capable of recognizing virtually any infecting pathogen. T and B cells are activated when they recognize small components of antigens, called epitopes, presented by APCs, illustrated in figure. Note that recognition occurs at a specific epitope rather than on the entire antigen; for this reason, epitopes are known as "antigenic determinants." In the absence of information from APCs, T and B cells remain inactive, or naïve, and are unable to prepare an immune response. The requirement for information from the APCs of innate immunity to trigger B cell or T cell activation illustrates the essential nature of the innate immune response to the functioning of the entire immune system.

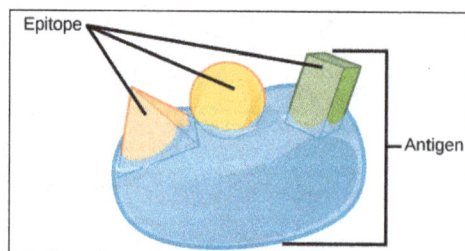

An antigen is a macromolecule that reacts with components of the immune system. A given antigen may contain several motifs that are recognized by immune cells. Each motif is an epitope. In this figure, the entire structure is an antigen, and the orange, salmon and green components projecting from it represent potential epitopes.

Naïve T cells can express one of two different molecules, CD4 or CD8, on their surface, as shown in figure, and are accordingly classified as CD4+ or CD8+ cells. These molecules are important because they regulate how a T cell will interact with and respond to an APC. Naïve CD4+ cells bind APCs via their antigen-embedded MHC II molecules and are stimulated to become helper T (T_H) lymphocytes, cells that go on to stimulate B cells (or cytotoxic T cells) directly or secrete cytokines to inform more and various target cells about the pathogenic threat. In contrast, CD8+ cells engage antigen-embedded MHC I molecules on APCs and are stimulated to become cytotoxic T lympho-cytes (CTLs), which directly kill infected cells by apoptosis and emit cytokines to amplify the immune response. The two populations of T cells have different mechanisms of immune protection, but both bind MHC molecules via their antigen receptors called T cell receptors (TCRs). The CD4 or CD8 surface molecules differentiate whether the TCR will engage an MHC II or an MHC I molecule. Because they assist in binding specificity, the CD4 and CD8 molecules are described as coreceptors.

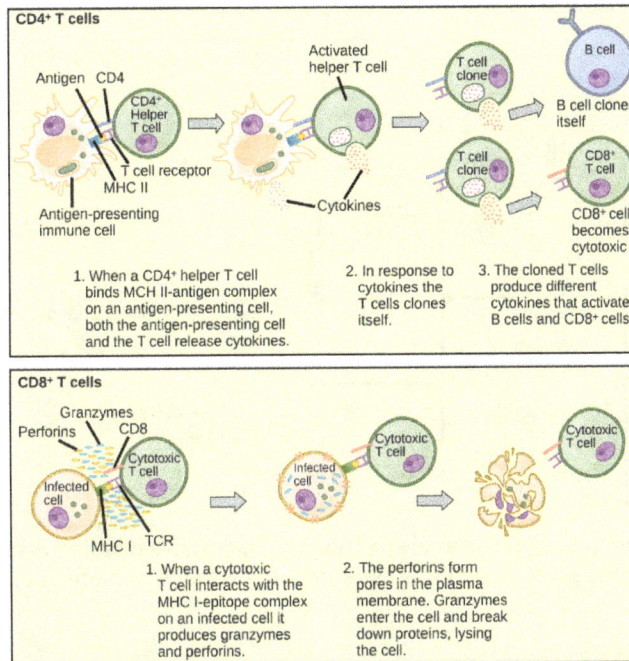

Naïve CD4$^+$ T cells engage MHC II molecules on antigen-presenting cells (APCs) and become activated. Clones of the activated helper T cell, in turn, activate B cells and CD8$^+$ T cells, which become cytotoxic T cells. Cytotoxic T cells kill infected cells.

Which of the following statements about T cells is false?

1. Helper T cells release cytokines while cytotoxic T cells kill the infected cell.

2. Helper T cells are CD4$^+$, while cytotoxic T cells are CD8$^+$.

3. MHC II is a receptor found on most body cells, while MHC I is a receptor found on immune cells only.

4. The T cell receptor is found on both CD4$^+$ and CD8$^+$ T cells.

Consider the innumerable possible antigens that an individual will be exposed to during a lifetime. The mammalian adaptive immune system is adept in responding appropriately to each antigen. Mammals have an enormous diversity of T cell populations, resulting from the diversity of TCRs. Each TCR consists of two polypeptide chains that span the T cell membrane, as illustrated in figure the chains are linked by a disulfide bridge. Each polypeptide chain is comprised of a constant domain and a variable domain: a domain, in this sense, is a specific region of a protein that may be regulatory or structural. The intracellular domain is involved in intracellular signaling. A single T cell will express thousands of identical copies of one specific TCR variant on its cell surface. The specificity of the adaptive immune system occurs because it synthesizes millions of different T cell populations, each expressing a TCR that differs in its variable domain. This TCR diversity is achieved by the mutation and recombination of genes that encode these receptors in stem cell precursors of T cells. The binding between an antigen-displaying MHC molecule and a complementary TCR "match" indicates that the adaptive immune system needs to activate and produce that specific T cell because its structure is appropriate to recognize and destroy the invading pathogen.

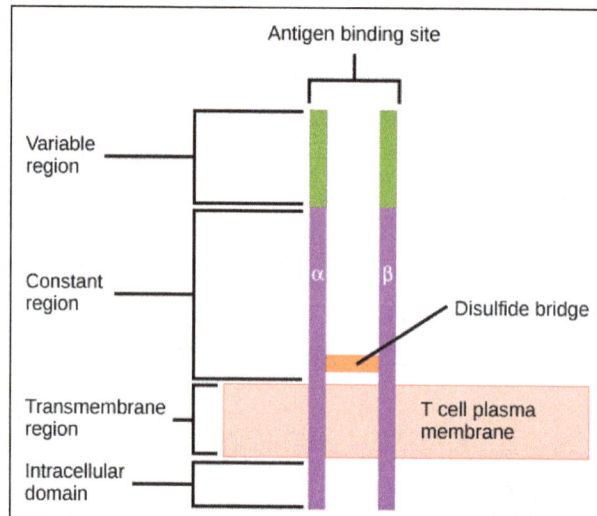

A T cell receptor spans the membrane and projects variable binding regions into the extracellular space to bind processed antigens via MHC molecules on APCs.

Helper T Lymphocytes

The T_H lymphocytes function indirectly to identify potential pathogens for other cells of the immune system. These cells are important for extracellular infections, such as those caused by certain bacteria, helminths, and protozoa. T_H lymphocytes recognize specific antigens displayed in the MHC II complexes of APCs. There are two major populations of T_H cells: T_H1 and T_H2. T_H1 cells secrete cytokines to enhance the activities of macrophages and other T cells. T_H1 cells activate the action of cyotoxic T cells, as well as macrophages. T_H2 cells stimulate naïve B cells to destroy foreign invaders via antibody secretion. Whether a T_H1 or a T_H2 immune response develops depends on the specific types of cytokines secreted by cells of the innate immune system, which in turn depends on the nature of the invading pathogen.

The T_H1-mediated response involves macrophages and is associated with inflammation. Recall the frontline defenses of macrophages involved in the innate immune response. Some intracellular bacteria, such as *Mycobacterium tuberculosis*, have evolved to multiply in macrophages after they have been engulfed. These pathogens evade attempts by macrophages to destroy and digest the pathogen. When *M. tuberculosis* infection occurs, macrophages can stimulate naïve T cells to become T_H1 cells. These stimulated T cells secrete specific cytokines that send feedback to the macrophage to stimulate its digestive capabilities and allow it to destroy the colonizing *M. tuberculosis*. In the same manner, T_H1-activated macrophages also become better suited to ingest and kill tumor cells. In summary; T_H1 responses are directed toward intracellular invaders while T_H2 responses are aimed at those that are extracellular.

B Lymphocytes

When stimulated by the T_H2 pathway, naïve B cells differentiate into antibody-secreting plasma cells. A plasma cell is an immune cell that secrets antibodies; these cells arise from B cells that were stimulated by antigens. Similar to T cells, naïve B cells initially are coated in thousands of B cell receptors (BCRs), which are membrane-bound forms of Ig (immunoglobulin, or an antibody). The B cell receptor has two heavy chains and two light chains connected by disulfide linkages. Each chain has a constant and a variable region; the latter is involved in antigen binding. Two other membrane proteins, Ig alpha and Ig beta, are involved in signaling. The receptors of any particular B cell, as shown in figure are all the same, but the hundreds of millions of different B cells in an individual have distinct recognition domains that contribute to extensive diversity in the types of molecular structures to which they can bind. In this state, B cells function as APCs. They bind and engulf foreign antigens via their BCRs and then display processed antigens in the context of MHC II molecules to T_H2 cells. When a T_H2 cell detects that a B cell is bound to a relevant antigen, it secretes specific cytokines that induce the B cell to proliferate rapidly, which makes thousands of identical (clonal) copies of it, and then it synthesizes and secretes antibodies with the same antigen recognition pattern as the BCRs. The activation of B cells corresponding to one specific BCR variant and the dramatic proliferation of that variant is known as clonal selection. This phenomenon drastically, but briefly, changes the proportions of BCR variants expressed by the immune system, and shifts the balance toward BCRs specific to the infecting pathogen.

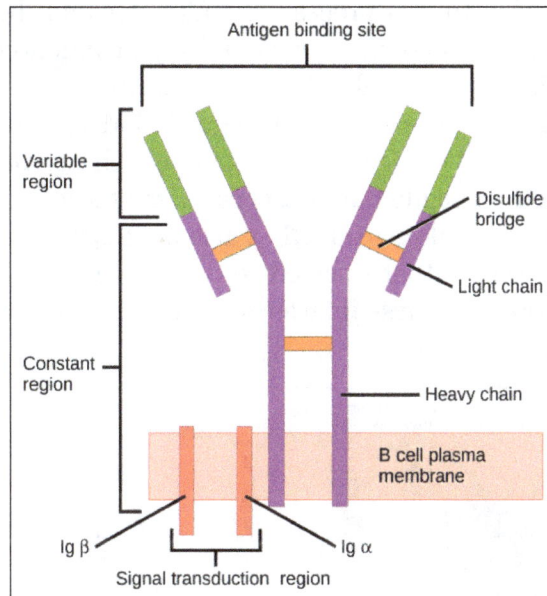

B cell receptors are embedded in the membranes of B cells and bind a variety of antigens through their variable regions. The signal transduction region transfers the signal into the cell.

T and B cells differ in one fundamental way: whereas T cells bind antigens that have been digested and embedded in MHC molecules by APCs, B cells function as APCs that bind intact antigens that have not been processed. Although T and B cells both react with molecules that are termed "antigens," these lymphocytes actually respond to very different types of molecules. B cells must be able to bind intact antigens because they secrete antibodies that must recognize the pathogen directly, rather than digested remnants of the pathogen. Bacterial carbohydrate and lipid molecules can activate B cells independently from the T cells.

Cytotoxic T Lymphocytes

CTLs, a subclass of T cells, function to clear infections directly. The cell-mediated part of the adaptive immune system consists of CTLs that attack and destroy infected cells. CTLs are particularly important in protecting against viral infections; this is because viruses replicate within cells where they are shielded from extracellular contact with circulating antibodies. When APCs phagocytize pathogens and present MHC I-embedded antigens to naïve CD8[+] T cells that express complementary TCRs, the CD8[+] T cells become activated to proliferate according to clonal selection. These resulting CTLs then identify non-APCs displaying the same MHC I-embedded antigens (for example, viral proteins)—for example, the CTLs identify infected host cells.

Intracellularly, infected cells typically die after the infecting pathogen replicates to a sufficient concentration and lyses the cell, as many viruses do. CTLs attempt to identify and destroy infected cells before the pathogen can replicate and escape, thereby halting the progression of intracellular infections. CTLs also support NK lymphocytes to destroy early cancers. Cytokines secreted by the T_H1 response that stimulates macrophages also stimulate CTLs and enhance their ability to identify and destroy infected cells and tumors.

CTLs sense MHC I-embedded antigens by directly interacting with infected cells via their TCRs. Binding of TCRs with antigens activates CTLs to release perforin and granzyme, degradative enzymes that will induce apoptosis of the infected cell. Recall that this is a similar destruction mechanism to that used by NK cells. In this process, the CTL does not become infected and is not harmed by the secretion of perforin and granzymes. In fact, the functions of NK cells and CTLs are complementary and maximize the removal of infected cells, as illustrated in figure. If the NK cell cannot identify the "missing self" pattern of down-regulated MHC I molecules, then the CTL can identify it by the complex of MHC I with foreign antigens, which signals "altered self." Similarly, if the CTL cannot detect antigen-embedded MHC I because the receptors are depleted from the cell surface, NK cells will destroy the cell instead. CTLs also emit cytokines, such as interferons, that alter surface protein expression in other infected cells, such that the infected cells can be easily identified and destroyed. Moreover, these interferons can also prevent virally infected cells from releasing virus particles.

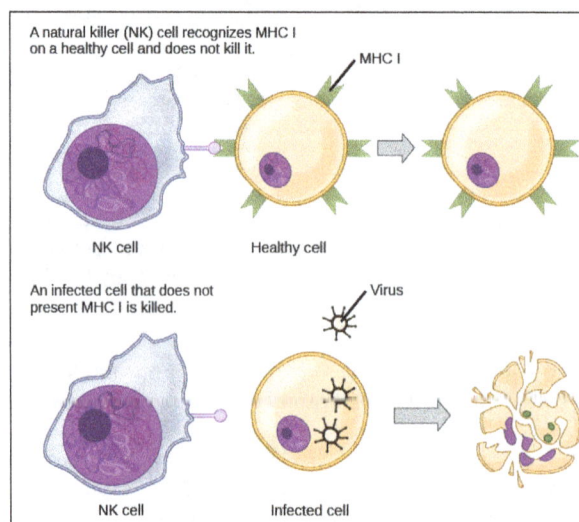

Natural killer (NK) cells recognize the MHC I receptor on healthy cells. If MHC I is absent, the cell is lysed.

Plasma cells and CTLs are collectively called effector cells: they represent differentiated versions of their naïve counterparts, and they are involved in bringing about the immune defense of killing pathogens and infected host cells.

Mucosal Surfaces and Immune Tolerance

The innate and adaptive immune responses discussed thus far comprise the systemic immune system (affecting the whole body), which is distinct from the mucosal immune system. Mucosal immunity is formed by mucosa-associated lymphoid tissue, which functions independently of the systemic immune system, and which has its own innate and adaptive components. Mucosa-associated lymphoid tissue (MALT), illustrated in figure, is a collection of lymphatic tissue that combines with epithelial tissue lining the mucosa throughout the body. This tissue functions as the immune barrier and response in areas of the body with direct contact to the external environment. The systemic and mucosal immune systems use many of the same cell types. Foreign particles that make their way to MALT are taken up by absorptive epithelial cells called M cells and delivered to APCs located directly below the mucosal tissue. M cells function in the transport described, and are located in the Peyer's patch, a lymphoid nodule. APCs of the mucosal immune system are primarily dendritic cells, with B cells and macrophages having minor roles. Processed antigens displayed on APCs are detected by T cells in the MALT and at various mucosal induction sites, such as the tonsils, adenoids, appendix, or the mesenteric lymph nodes of the intestine. Activated T cells then migrate through the lymphatic system and into the circulatory system to mucosal sites of infection.

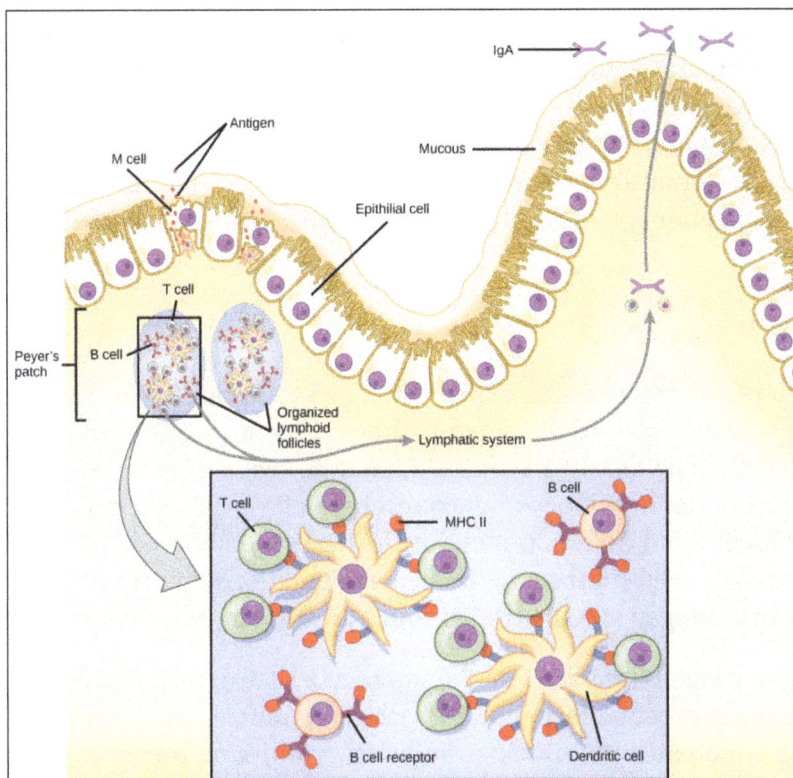

The topology and function of intestinal MALT is shown.

In figure, pathogens are taken up by M cells in the intestinal epithelium and excreted into a pocket formed by the inner surface of the cell. The pocket contains antigen-presenting cells such as dendritic cells, which engulf the antigens, then present them with MHC II molecules on the cell surface. The dendritic cells migrate to an underlying tissue called a Peyer's patch. Antigen-presenting cells, T cells, and B cells aggregate within the Peyer's patch, forming organized lymphoid follicles. There, some T cells and B cells are activated. Other antigen-loaded dendritic cells migrate through the lymphatic system where they activate B cells, T cells, and plasma cells in the lymph nodes. The activated cells then return to MALT tissue effector sites. IgA and other antibodies are secreted into the intestinal lumen.

MALT is a crucial component of a functional immune system because mucosal surfaces, such as the nasal passages, are the first tissues onto which inhaled or ingested pathogens are deposited. The mucosal tissue includes the mouth, pharynx, and esophagus, and the gastrointestinal, respiratory, and urogenital tracts.

The immune system has to be regulated to prevent wasteful, unnecessary responses to harmless substances, and more importantly so that it does not attack "self." The acquired ability to prevent an unnecessary or harmful immune response to a detected foreign substance known not to cause disease is described as immune tolerance. Immune tolerance is crucial for maintaining mucosal homeostasis given the tremendous number of foreign substances (such as food proteins) that APCs of the oral cavity, pharynx, and gastrointestinal mucosa encounter. Immune tolerance is brought about by specialized APCs in the liver, lymph nodes, small intestine, and lung that present harmless antigens to an exceptionally diverse population of regulatory T (T_{reg}) cells, specialized lymphocytes that suppress local inflammation and inhibit the secretion of stimulatory immune factors. The combined result of T_{reg} cells is to prevent immunologic activation and inflammation in undesired tissue compartments and to allow the immune system to focus on pathogens instead. In addition to promoting immune tolerance of harmless antigens, other subsets of T_{reg} cells are involved in the prevention of the autoimmune response, which is an inappropriate immune response to host cells or self-antigens. Another T_{reg} class suppresses immune responses to harmful pathogens after the infection has cleared to minimize host cell damage induced by inflammation and cell lysis.

Immunological Memory

The adaptive immune system possesses a memory component that allows for an efficient and dramatic response upon reinvasion of the same pathogen. Memory is handled by the adaptive immune system with little reliance on cues from the innate response. During the adaptive immune response to a pathogen that has not been encountered before, called a primary response, plasma cells secreting antibodies and differentiated T cells increase, then plateau over time. As B and T cells mature into effector cells, a subset of the naïve populations differentiates into B and T memory cells with the same antigen specificities, as illustrated in figure.

A memory cell is an antigen-specific B or T lymphocyte that does not differentiate into effector cells during the primary immune response, but that can immediately become effector cells upon re-exposure to the same pathogen. During the primary immune response, memory cells do not respond to antigens and do not contribute to host defenses. As the infection is cleared and pathogenic stimuli subside, the effectors are no longer needed, and they undergo apoptosis. In contrast, the memory cells persist in the circulation.

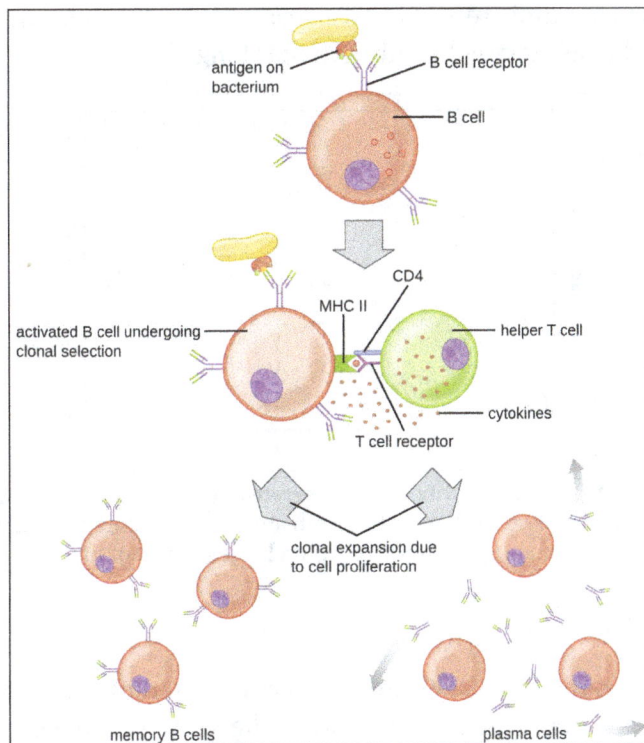

After initially binding an antigen to the B cell receptor (BCR), a B cell internalizes the antigen and presents it on MHC II. A helper T cell recognizes the MHC II–antigen complex and activates the B cell. As a result, memory B cells and plasma cells are made.

The Rh antigen is found on Rh-positive red blood cells. An Rh-negative female can usually carry an Rh-positive fetus to term without difficulty. However, if she has a second Rh-positive fetus, her body may launch an immune attack that causes hemolytic disease of the newborn. Why do you think hemolytic disease is only a problem during the second or subsequent pregnancies.

If the pathogen is never encountered again during the individual's lifetime, B and T memory cells will circulate for a few years or even several decades and will gradually die off, having never functioned as effector cells. However, if the host is re-exposed to the same pathogen type, circulating memory cells will immediately differentiate into plasma cells and CTLs without input from APCs or T_H cells. One reason the adaptive immune response is delayed is because it takes time for naïve B and T cells with the appropriate antigen specificities to be identified and activated. Upon reinfection, this step is skipped, and the result is a more rapid production of immune defenses. Memory B cells that differentiate into plasma cells output tens to hundreds-fold greater antibody amounts than were secreted during the primary response, as the graph in figure illustrates. This rapid and dramatic antibody response may stop the infection before it can even become established, and the individual may not realize they had been exposed.

Vaccination is based on the knowledge that exposure to non-infectious antigens, derived from known pathogens, generates a mild primary immune response. The immune response to vaccination may not be perceived by the host as illness but still confers immune memory. When exposed to the corresponding pathogen to which an individual was vaccinated, the reaction is similar to a secondary exposure. Because each reinfection generates more memory cells and increased resistance to the pathogen, and because some memory cells die, certain vaccine courses involve one or more booster vaccinations to mimic repeat exposures: for instance, tetanus boosters are necessary every ten years because the memory cells only live that long.

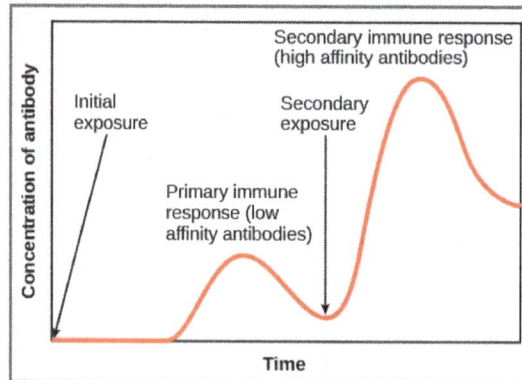

In the primary response to infection, antibodies are secreted first from plasma cells. Upon re-exposure to the same pathogen, memory cells differentiate into antibody-secreting plasma cells that output a greater amount of antibody for a longer period of time.

Mucosal Immune Memory

A subset of T and B cells of the mucosal immune system differentiates into memory cells just as in the systemic immune system. Upon reinvasion of the same pathogen type, a pronounced immune response occurs at the mucosal site where the original pathogen deposited, but a collective defense is also organized within interconnected or adjacent mucosal tissue. For instance, the immune memory of an infection in the oral cavity would also elicit a response in the pharynx if the oral cavity was exposed to the same pathogen.

Vaccinologist

Vaccination (or immunization) involves the delivery, usually by injection as shown in figure, of non-infectious antigen(s) derived from known pathogens. Other components, called adjuvants, are delivered in parallel to help stimulate the immune response. Immunological memory is the reason vaccines work. Ideally, the effect of vaccination is to elicit immunological memory, and thus resistance to specific pathogens without the individual having to experience an infection.

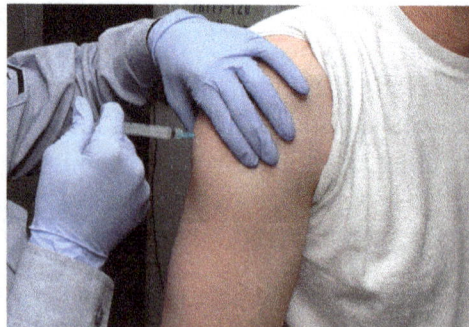

Vaccines are often delivered by injection into the arm.

Vaccinologists are involved in the process of vaccine development from the initial idea to the availability of the completed vaccine. This process can take decades, can cost millions of dollars, and can involve many obstacles along the way. For instance, injected vaccines stimulate the systemic immune system, eliciting humoral and cell-mediated immunity, but have little effect on the mucosal response, which presents a challenge because many pathogens are deposited and replicate in mucosal compartments, and the injection does not provide the most efficient immune memory for these disease agents. For this reason, vaccinologists are actively involved in developing new vaccines that are applied via intranasal, aerosol, oral, or transcutaneous (absorbed through the skin) delivery methods. Importantly, mucosal-administered vaccines elicit both mucosal and systemic immunity and produce the same level of disease resistance as injected vaccines.

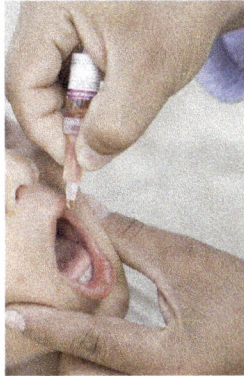

The polio vaccine can be administered orally.

Currently, a version of intranasal influenza vaccine is available, and the polio and typhoid vaccines can be administered orally, as shown in figure. Similarly, the measles and rubella vaccines are being adapted to aerosol delivery using inhalation devices. Eventually, transgenic plants may be engineered to produce vaccine antigens that can be eaten to confer disease resistance. Other vaccines may be adapted to rectal or vaginal application to elicit immune responses in rectal, genitourinary, or reproductive mucosa. Finally, vaccine antigens may be adapted to transdermal application in which the skin is lightly scraped and microneedles are used to pierce the outermost layer. In addition to mobilizing the mucosal immune response, this new generation of vaccines may end the anxiety associated with injections and, in turn, improve patient participation.

Primary Centers of the Immune System

Although the immune system is characterized by circulating cells throughout the body, the regulation, maturation, and intercommunication of immune factors occur at specific sites. The blood circulates immune cells, proteins, and other factors through the body. Approximately 0.1 percent of all cells in the blood are leukocytes, which encompass monocytes (the precursor of macrophages) and lymphocytes. The majority of cells in the blood are erythrocytes (red blood cells). Lymph is a watery fluid that bathes tissues and organs with protective white blood cells and does not contain erythrocytes. Cells of the immune system can travel between the distinct lymphatic and blood circulatory systems, which are separated by interstitial space, by a process called extravasation (passing through to surrounding tissue).

The cells of the immune system originate from hematopoietic stem cells in the bone marrow. Cytokines stimulate these stem cells to differentiate into immune cells. B cell maturation occurs in the bone marrow, whereas naïve T cells transit from the bone marrow to the thymus for maturation. In the thymus, immature T cells that express TCRs complementary to self-antigens are destroyed. This process helps prevent autoimmune responses.

On maturation, T and B lymphocytes circulate to various destinations. Lymph nodes scattered throughout the body, as illustrated in figure, house large populations of T and B cells, dendritic cells, and macrophages. Lymph gathers antigens as it drains from tissues. These antigens then are filtered through lymph nodes before the lymph is returned to circulation. APCs in the lymph nodes capture and process antigens and inform nearby lymphocytes about potential pathogens.

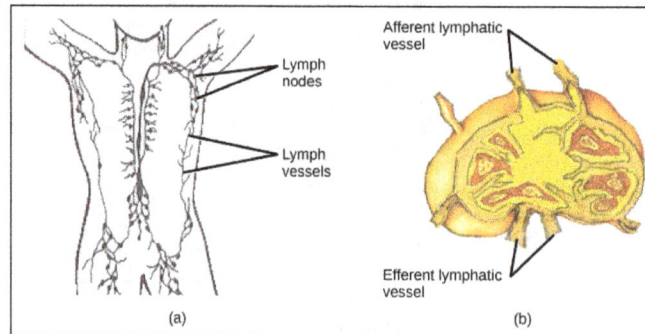

(a) Lymphatic vessels carry a clear fluid called lymph throughout the body. The liquid enters (b) lymph nodes through afferent vessels. Lymph nodes are filled with lymphocytes that purge infecting cells. The lymph then exits through efferent vessels.

The spleen houses B and T cells, macrophages, dendritic cells, and NK cells. The spleen, shown in figure, is the site where APCs that have trapped foreign particles in the blood can communicate with lymphocytes. Antibodies are synthesized and secreted by activated plasma cells in the spleen, and the spleen filters foreign substances and antibody-complexed pathogens from the blood. Functionally, the spleen is to the blood as lymph nodes are to the lymph.

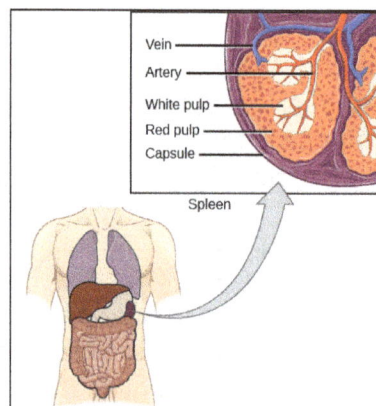

Figure shows the spleen is similar to a lymph node but is much larger and filters blood instead of lymph. Blood enters the spleen through arteries and exits through veins. The spleen contains two types of tissue: red pulp and white pulp. Red pulp consists of cavities that store blood. Within the red pulp, damaged red blood cells are removed and replaced by new ones. White pulp is rich in lymphocytes that remove antigen-coated bacteria from the blood.

In conclusion, the adaptive immune response is a slower-acting, longer-lasting, and more specific response than the innate response. However, the adaptive response requires information from the innate immune system to function. APCs display antigens via MHC molecules to complementary naïve T cells. In response, the T cells differentiate and proliferate, becoming T_H cells or CTLs. T_H cells stimulate B cells that have engulfed and presented pathogen-derived antigens. B cells differentiate into plasma cells that secrete antibodies, whereas CTLs induce apoptosis in intracellularly infected or cancerous cells. Memory cells persist after a primary exposure to a pathogen. If re-exposure occurs, memory cells differentiate into effector cells without input from the innate immune system. The mucosal immune system is largely independent from the systemic immune system but functions in a parallel fashion to protect the extensive mucosal surfaces of the body.

Boosting your Immunity

The idea of boosting your immunity is enticing, but the ability to do so has proved elusive for several reasons. The immune system is precisely that — a system, not a single entity. To function well, it requires balance and harmony. There is still much that researchers don't know about the intricacies and interconnectedness of the immune response. For now, there are no scientifically proven direct links between lifestyle and enhanced immune function.

But that doesn't mean the effects of lifestyle on the immune system aren't intriguing and shouldn't be studied. Researchers are exploring the effects of diet, exercise, age, psychological stress, and other factors on the immune response, both in animals and in humans. In the meantime, general healthy-living strategies are a good way to start giving your immune system the upper hand.

Increase Immunity the Healthy way

Many products on store shelves claim to boost or support immunity. But the concept of boosting immunity actually makes little sense scientifically. In fact, boosting the number of cells in your body — immune cells or others — is not necessarily a good thing. For example, athletes who engage in "blood doping" — pumping blood into their systems to boost their number of blood cells and enhance their performance — run the risk of strokes.

Attempting to boost the cells of your immune system is especially complicated because there are so many different kinds of cells in the immune system that respond to so many different microbes in so many ways. Which cells should you boost, and to what number? So far, scientists do not know the answer. What is known is that the body is continually generating immune cells. Certainly it produces many more lymphocytes than it can possibly use. The extra cells remove themselves through a natural process of cell death called apoptosis — some before they see any action, some after the battle is won. No one knows how many cells or what the best mix of cells the immune system needs to function at its optimum level.

Immune System and Age

As we age, our immune response capability becomes reduced, which in turn contributes to more infections and more cancer. As life expectancy in developed countries has increased, so too has the incidence of age-related conditions.

While some people age healthily, the conclusion of many studies is that, compared with younger people, the elderly are more likely to contract infectious diseases and, even more importantly, more likely to die from them. Respiratory infections, influenza, and particularly pneumonia are a leading cause of death in people over 65 worldwide. No one knows for sure why this happens, but some scientists observe that this increased risk correlates with a decrease in T cells, possibly from the thymus atrophying with age and producing fewer T cells to fight off infection. Whether this decrease in thymus function explains the drop in T cells or whether other changes play a role is not fully understood. Others are interested in whether the bone marrow becomes less efficient at producing the stem cells that give rise to the cells of the immune system.

A reduction in immune response to infections has been demonstrated by older people's response to vaccines. For example, studies of influenza vaccines have shown that for people over age 65, the vaccine is much less effective compared to healthy children (over age 2). But despite the reduction in efficacy, vaccinations for influenza and *S. pneumoniae* have significantly lowered the rates of sickness and death in older people when compared with no vaccination.

There appears to be a connection between nutrition and immunity in the elderly. A form of malnutrition that is surprisingly common even in affluent countries is known as "micronutrient malnutrition." Micronutrient malnutrition, in which a person is deficient in some essential vitamins and trace minerals that are obtained from or supplemented by diet, can be common in the elderly. Older people tend to eat less and often have less variety in their diets. One important question is whether dietary supplements may help older people maintain a healthier immune system. Older people should discuss this question with a physician who is well versed in geriatric nutrition, because while some dietary supplementation may be beneficial for older people, even small changes can have serious repercussions in this age group.

Diet and your Immune System

Like any fighting force, the immune system army marches on its stomach. Healthy immune system warriors need good, regular nourishment. Scientists have long recognized that people who live in poverty and are malnourished are more vulnerable to infectious diseases. Whether the increased rate of disease is caused healthy immune system by malnutrition's effect on the immune system, however, is not certain. There are still relatively few studies of the effects of nutrition on the immune system of humans, and even fewer studies that tie the effects of nutrition directly to the development (versus the treatment) of diseases.

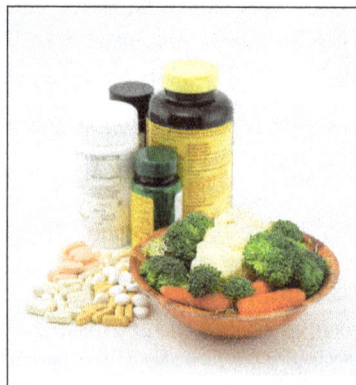

Like any fighting force, the immune system army marches on its stomach. Healthy immune system warriors need good, regular nourishment. Scientists have long recognized that people who live in poverty and are malnourished are more vulnerable to infectious diseases.

There is some evidence that various micronutrient deficiencies — for example, deficiencies of zinc, selenium, iron, copper, folic acid, and vitamins A, B6, C, and E — alter immune responses in animals, as measured in the test tube. However, the impact of these immune system changes on the health of animals is less clear, and the effect of similar deficiencies on the human immune response has yet to be assessed.

So what can you do? If you suspect your diet is not providing you with all your micronutrient needs — maybe, for instance, you don't like vegetables — taking a daily multivitamin and mineral supplement may bring other health benefits, beyond any possibly beneficial effects on the immune system. Taking megadoses of a single vitamin does not. More is not necessarily better.

Improving Immunity with Herbs and Supplements

Walk into a store, and you will find bottles of pills and herbal preparations that claim to "support immunity" or otherwise boost the health of your immune system. Although some preparations have been found to alter some components of immune function, thus far there is no evidence that they actually bolster immunity to the point where you are better protected against infection and disease. Demonstrating whether an herb — or any substance, for that matter — can enhance immunity is, as yet, a highly complicated matter. Scientists don't know, for example, whether an herb that seems to raise the levels of antibodies in the blood is actually doing anything beneficial for overall immunity.

Stress and Immune Function

Modern medicine has come to appreciate the closely linked relationship of mind and body. A wide variety of maladies, including stomach upset, hives, and even heart disease, are linked to the effects of emotional stress. Despite the challenges, scientists are actively studying the relationship between stress and immune function.

For one thing, stress is difficult to define. What may appear to be a stressful situation for one person is not for another. When people are exposed to situations they regard as stressful, it is difficult for them to measure how much stress they feel, and difficult for the scientist to know if a person's subjective impression of the amount of stress is accurate. The scientist can only measure things that may reflect stress, such as the number of times the heart beats each minute, but such measures also may reflect other factors.

Most scientists studying the relationship of stress and immune function, however, do not study a sudden, short-lived stressor; rather, they try to study more constant and frequent stressors known as chronic stress, such as that caused by relationships with family, friends, and co-workers, or sustained challenges to perform well at one's work. Some scientists are investigating whether on-going stress takes a toll on the immune system.

But it is hard to perform what scientists call "controlled experiments" in human beings. In a controlled experiment, the scientist can change one and only one factor, such as the amount of a particular chemical, and then measure the effect of that change on some other measurable phenomenon, such as the amount of antibodies produced by a particular type of immune system cell when it is exposed to the chemical. In a living animal, and especially in a human being, that kind of control is just not possible, since there are so many other things happening to the animal or person at the time that measurements are being taken.

Despite these inevitable difficulties in measuring the relationship of stress to immunity, scientists are making progress.

Does being Cold give you a Weak Immune System?

Almost every mother has said it: "Wear a jacket or you'll catch a cold!" Is she right? So far, researchers who are studying this question think that normal exposure to moderate cold doesn't increase your susceptibility to infection. Most health experts agree that the reason winter is "cold and flu season" is not that people are cold, but that they spend more time indoors, in closer contact with other people who can pass on their germs.

But researchers remain interested in this question in different populations. Some experiments with mice suggest that cold exposure might reduce the ability to cope with infection. But what about humans? Scientists have dunked people in cold water and made others sit nude in subfreezing temperatures. They've studied people who lived in Antarctica and those on expeditions in the Canadian Rockies. The results have been mixed. For example, researchers documented an increase in upper respiratory infections in competitive cross-country skiers who exercise vigorously in the cold, but whether these infections are due to the cold or other factors — such as the intense exercise or the dryness of the air — is not known.

A group of Canadian researchers that has reviewed hundreds of medical studies on the subject and conducted some of its own research concludes that there's no need to worry about moderate cold exposure — it has no detrimental effect on the human immune system. Should you bundle up when it's cold outside? The answer is "yes" if you're uncomfortable, or if you're going to be outdoors for an extended period where such problems as frostbite and hypothermia are a risk. But don't worry about immunity.

Exercise: Good or Bad for Immunity

Regular exercise is one of the pillars of healthy living. It improves cardiovascular health, lowers blood pressure, helps control body weight, and protects against a variety of diseases. But does it help to boost your immune system naturally and keep it healthy? Just like a healthy diet, exercise can contribute to general good health and therefore to a healthy immune system. It may contribute even more directly by promoting good circulation, which allows the cells and substances of the immune system to move through the body freely and do their job efficiently.

Some scientists are trying to take the next step to determine whether exercise directly affects a person's susceptibility to infection. For example, some researchers are looking at whether extreme amounts of intensive exercise can cause athletes to get sick more often or somehow impairs their immune function. To do this sort of research, exercise scientists typically ask athletes to exercise intensively; the scientists test their blood and urine before and after the exercise to detect any changes in immune system components. While some changes have been recorded, immunologists do not yet know what these changes mean in terms of human immune response.

But these subjects are elite athletes undergoing intense physical exertion. What about moderate exercise for average people? Does it help keep the immune system healthy? For now, even though a direct beneficial link hasn't been established, it's reasonable to consider moderate regular exercise to be a beneficial arrow in the quiver of healthy living, a potentially important means for keeping your immune system healthy along with the rest of your body.

One approach that could help researchers get more complete answers about whether lifestyle factors such as exercise help improve immunity takes advantage of the sequencing of the human genome. This opportunity for research based on updated biomedical technology can be employed to give a more complete answer to this and similar questions about the immune system. For example, microarrays or "gene chips" based on the human genome allow scientists to look simultaneously at how thousands of gene sequences are turned on or off in response to specific physiological conditions — for example, blood cells from athletes before and after exercise. Researchers hope to use these tools to analyze patterns in order to better understand how the many pathways involved act at once.

Immunology

Immunology is the study of the immune system and is a very important branch of the medical and biological sciences. The immune system protects us from infection through various lines of defence. If the immune system is not functioning as it should, it can result in disease, such as autoimmunity, allergy and cancer. It is also now becoming clear that immune responses contribute to the development of many common disorders not traditionally viewed as immunologic, including metabolic, cardiovascular, and neurodegenerative conditions such as Alzheimer's.

Importance of Immunology

From Edward Jenner's pioneering work in the 18th Century that would ultimately lead to vaccination in its modern form (an innovation that has likely saved more lives than any other medical advance), to the many scientific breakthroughs in the 19th and 20th centuries that would lead to, amongst other things, safe organ transplantation, the identification of blood groups, and the now ubiquitous use of monoclonal antibodies throughout science and healthcare, immunology has changed the face of modern medicine. Immunological research continues to extend horizons in our understanding of how to treat significant health issues, with ongoing research efforts in immunotherapy, autoimmune diseases, and vaccines for emerging pathogens, such as Ebola. Advancing our understanding of basic immunology is essential for clinical and commercial application and has facilitated the discovery of new diagnostics and treatments to manage a wide array of diseases. In addition to the above, coupled with advancing technology, immunological research has provided critically important research techniques and tools, such as flow cytometry and antibody technology.

Immune Dysfunction and Clinical Immunology

The immune system is a highly regulated and balanced system and when the balance is disturbed, disease can result. Research in this area involves studying disease that is caused by immune system dysfunction. Much of this work has significance in the development of new therapies and treatments that can manage or cure the condition by altering the way the immune system is working or, in the case of vaccines, priming the immune system and boosting the immune reaction to specific pathogens.

Immunodeficiency disorders involve problems with the immune system that impair its ability to mount an appropriate defence. As a result, these are almost always associated with severe infections that persist, recur and/or lead to complications, making these disorders severely debilitating and even fatal. There are two types of immunodeficiency disorders: primary immunodeficiencies are typically present from birth, are generally hereditary and are relatively rare. Such an example is common variable immunodeficiency (CVID). Secondary immunodeficiencies generally develop later in life and may result following an infection, as is the case with AIDS following HIV infection.

Autoimmune diseases occur when the immune system attacks the body it is meant to protect. People suffering from autoimmune diseases have a defect that makes them unable to distinguish 'self' from 'non-self' or 'foreign' molecules. The principles of immunology have provided a wide variety of laboratory tests for the detection of autoimmune diseases. Autoimmune diseases may be described as 'primary' autoimmune diseases, like type-1 diabetes, which may be manifested from birth or during early life; or as 'secondary' autoimmune diseases, which manifest later in life due to various factors. Rheumatoid arthritis and multiple sclerosis are thought to belong to this type of autoimmunity. Also, autoimmune diseases can be localised, such as Crohn's Disease affecting the GI tract, or systemic, such as systemic lupus erythematosus (SLE).

Allergies are hypersensitivity disorders that occur when the body's immune system reacts against harmless foreign substances, resulting in damage to the body's own tissues. Almost any substance can cause allergies (an allergen), but most commonly, allergies arise after eating certain types of food, such as peanuts, or from inhaling airborne substances, such as pollen, or dust. In allergic reactions, the body believes allergens are dangerous and immediately produces substances to attack them. This causes cells of the immune system to release potent chemicals like histamine, which causes inflammation and many of the symptoms associated with allergies. Immunology strives to understand what happens to the body during an allergic response and the factors responsible for causing them. This should lead to better methods of diagnosing, preventing and controlling allergic diseases.

Asthma is a debilitating and sometimes fatal disease of the airways. It generally occurs when the immune system responds to inhaled particles from the air, and can lead to thickening of the airways in patients over time. It is a major cause of illness and is particularly prevalent in children. In some cases it has an allergic component, however in a number of cases the origin is more complex and poorly understood.

Cancer is a disease of abnormal and uncontrolled cell growth and proliferation and is defined by a set of hallmarks, one of which is the capacity for cancer cells to avoid immune destruction. With the knowledge that evasion of the immune system can contribute to cancer, researchers have turned to manipulating the immune system to defeat cancer (immunotherapy). Cancer immunotherapy seeks to stimulate the immune system's innate powers to fight cancerous tissue and has shown extraordinary promise as a new weapon in our arsenal against the disease. Other applications of immunological knowledge against cancer include the use of monoclonal antibodies (proteins that seek and directly bind to a specific target protein called an antigen. An example is Herceptin, which is a monoclonal antibody used to treat breast and stomach cancer). Moreover, a number of successful cancer vaccines have been developed, most notably the HPV vaccine.

Transplants involve transferring cells, tissues or organs from a donor to a recipient. The most formidable barrier to transplants is the immune system's recognition of the transplanted organs as foreign. Understanding the mechanisms and clinical features of rejection is important in determining a diagnosis, advising treatment and is critical for developing new strategies and drugs to manage transplants and limit the risk of rejection.

Vaccines are agents that teach the body to recognise and defend itself against infections from harmful pathogens, such as bacteria, viruses and parasites. Vaccines provide a sneak 'preview' of a specific pathogen, which stimulates the body's immune system to prepare itself in the event that infection occurs. Vaccines contain a harmless element of the infectious agent that stimulates the immune system to mount a response, beginning with the production of antibodies. Cells responsive to the vaccine proliferate both in order to manufacture antibodies specific to the provoking agent and also to form 'memory cells'. Upon encountering the infectious agent a second time, these memory cells are quickly able to deal with the threat by producing sufficient quantities of antibody. Pathogens inside the body are eventually destroyed, thereby thwarting further infection. Several infectious diseases including smallpox, measles, mumps, rubella, diphtheria, tetanus, whooping cough, tuberculosis and polio are no longer a threat in Europe due to the successful application of vaccines.

References

- Immune: kidshealth.org, Retrieved 4 March, 2019

- Immune-system: microrao.com, Retrieved 11 June, 2019

- Innate-immunity, the-immune-system, organ-systems: khanacademy.org, Retrieved 14 January, 2019

- Inflammation, health: healthline.com, Retrieved 20 May, 2019

- Adaptive-immune-response, biology: opentextbc.ca, Retrieved 8 February, 2019

- How-to-boost-your-immune-system, staying-healthy: health.harvard.edu, Retrieved 17 April, 2019

- What-is-immunology: immunology.org, Retrieved 19 July, 2019

Chapter 2

Antigen, Antibody and Major Histocompatibility Complex

The protein which is used by the immune system for neutralizing various pathogens is known as an antibody. The structures which are bound by antibodies are known as antigens. The set of genes which are integral for the recognition of foreign molecules by the acquired immune system is termed as major histocompatibility complex. This chapter discusses in detail the concepts related to antigens, antibodies and major histocompatibility complex.

Antigen

Antigen is a substances usually protein in nature and sometimes polysaccharide, that generates a specific immune response and induces the formation of a specific antibody or specially sensitized T cells or both.

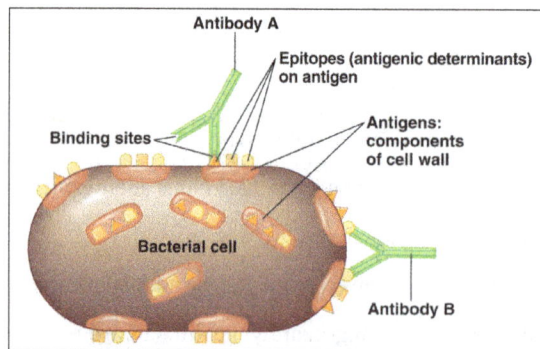

Diagram showing an antigen with epitopes (antigenic determinants).

Although all antigens are recognized by specific lymphocytes or by antibodies, only some antigens are capable of activating lymphocytes. Molecules that stimulate immune responses are called Immunogens.

Epitope is immunologically active regions of an immunogen (or antigen) that binds to antigen-specific membrane receptors on lymphocytes or to secreted antibodies. It is also called antigenic determinants. Autoantigens, for example, are a person's own self antigens. Examples: Thyroglobulin, DNA, Corneal tissue, etc.

Alloantigens are antigens found in different members of the same species (the red blood cell antigens A and B are examples).

Heterophile antigens are identical antigens found in the cells of different species. Examples: Forrssman antigen, Cross-reacting microbial antigens, etc. Adjuvants are substances that are non-immunogenic alone but enhance the immunogenicity of any added immunogen.

Chemical Nature of Antigens (Immunogens)

1. Proteins: The vast majority of immunogens are proteins. These may be pure proteins or they may be glycoproteins or lipoproteins. In general, proteins are usually very good immunogens.

2. Polysaccharides: Pure polysaccharides and lipopolysaccharides are good immunogens.

3. Nucleic Acids: Nucleic acids are usually poorly immunogenic. However, they may become immunogenic when single stranded or when complexed with proteins.

Lipids

In General Lipids are Non-immunogenic, Although They may be Haptens.

Types of Antigen on the Basis of Order of their Class (Origin)

- Exogenous antigens:
  - This antigen enters the body or system and starts circulating in the body fluids and trapped by the APCs (Antigen processing cells such as macrophages, dendritic cells, etc).
  - The uptakes of these exogenous antigens by APCs are mainly mediated by the phagocytosis.
  - Examples: bacteria, viruses, fungi etc.
  - Some antigens start out as exogenontigens, and later become endogenous (for example, intracellular viruses).
- Endogenous antigens:
  - These are body's own cells or sub fragments or compounds or the antigenic products that are produced.
  - The endogenous antigens are processed by the macrophages which are later accepted by the cytotoxic T – cells.
  - Endogenous antigens include xenogenic (heterologous), autologous and idiotypic or allogenic (homologous) antigens.
  - Examples: Blood group antigens, HLA (Histocompatibility Leukocyte antigens), etc.
- Autoantigens:
  - An autoantigen is usually a normal protein or complex of proteins (and sometimes DNA or RNA) that is recognized by the immune system of patients suffering from a specific autoimmune disease.
  - These antigens should not be, under normal conditions, the target of the immune system, but, due mainly to genetic and environmental factors, the normal immunological tolerance for such an antigen has been lost in these patients.

- Examples: Nucleoproteins, Nucleic acids, etc.

On the basis of Immune Response

- Complete Antigen or Immunogen:

  ○ Possess antigenic properties denovo, i.e. there are able to generate an immune response by them.

  ○ High molecular weight (more than 10,000).

  ○ May be proteins or polysaccharides.

- Incomplete Antigen or Hapten

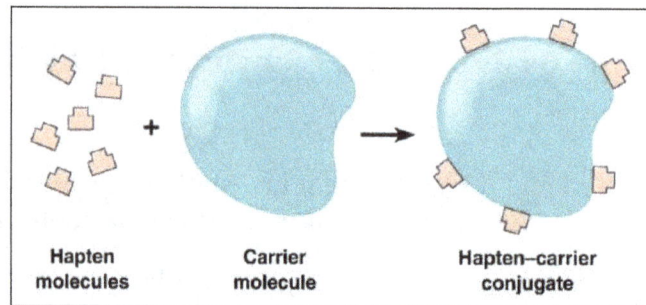

Hapten   Carrier   Hapten–carrier
molecules   molecule   conjugate

  ○ These are the foreign substance, usually non-protein substances.

  ○ Unable to induce an immune response by itself, they require carrier molecule to act as a complete antigen.

  ○ The carrier molecule is a non-antigenic component and helps in provoking the immune response. Example: Serum Protein such as Albumin or Globulin.

  ○ Low Molecular Weight (Less than 10,000).

  ○ Haptens can react specifically with its corresponding antibody.

  ○ Examples: Capsular polysaccharide of pneumococcus, polysaccharide "C" of beta haemolytic streptococci, cardiolipin antigens, etc.

Property of Antigens/Factors Influencing Immunogenicity

Immunogenicity is determined by:

- Foreignness

  ○ An antigen must be a foreign substances to the animal to elicit an immune response.

- Molecular Size

  ○ The most active immunogens tend to have a molecular mass of 14,000 to 6,00,000 Da.

  ○ Examples: tetanus toxoid, egg albumin, thyroglobulin are highly antigenic.

- Insulin (5700) are either non-antigenic or weakly antigenic.

- Chemical Nature and Composition:

  - In general, the more complex the substance is chemically the more immunogenic it will be.

  - Antigens are mainly proteins and some are polysaccharides.

  - It is presumed that presence of an aromatic radical is essential for rigidity and antigenicity of a substance.

- Physical Form:

  - In general particulate antigens are more immunogenic than soluble ones.

  - Denatured antigens are more immunogenic than the native form.

- Antigen Specificity:

  - Antigen Specificity depends on the specific actives sites on the antigenic molecules (Antigenic determinants).

  - Antigenic determinants or epitopes are the regions of antigen which specifically binds with the antibody molecule.

- Species Specificity:

  - Tissues of all individuals in a particular species possess, species specific antigen.

  - Human Blood proteins can be differentiated from animal protein by specific antigen-antibody reaction.

- Organ Specificity:

  - Organ specific antigens are confined to particular organ or tissue.

  - Certain proteins of brain, kidney, and thyroglobulin and lens protein of one species share specificity with that of another species.

- Auto-specificity:

  - The autologous or self-antigens are ordinarily not immunogenic, but under certain circumstances lens protein, thyroglobulin and others may act as autoantigens.

- Genetic Factors:

  - Some substances are immunogenic in one species but not in another .Similarly, some substances are immunogenic in one individual but not in others (i.e. responders and non-responders).

  - The species or individuals may lack or have altered genes that code for the receptors for antigen on B cells and T cells.

- ○ They may not have the appropriate genes needed for the APC to present antigen to the helper T cells.

- Age:

  - ○ Age can also influence immunogenicity.

  - ○ Usually the very young and the very old have a diminished ability to elicit and immune response in response to an immunogen.

- Degradability:

  - ○ Antigens that are easily phagocytosed are generally more immunogenic.

  - ○ This is because for most antigens (T-dependant antigens) the development of an immune response requires that the antigen be phagocytosed, processed and presented to helper T cells by an antigen presenting cell (APC).

- Dose of the antigen:

  - ○ The dose of administration of an immunogen can influence its immunogenicity.

  - ○ There is a dose of antigen above or below which the immune response will not be optimal.

- Route of Administration:

  - ○ Generally the subcutaneous route is better than the intravenous or intragastric routes.

  - ○ The route of antigen administration can also alter the nature of the response.

  - ○ Antigen administered intravenously is carried first to the spleen, whereas antigen administered subcutaneously moves first to local lymph nodes.

- Adjuvants:

  - ○ Substances that can enhance the immune response to an immunogen are called adjuvants.

  - ○ The use of adjuvants, however, is often hampered by undesirable side effects such as fever and inflammation.

  - ○ Example: aluminum hydroxide.

Superantigens

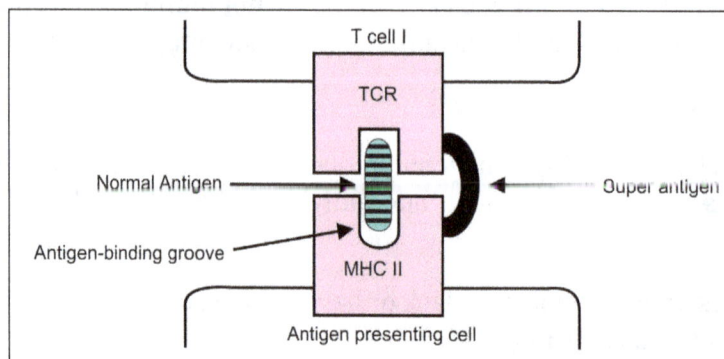

- When the immune system encounters a conventional T-dependent antigen, only a small fraction (1 in 104 -105) of the T cell population is able to recognize the antigen and become activated (monoclonal/oligoclonal response).

- However, there are some antigens which polyclonally activate a large fraction of the T cells (up to 25%). These antigens are called superantigens.

- Examples of superantigens include: Staphylococcal enterotoxins (food poisoning), Staphylococcal toxic shock toxin (toxic shock syndrome), Staphylococcal exfoliating toxins (scalded skin syndrome) and Streptococcal pyrogenic exotoxins (shock).

- Although the bacterial superantigens are the best studied there are superantigens associated with viruses and other microorganisms as well.

- The diseases associated with exposure to superantigens are, in part, due to hyper activation of the immune system and subsequent release of biologically active cytokines by activated T cells

Antigenic Determinants and Processing Pathways

Antigen epitopes make it possible for the immune system to recognize pathogens. An epitope, also known as an antigenic determinant, is the part of an antigen that is recognized by the immune system, specifically by antibodies, B cells, and T cells. The latter can use epitopes to distinguish between different antigens, and only binds to their specific antigen. In antibodies, the binding site for an epitope is called a paratope. Although epitopes are usually derived from non-self-proteins, sequences derived from the host that can be recognized are also classified as epitopes. Epitopes determine how antigen binding and antigen presentation occur.

Types of Antigenic Determinants

The epitopes of protein antigens are divided into two categories based on their structures and interaction with the paratope:

- A conformational epitope is composed of discontinuous sections of the antigen's amino acid sequence. These epitopes interact with the paratope based on the 3-D surface features and tertiary structure (overall shape) of the antigen. Most epitopes are conformational.

- Linear epitopes interact with the paratope based on their primary structure (shape of the protein's components). A linear epitope is formed by a continuous sequence of amino acids from the antigen, which creates a "line" of sorts that builds the protein structure.

Antigenic determinants recognized by B cells and the antibodies secreted by B cells can be either conformational or linear epitopes. Antigenic determinants recognized by T cells are typically linear epitopes. T cells do not recognize polysaccharide or nucleic acid antigens. This is why polysaccharides are generally T-independent antigens and proteins are generally T-dependent antigens. The determinants need not be located on the exposed surface of the antigen in its original form, since recognition of the determinant by T cells requires that the antigen be first processed by antigen presenting cells. Free peptides flowing through the body are not recognized by T cells, but the peptides associate with molecules coded for by the major histocompatibility complex (MHC). This combination of MHC molecules and peptide is recognized by T cells.

Antigen-processing Pathways

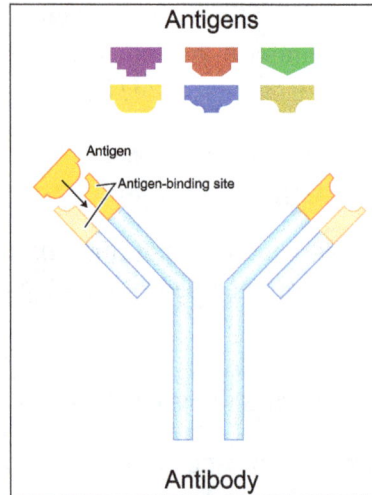

Antigen-Binding Site of an Antibody: Antigen-binding sites can recognize different epitopes on an antigen.

In order for an antigen-presenting cell (APC) to present an antigen to a naive T cell, it must first be processed so itacan be recognized by the T cell receptor. This occurs within an APC that phagocytizes an antigen and then digests it through fragmentation (proteolysis) of the antigen protein, association of the fragments with MHC molecules, and expression of the peptide-MHC molecules at the cell surface. There, they are recognized by the T cell receptor on a T cell during antigen presentation. MHC molecules must move between the cell membrane and cytoplasm in order for antigen processing to occur properly. However, the pathway leading to the association of protein fragments with MHC molecules differs between class I and class II MHC, which are presented to cytotoxic or helper T cells respectively. There are two different pathways for antigen processing:

- The endogenous pathway occurs when MHC class I molecules present antigens derived from intracellular (endogenous) proteins in the cytoplasm, such as the proteins produced within virus-infected cells. Generally, proteosomes are used to break up the viral proteins and combine them with MHC I.

- The exogenous pathway occurs when MHC class II molecules present fragments derived from extracellular (exogenous) proteins that are located within the cell. First, pathogens are phagocytized, and then endosomes within the cell break down antigens with proteases, which then combine with MHC II.

Some viral pathogens have developed ways to evade antigen processing. For example, cytomegalovirus and HIV-infected cells sometimes disrupt MHC movement through the cytoplasm, which may prevent them from binding to antigens or from moving back to the cell membrane after binding with an antigen.

Antibody

An antibody is a protein produced by the immune system that is capable of binding with high specificity to an antigen. These antigens are typically other proteins, but may be carbohydrates, small molecules or even nucleotides. Antibodies are powerful research tools because they bind specifically to a unique epitope on the antigen, thereby allowing the detection of a specific protein in an assay while avoiding detection of unrelated proteins. This specific binding capability also allows antibodies to be used in diagnostic applications such as pregnancy tests and in therapeutic applications such as cancer treatments. The antibody itself is a Y-shaped protein that contains a constant region common to all antibodies produced by a particular species and a variable region that is unique and specific to a particular epitope. The following diagram illustrates this structure:

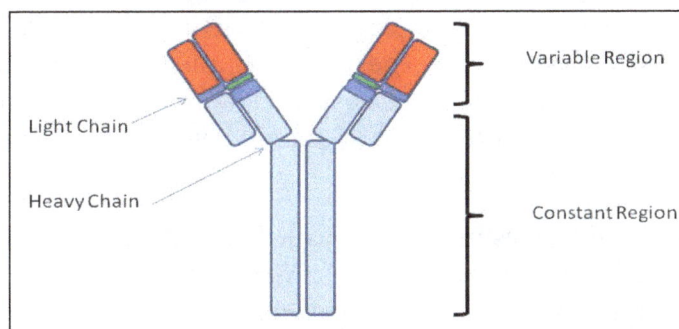

Antibodies that bind specifically to the antigen of interest can be used in a number of immuno-assays. For example, Western Blot and ELISA assays allow for detection and quantification of specific proteins. Immunohistochemistry allows for the localization of a specific protein within a cell or tissue. And, Immunoprecipitation allows for the isolation of a specific protein from within a mixture of proteins.

Major Histocompatibility Complex

The function of MHC molecules is to bind peptide fragments derived from pathogens and display them on the cell surface for recognition by the appropriate T cells. The consequences are almost always deleterious to the pathogen—virus-infected cells are killed, macrophages are activated to kill bacteria living in their intracellular vesicles, and B cells are activated to produce antibodies that eliminate or neutralize extracellular pathogens. Thus, there is strong selective pressure in favor of any pathogen that has mutated in such a way that it escapes presentation by an MHC molecule.

Two separate properties of the MHC make it difficult for pathogens to evade immune responses in this way. First, the MHC is polygenic: it contains several different MHC class I and MHC class II genes, so that every individual possesses a set of MHC molecules with different ranges of peptide-binding specificities. Second, the MHC is highly polymorphic; that is, there are multiple variants of each gene within the population as a whole. The MHC genes are, in fact, the most polymorphic genes known. Here, we will describe the organization of the genes in the MHC and discuss how the variation in MHC molecules arises. We will also see how the effect of polygeny and polymorphism on the range of peptides that can be bound contributes to the ability of the immune system to respond to the multitude of different and rapidly evolving pathogens.

1. Many proteins involved in antigen processing and presentation are encoded by genes within the major histocompatibility complex:

The major histocompatibility complex is located on chromosome 6 in humans and chromosome 17 in the mouse and extends over some 4 centimorgans of DNA, about 4×10^6 base pairs. In humans it contains more than 200 genes. As work continues to define the genes within and around the MHC, both its extent and the number of genes are likely to grow; in fact, recent studies suggest that the MHC may span at least 7×10^6 base pairs. The genes encoding the α chains of MHC class I molecules and the α and β chains of MHC class II molecules are linked within the complex; the genes for β_2-microglobulin and the invariant chain are on different chromosomes (chromosomes 15 and 5, respectively, in humans and chromosomes 2 and 18 in the mouse). Figure shows the general organization of the MHC class I and II genes in human and mouse. In humans these genes are called *Human Leukocyte Antigen* or HLA genes, as they were first discovered through antigenic differences between white blood cells from different individuals; in the mouse they are known as the H-2 genes.

There are three class I α-chain genes in humans, called HLA-A, -B, and -C. There are also three pairs of MHC class II α- and β-chain genes, called HLA-DR, -DP, and -DQ. However, in many cases the HLA-DR cluster contains an extra β-chain gene whose product can pair with the DRα chain. This means that the three sets of genes can give rise to four types of MHC class II molecule. All the MHC class I and class II molecules can present peptides to T cells, but each protein binds a different range of peptides. Thus, the presence of several different genes of each MHC class means that any one individual is equipped to present a much broader range of peptides than if only one MHC molecule of each class were expressed at the cell surface.

The two TAP genes lie in the MHC class II region, in close association with the LMP genes that encode components of the proteasome, whereas the gene for tapasin, which binds to both TAP and empty MHC class I molecules, lies at the edge of the MHC nearest the centromere. The genetic linkage of the MHC class I genes, whose products deliver cytosolic peptides to the cell surface, with the TAP, tapasin, and proteasome genes, which encode the molecules that generate peptides in the cytosol and transport them into the endoplasmic reticulum, suggests that the entire MHC has been selected during evolution for antigen processing and presentation.

When cells are treated with the interferons IFN-α, -β, or -γ, there is a marked increase in transcription of MHC class I α-chain and β_2-microglobulin genes, and of the proteasome, tapasin, and TAP genes. Interferons are produced early in viral infections as part of the innate immune response, and so this effect increases the ability of cells to process viral proteins and present the resulting peptides at the cell surface. This helps to activate the appropriate T cells and initiate the adaptive immune response in response to the virus. The coordinated regulation of the genes encoding these components may be facilitated by the linkage of many of them in the MHC.

The HLA-DM genes, which encode the DM molecule whose function is to catalyze peptide binding to MHC class II molecules, are clearly related to the MHC class II genes. The DNα and DOβ genes, which encode the DO molecule, a negative regulator of DM, are also clearly related to the MHC class II genes. The classical MHC class II genes, along with the invariant-chain gene and the genes for DMα, β, and DNα, but not DOβ, are coordinately regulated. This distinct regulation of MHC class II genes by IFN-γ, which is made by activated T cells of T_H1 type as well as by activated CD8 and NK cells, allows T cells responding to bacterial infections to upregulate those molecules concerned in the processing and presentation of intravesicular antigens. Expression of all of these molecules is induced by IFN-γ (but not by IFN-α or -β), via the production of a transcriptional activator known as MHC class *II* trans*activator (CIITA). An absence of CIITA causes severe immunodeficiency due to nonproduction of MHC class II molecules.

2. A variety of genes with specialized functions in immunity are also encoded in the MHC:

Although the most important known function of the gene products of the MHC is the processing and presentation of antigens to T cells, many other genes map within this region; some of these are known to have other roles in the immune system, but many have yet to be characterized functionally. Figure shows the detailed organization of the human MHC.

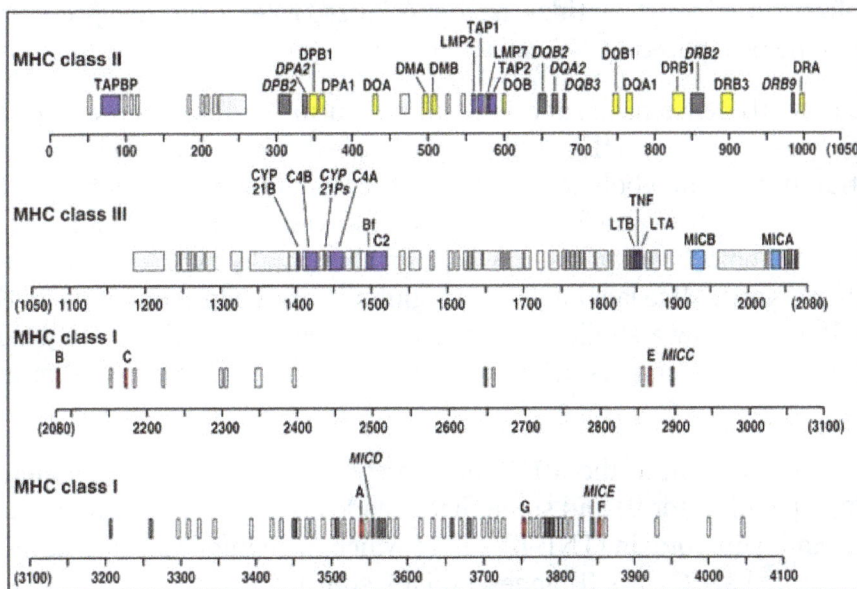

Detailed map of the human MHC.

In figure, the organization of the class I, class II, and class III regions of the human MHC are shown, with approximate genetic distances given in thousands of base pairs (kb). Most of the genes in the class I and class II regions are mentioned in the text. The additional genes indicated in the class I region (for example, E, F, and G) are class I-like genes, encoding class IB molecules; the additional class II genes are pseudogenes. The genes shown in the class III region encode the complement proteins C4 (two genes, shown as C4A and C4B), C2 and factor B (shown as Bf) as well as genes that encode the cytokines tumor necrosis factor-α (TNF) and lymphotoxin (LTA, LTB). Closely linked to the C4 genes is the gene encoding 21-hydroxylase (shown as CYP 21B), an enzyme involved in steroid synthesis. Genes shown in gray and named in italic are pseudogenes. The genes are colour coded, with the MHC class I genes being shown in red, except for the MIC genes, which are shown in blue; these are distinct from the other class I-like genes and are under different transcriptional control. The MHC class II genes are shown in yellow. Genes in the MHC region which have immune functions but are not related to the MHC class I and class II genes are shown in purple.

In addition to the highly polymorphic 'classical' MHC class I and class II genes, there are many genes encoding MHC class I-type molecules that show little polymorphism; most of these have yet to be assigned a function. They are linked to the class I region of the MHC and their exact number varies greatly between species and even between members of the same species. These genes have been termed MHC class IB genes; like MHC class I genes, they encode β_2-microglobulin-associated cell-surface molecules. Their expression on cells is variable, both in the amount expressed at the cell surface and in the tissue distribution.

One of the mouse MHC class IB molecules, H2-M3, can present peptides with N-formylated amino termini, which is of interest because all bacteria initiate protein synthesis with N-formylmethionine. Cells infected with cytosolic bacteria can be killed by CD8 T cells that recognize N-formylated bacterial peptides bound to H2-M3. Whether an equivalent MHC class IB molecule exists in humans is not known. The large number of MHC class IB genes (50 or more in the mouse) means that many different MHC class IB molecules can exist in a single animal. They may, like the protein that presents N-formylmethionyl peptides, have specialized roles in antigen presentation. Some of them are known to be recognized by NK cell receptors.

Yet other MHC class IB genes have functions unrelated to the immune system. The HFe gene lies some 3×10^6 base pairs from HLA-A. Its product is expressed on cells in the intestinal tract, and has a function in iron metabolism, regulating the uptake of iron into the body, most likely through interactions with the transferrin receptor. Individuals defective for this gene have an iron-storage disease, hemochromatosis, in which an abnormally high level of iron is retained in the liver and other organs. Mice lacking β_2-microglobulin, and hence defective in the expression of all class I molecules, show a similar iron overload. Exactly how this gene product regulates the levels of iron within the body is not known, but it is unlikely to involve an immunological mechanism.

The other genes that map within the MHC include some that encode complement components (for example, C2, C4, and factor B) and some that encode cytokines—for example, tumor necrosis factor-α (TNF-α) and lymphotoxin (TNF-β)—all of which have important functions in immunity. These have been termed MHC class III genes, and are shown in figure.

Many studies have established associations between susceptibility to certain diseases and particular alleles of MHC genes, and we now have considerable insight into how polymorphism in the classical MHC class I and class II genes can affect resistance or susceptibility. But although most of these MHCinfluenced diseases are known or suspected to have an immune etiology, this is not true of all of them, and it is important to remember that there are many genes lying within the MHC that have no known or suspected immunological function. One of these is the enzyme 21-hydroxylase which, when deficient, causes congenital adrenal hyperplasia and, in severe cases, salt-wasting syndrome. Even where a disease-related gene is clearly homologous to immune system genes, as is the case with HFe, the disease mechanism may not be immune related. Disease associations mapping to the MHC must therefore be interpreted with caution, in the light of a detailed understanding of its genetic structure and the functions of its individual genes. Much remains to be learned about the latter and about the significance of all the genetic variation localized within the MHC. For instance, the C4 genes are highly polymorphic, but the adaptive significance of this genetic variability is not well understood.

3. Specialized MHC class I molecules act as ligands for activation and inhibition of NK cells:

Some class IB genes, for example the members of the MIC gene family, are under a different regulatory control from the classical MHC class I genes and are induced in response to cellular stress (such as heat shock). There are five MIC genes, but only two—*MICA* and *MICB*—are expressed and produce protein products. They are expressed in fibroblasts and epithelial cells, particularly in intestinal epithelial cells, and may play a part in innate immunity or in the induction of immune responses in circumstances where interferons are not produced. The MICA and MICB molecules are recognized by a receptor that is present on NK cells, γ : δ T cells and some CD8 T cells and is capable of activating these cells to kill MIC-expressing targets. The MIC receptor is composed of two chains. One is NKG2D, an 'activating' member of the NKG2 family of NK-cell receptors whose cytoplasmic domain lacks an inhibitory sequence motif found in other members of this family that act as inhibitory receptors; the other is a protein called DAP10, which transmits the signal into the interior of the cell by interacting with and activating intracellular protein tyrosine kinases.

Other MHC class IB molecules may inhibit cell killing by NK cells, such a role has been suggested for the MHC class IB molecule HLA-G, which is expressed on fetus-derived placental cells that migrate into the uterine wall. These cells express no classical MHC class I molecules and cannot be recognized by CD8 T cells but, unlike other cells lacking classical MHC class I molecules, they are not killed by NK cells. This appears to be because HLA-G is recognized by an inhibitory receptor, ILT-2, on the NK cell, which prevents the NK cell killing the placental cell.

Another MHC class IB molecule, HLA-E, also has a specialized role in cell recognition by NK cells. HLA-E binds a very restricted subset of peptides, derived from the leader peptides of other HLA class I molecules. This peptide: HLA-E complexes can bind to the receptor NKG2A, which is present on NK cells in a complex with the cell-surface molecule CD94. NKG2A is an inhibitory member of the NKG2 family and on stimulation inhibits the cytotoxic activity of the NK cell. Thus a cell that expresses either HLA-E or HLA-G is not killed by NK cells.

4. The protein products of MHC class I and class II genes are highly polymorphic:

Because of the polygeny of the MHC, every person will express at least three different antigen-presenting MHC class I molecules and three (or sometimes four) MHC class II molecules on his or her cells. In fact, the number of different MHC molecules expressed on the cells of most people is greater because of the extreme polymorphism of the MHC and the codominant expression of MHC gene products.

The term polymorphism comes from the Greek *poly*, meaning many, and *morphe*, meaning shape or structure. As used here, it means within-species variation at a gene locus, and thus in its protein product; the variant genes that can occupy the locus are termed alleles. There are more than 200 alleles of some human MHC class I and class II genes, each allele being present at a relatively high frequency in the population. So there is only a small chance that the corresponding MHC locus on both the homologous chromosomes of an individual will have the same allele; most individuals will be heterozygous at MHC loci. The particular combination of MHC alleles found on a single chromosome is known as an MHC haplotype. Expression of MHC alleles is codominant, with the protein products of both the alleles at a locus being expressed in the cell, and both gene products being able to present antigens to T cells. The extensive polymorphism at each locus thus has the potential to double the number of different MHC molecules expressed in an individual and thereby increases the diversity already available through polygeny.

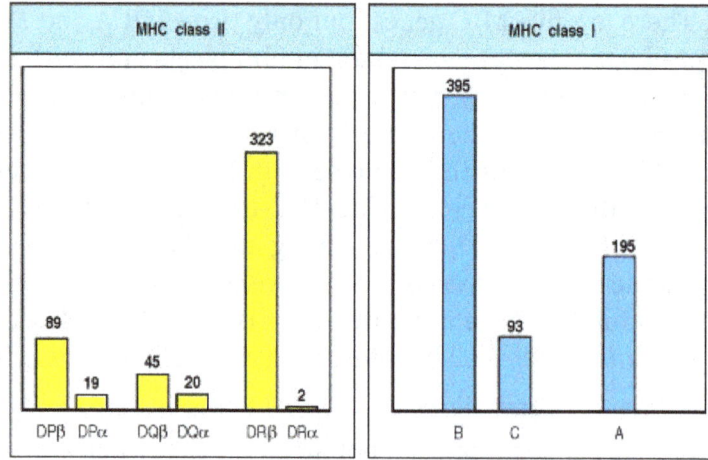

Figure: Human MHC genes are highly polymorphic.

In figure, with the notable exception of the DRα locus, which is functionally monomorphic, each locus has many alleles. The number of different alleles is shown in this figure by the height of the bars. The figures are the numbers of HLA alleles currently officially assigned by the WHO Nomenclature Committee for Factors of the HLA System as of August 2000.

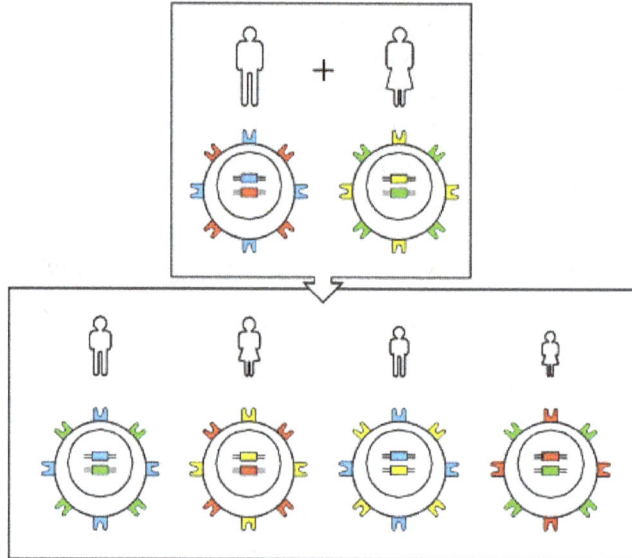

Expression of MHC alleles is codominant.

In figure, the MHC is so polymorphic that most individuals are likely to be heterozygous at each locus. Alleles are expressed from both MHC haplotypes in any one individual, and the products of all alleles are found on all expressing cells. In any mating, four possible combinations of haplotypes can be found in the offspring; thus siblings are also likely to differ in the MHC alleles they express, there being one chance in four that an individual will share both haplotypes with a sibling. One consequence of this is the difficulty of finding suitable donors for tissue transplantation.

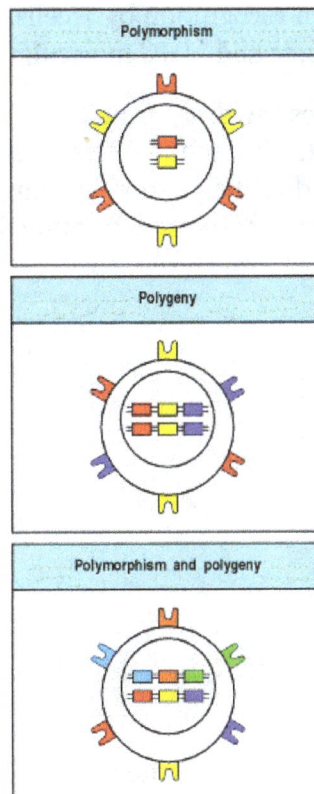

Figure shows polymorphism and polygeny both contribute to the diversity of MHC molecules expressed by an individual. The high polymorphism of the classical MHC loci ensures a diversity in MHC gene expression in the population as a whole. However, no matter how polymorphic a gene, no individual can express more than two alleles at a single gene locus. Polygeny, the presence of several different related genes with similar functions ensures that each individual produces a number of different MHC molecules. Polymorphism and polygeny combine to produce the diversity of MHC molecules seen both within an individual and in the population at large.

Thus, with three MHC class I genes and a possible four sets of MHC class II genes on each chromosome 6, a human typically expresses six different MHC class I molecules and eight different MHC class II molecules on his or her cells. For the MHC class II genes, the number of different MHC molecules may be increased still further by the combination of α and β chains encoded by different chromosomes (so that two α chains and two β chains can give rise to four different proteins, for example). In mice it has been shown that not all combinations of α and β chains can form stable dimers and so, in practice, the exact number of different MHC class II molecules expressed depends on which alleles are present on each chromosome.

All MHC products are polymorphic to a greater or lesser extent, with the exception of the DRα chain and its mouse homologue Eα. These chains do not vary in sequence between different individuals and are said to be monomorphic. This might indicate a functional constraint that prevents variation in the DRα and Eα proteins, but no such special function has been found. Many mice, both domestic and wild, have a mutation in the Eα gene that prevents synthesis of the Eα protein. They thus lack cell-surface H-2E molecules, so if H2-E molecules do have a special function it is unlikely to be an essential one. All other MHC classes I and class II genes are polymorphic.

5. MHC polymorphism affects antigen recognition by T cells by influencing both peptide binding and the contacts between T-cell receptor and MHC molecule:

The products of individual MHC alleles can differ from one another by up to 20 amino acids, making each variant protein quite distinct. Most of the differences are localized to exposed surfaces of the outer domain of the molecule, and to the peptide-binding groove in particular. The polymorphic residues that line the peptide-binding groove determine the peptide-binding properties of the different MHC molecules.

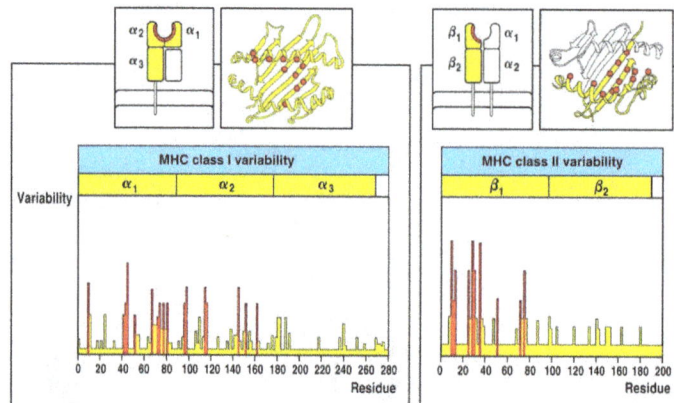

Figure shows allelic variation occurs at specific sites within MHC molecules. Variability plots of the amino acid sequences of MHC molecules show that the variation arising from genetic polymorphism is restricted to the amino-terminal domains (α_1 and α_2 domains of class I molecules, and α_1 and β_1 domains of MHC class II molecules). These are the domains that form the peptide-binding cleft. Moreover, allelic variability is clustered in specific sites within the amino-terminal domains, lying in positions that line the peptide-binding cleft, either on the floor of the groove or directed inward from the walls. For the MHC class II molecule, the variability of the HLA-DR alleles is shown. For HLA-DR, and its homologues in other species, the α chain is essentially invariant and only the β chain shows significant polymorphism.

We have seen that peptides bind to MHC class I molecules through specific anchor residues, and that the amino acid side chains of these residues anchor the peptide by binding in pockets that line the peptide-binding groove. Polymorphism in MHC class I molecules affects which amino acids line these pockets and thus their binding specificity. In consequence, the anchor residues of peptides that bind to each allelic variant are different. The set of anchor residues that allows binding to a given MHC class I molecule is called a sequence motif. These sequence motifs make it possible to identify peptides within a protein that can potentially bind the appropriate MHC molecule, which may be very important in designing peptide vaccines. Different allelic variants of MHC class II molecules also bind different peptides, but the more open structure of the MHC class II peptide-binding groove and the greater length of the peptides bound in it allow greater flexibility in peptide binding . It is therefore more difficult to predict which peptides will bind to MHC class II molecules.

In rare cases, processing of a protein will not generate any peptides with a suitable motif for binding to any of the MHC molecules expressed by an individual. When this happens, the individual fails to respond to the antigen. Such failures in responsiveness to simple antigens were first reported in inbred animals, where they were called immune response (Ir) gene defects. These defects were identified and mapped to genes within the MHC long before the function of MHC molecules was understood. Indeed, they were the first clue to the antigen-presenting function of MHC molecules, although it was only much later that the 'Ir genes' were shown to encode MHC class II molecules. Ir gene defects are common in inbred strains of mice because the mice are homozygous at all their MHC loci and thus express only one type of MHC molecule from each gene locus. This limits the range of peptides they can present to T cells. Ordinarily, MHC polymorphism guarantees a sufficient number of different MHC molecules in a single individual to make this type of non-responsiveness unlikely, even to relatively simple antigens such as small toxins. This has obvious importance for host defense.

Initially, the only evidence linking Ir gene defects to the MHC was genetic—mice of one MHC genotype could make antibody in response to a particular antigen, whereas mice of a different MHC genotype, but otherwise genetically identical, could not. The MHC genotype was somehow controlling the ability of the immune system to detect or respond to specific antigens, but it was not clear at the time that direct recognition of MHC molecules was involved.

Later experiments showed that the antigen specificity of T-cell recognition was controlled by MHC molecules. The immune responses affected by the Ir genes were known to be dependent on T cells, and this led to a series of experiments in mice to ascertain how MHC polymorphism might control T-cell responses. The earliest of these experiments showed that T cells could only be activated by macrophages or B cells that shared MHC alleles with the mouse in which the T cells originated. This was the first evidence that antigen recognition by T cells depends on the presence of specific MHC molecules in the antigen-presenting cell. The clearest example of this feature of T-cell recognition came, however, from studies of virus-specific cytotoxic T cells, for which Peter Doherty and Rolf Zinkernagel were awarded the Nobel Prize in 1996.

When mice are infected with a virus, they generate cytotoxic T cells that kill self-cells infected with the virus, while sparing uninfected cells or cells infected with unrelated viruses. The cytotoxic T cells are thus virus-specific. A particularly striking outcome of these experiments was that the specificity of the cytotoxic T cells was also affected by the polymorphism of MHC molecules. Cytotoxic T cells induced by viral infection in mice of MHC genotype a (MHC^a) would kill any MHC^a cell infected with that virus but would not kill cells of MHC genotype b, or c, and so on, even if they were infected with the same virus. Because the MHC genotype restricts the antigen specificity of T cells, this effect is called MHC restriction. Together with the earlier studies on both B cells and macrophages, this work showed that MHC restriction is a critical feature of antigen recognition by all functional classes of T cells.

Because different MHC molecules bind different peptides, MHC restriction in immune responses to viruses and other complex antigens might be explained solely on this indirect basis. However, it can be seen from figure that some of the polymorphic amino acids in MHC molecules are located in the α helices flanking the peptide-binding cleft in such a way that they are exposed on the outer surface of the peptide: MHC complex and can be directly contacted by the T-cell receptor . It is therefore not surprising that when T cells are tested for their ability to recognize the same peptide bound to different MHC molecules, they readily distinguish the peptide bound to MHC^a from the same peptide bound to MHC^b. Thus, the specificity of a T-cell receptor is defined both by the peptide it recognizes and by the MHC molecule bound to it. This restricted recognition may sometimes be caused by differences in the conformation of the bound peptide imposed by the different MHC molecules rather than by direct recognition of polymorphic amino acids in the MHC molecule itself. MHC restriction in antigen recognition therefore reflects the combined effect of differences in peptide binding and of direct contact between the MHC molecule and the T-cell receptor.

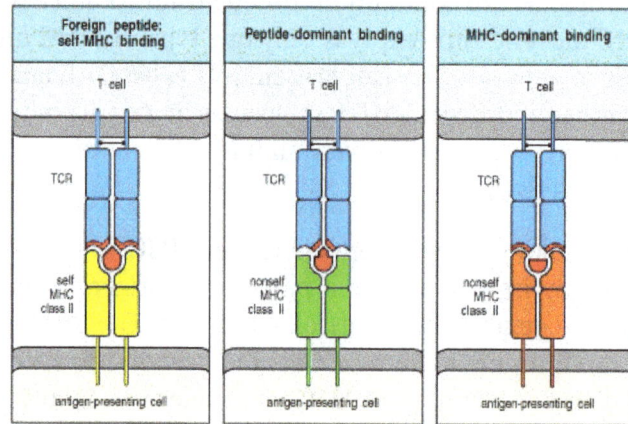

Figure shows two modes of crossreactive recognition that may explain alloreactivity. A T cell that is specific for one peptide: MHC combination (left panel) may cross-react with peptides presented by other, nonself (allogeneic), MHC molecules. This may come about in either of two ways. Most commonly, the peptides bound to the allogeneic MHC molecule fit well to the T-cell receptor (TCR), allowing binding even if there is not a good fit with the MHC molecule (center panel). Alternatively, but less often, the allogeneic MHC molecule may provide a better fit to the T-cell receptor, giving a tight binding that is thus less dependent on the peptide that is bound to the MHC molecule (right panel).

6. Nonself MHC molecules are recognized by 1–10% of T cells:

The discovery of MHC restriction, by revealing the physiological function of the MHC molecules, also helped explain the otherwise puzzling phenomenon of recognition of nonself MHC in the rejection of organs and tissues transplanted between members of the same species. Transplanted organs from donors bearing MHC molecules that differ from those of the recipient—even by as little as one amino acid—are invariably rejected. The rapid and very potent cell-mediated immune response to the transplanted tissue results from the presence in any individual of large numbers of T cells that are specifically reactive to nonself, or allogeneic, MHC molecules. Early studies on T-cell responses to allogeneic MHC molecules used the mixed lymphocyte reaction. In this reaction T cells from one individual are mixed with lymphocytes from a second individual. If the T cells of one individual recognize the other individual's MHC molecules as 'foreign,' the T cells will divide and proliferate. (The lymphocytes from the second individual are usually prevented from dividing by irradiation or treatment with the cytostatic drug mitomycin C.) Such studies have shown that roughly 1–10% of all T cells in an individual will respond to stimulation by cells from another, unrelated, member of the same species. This type of T-cell response is called alloreactivity because it represents the recognition of allelic polymorphism in allogeneic MHC molecules.

Before the role of the MHC molecules in antigen presentation was understood, it was a mystery why so many T cells should recognize nonself MHC molecules, as there is no reason the immune system should have evolved a defense against tissue transplants. However, once it was appreciated that T-cell receptors have evolved to recognize foreign peptides in combination with polymorphic

MHC molecules, alloreactivity became easier to explain. From experiments in which T cells from animals lacking MHC class I and class II molecules have been artificially driven to mature, it has been shown that the ability to recognize MHC molecules is inherent in the genes that encode the T-cell receptor, rather than being dependent on selection for MHC recognition during T-cell development. The high frequency of alloreactive T cells clearly reflects the commitment of the T-cell receptor to the recognition of MHC molecules in general.

Mature T cells have, however, survived a stringent selection process for the ability to respond to foreign, but not self, peptides bound to self MHC molecules. It is therefore thought that the alloreactivity of mature T cells reflects the cross-reactivity of T-cell receptors normally specific for a variety of foreign peptides bound by self MHC molecules. Given a T-cell receptor that normally binds a foreign peptide displayed by a self MHC molecule, there are two ways in which it may bind to nonself MHC molecules. In some cases, the peptide bound by the nonself MHC molecule interacts strongly with the T-cell receptor, and the T cells bearing this receptor are stimulated to respond. This type of cross-reactive recognition arises because the spectrum of peptides bound by nonself MHC molecules on the transplanted tissues differs from those bound by the host's own MHC, and it is known as peptide-dominant binding. In a second type of cross-reactive recognition, known as MHC-dominant binding, allo-reactive T cells respond because of direct binding of the T-cell receptor to distinctive features of the nonself MHC molecule (Figure, right panel). In these cases the recognition is less dependent on the particular peptide bound; T-cell receptor binding to unique features of the nonself MHC molecule generates a strong signal because of the high concentration of the nonself MHC molecule on the surface of the presenting cell. Both these mechanisms may contribute to the high frequency of T cells that can respond to nonself MHC molecules on transplanted tissue.

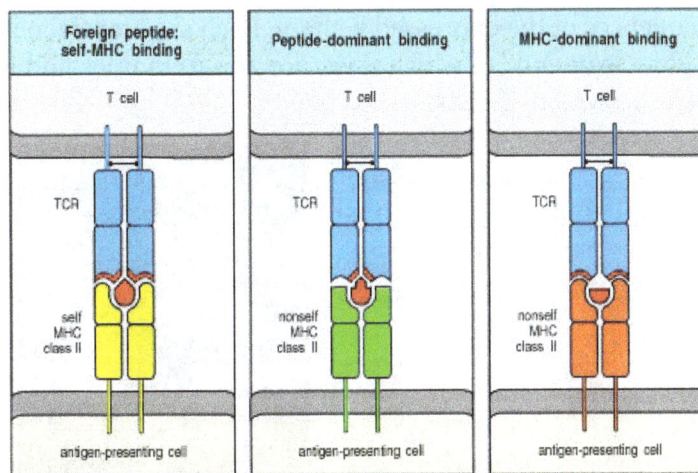

Figure shows two modes of crossreactive recognition that may explain alloreactivity. A T cell that is specific for one peptide:MHC combination (left panel) may cross-react with peptides presented by other, nonself (allogeneic), MHC molecules. This may come about in either of two ways. Most commonly, the peptides bound to the allogeneic MHC molecule fit well to the T-cell receptor (TCR), allowing binding even if there is not a good fit with the MHC molecule (center panel). Alternatively, but less often, the allogeneic MHC molecule may provide a better fit to the T-cell receptor, giving a tight binding that is thus less dependent on the peptide that is bound to the MHC molecule (right panel).

7. Many T cells respond to superantigens:

Superantigens are a distinct class of antigens that stimulate a primary T-cell response similar in magnitude to a response to allogeneic MHC. Such responses were first observed in mixed lymphocyte reactions using lymphocytes from strains of mice which were MHC identical but otherwise genetically distinct. The antigens provoking this reaction were originally designated minor lymphocyte stimulating (Mls) antigens, and it seemed reasonable to suppose that they might be functionally similar to the MHC molecules themselves. We now know that this is not the case, however. The Mls antigens found in these mice strains are encoded by retroviruses which have become stably integrated at various sites into the mouse chromosomes. They act as superantigens because they have a distinctive mode of binding to both MHC and T-cell receptor molecules that enables them to stimulate very large numbers of T cells. Superantigens are produced by many different pathogens, including bacteria, mycoplasmas, and viruses, and the responses they provoke are helpful to the pathogen rather than the host.

Superantigens are unlike other protein antigens, in that they are recognized by T cells without being processed into peptides that are captured by MHC molecules. Indeed, fragmentation of a superantigen destroys its biological activity, which depends on binding as an intact protein to the outside surface of an MHC class II molecule which has already bound peptide. In addition to binding MHC class II molecules, superantigens are able to bind the V_β region of many T-cell receptors. Bacterial superantigens bind mainly to the V_β CDR2 loop and to a smaller extent to the V_β CDR1 loop and an additional loop called the hypervariable 4 or HV4 loop. The HV4 loop is the predominant binding site for viral superantigens, at least for the Mls antigens encoded by the endogenous mouse mammary tumor viruses. Thus, the α-chain V region and the CDR3 of the β chain of the T-cell receptor have little effect on superantigen recognition, which is determined largely by the germline-encoded V sequences of the expressed β chain. Each superantigen is specific for one or a few of the different V_β gene segments, of which there are 20–50 in mice and humans; a superantigen can thus stimulate 2–20% of all T cells.

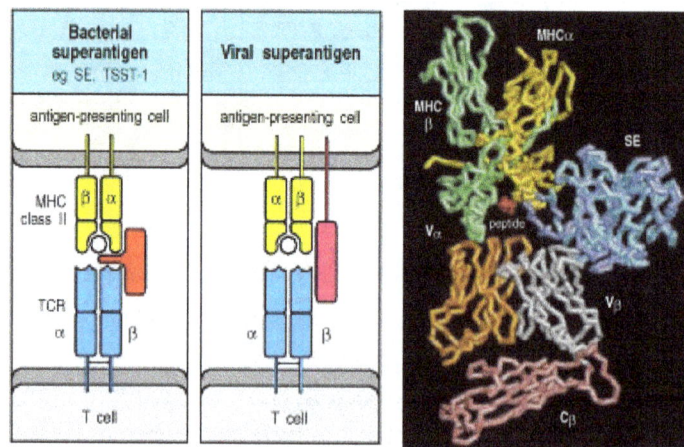

Figure shows superantigens bind directly to T-cell receptors and to MHC molecules. Superantigens can bind independently to MHC class II molecules and to T-cell receptors, binding to the Vβ domain of the T-cell receptor (TCR), away from the complementarity-determining regions, and to the outer faces of the MHC class II molecule, outside the peptide-binding site (top panels). The bottom panel shows a reconstruction of the interaction between a T-cell receptor, an MHC class II molecule and a staphylococcal enterotoxin (SE) superantigen, produced by superimposing separate structures of an enterotoxin: MHC class II complex onto an enterotoxin: T-cell receptor complex. The two enterotoxin molecules (actually SEC3 and SEB) are shown in turquoise and blue, binding to the α chain of the class II molecule (yellow) and to the β chain of the T-cell receptor (colored gray for the Vβ domain and pink for the Cβ domain).

This mode of stimulation does not prime an adaptive immune response specific for the pathogen. Instead, it causes a massive production of cytokines by CD4 T cells, the predominant responding population of T cells. These cytokines have two effects on the host: systemic toxicity and suppression of the adaptive immune response. Both these effects contribute to microbial pathogenicity. Among the bacterial superantigens are the staphylococcal enterotoxins (SEs), which cause food poisoning, and the toxic shock syndrome toxin-1 (TSST-1), the etiologic principle in toxic shock syndrome.

The role of viral superantigens in human disease is less clear. The T-cell responses to rabies virus and the Epstein-Barr virus indicate the existence of superantigens in these human pathogens but the genes encoding them have not yet been identified. The best characterized viral superantigens remain the mouse mammary tumor virus superantigens which are common as endogenous antigens in mice.

8. MHC polymorphism extends the range of antigens to which the immune system can respond:

Most polymorphic genes encode proteins that vary by only one or a few amino acids, whereas the different allelic variants of MHC proteins differ by up to 20 amino acids. The extensive polymorphism of the MHC proteins has almost certainly evolved to outflank the evasive strategies of pathogens. Pathogens can avoid an immune response either by evading detection or by suppressing the ensuing response. The requirement that pathogen antigens must be presented by an MHC molecule provides two possible ways of evading detection. One is through mutations that eliminate from its proteins all peptides able to bind MHC molecules. The Epstein-Barr virus provides an example of this strategy. In regions of south-east China and in Papua New Guinea there are small isolated populations in which about 60% of individuals carry the HLA-All allele. Many isolates of the Epstein-Barr virus obtained from these populations have mutations in a dominant peptide epitope normally presented by HLA-All; the mutant peptides no longer bind to HLA-All and cannot be recognized by HLA-All-restricted T cells. This strategy is plainly much more difficult to follow if there are many different MHC molecules, and the presence of different loci encoding functionally related proteins may have been an evolutionary adaptation by hosts to this strategy by pathogens.

In large outbred populations, polymorphisms at each locus can potentially double the number of different MHC molecules expressed by an individual, as most individuals will be heterozygotes. Polymorphism has the additional advantage that individuals in a population will differ in the combinations of MHC molecules they express and will therefore present different sets of peptides from each pathogen. This makes it unlikely that all individuals in a population will be equally susceptible to a given pathogen and its spread will therefore be limited. That exposure to pathogens over an evolutionary timescale can select for expression of particular MHC alleles is indicated by the strong association of the HLA-B53 allele with recovery from a potentially lethal form of malaria; this allele is very common in people from West Africa, where malaria is endemic, and rare elsewhere, where lethal malaria is uncommon.

Similar arguments apply to a second strategy for evading recognition. If pathogens can develop mechanisms to block the presentation of their peptides by MHC molecules, they can avoid the adaptive immune response. Adenoviruses encode a protein that binds to MHC class I molecules in the endoplasmic reticulum and prevents their transport to the cell surface, thus preventing the recognition of viral peptides by CD8 cytotoxic T cells. This MHC-binding protein must interact with a polymorphic region of the MHC class I molecule, as some allelic variants are retained in the endoplasmic reticulum by the adenoviral protein whereas others are not. Increasing the variety of MHC molecules expressed therefore reduces the likelihood that a pathogen will be able to block presentation by all of them and completely evade an immune response.

These arguments raise a question: if having three MHC class I loci is better than having one, why are there not far more MHC loci? The probable explanation is that each time a distinct MHC molecule is added to the MHC repertoire, all T cells that can recognize self-peptides bound to that molecule must be removed in order to maintain self-tolerance. It seems that the number of MHC loci present in humans and mice is about optimal to balance out the advantages of presenting an increased range of foreign peptides and the disadvantages of an increased loss of T cells from the repertoire.

9. Multiple genetic processes generate MHC polymorphism:

MHC polymorphism appears to have been strongly selected by evolutionary pressures. However, for selection to work efficiently in organisms that reproduce slowly, such as humans, there must also be powerful mechanisms for generating the variability on which selection can act. The generation of polymorphism in MHC molecules is an evolutionary problem not easily analyzed in the laboratory; however, it is clear that several genetic mechanisms contribute to the generation of new alleles. Some new alleles are the result of point mutations, but many arise from the combination of sequences from different alleles either by genetic recombination or by gene conversion, a process in which one sequence is replaced, in part, by another from a different gene.

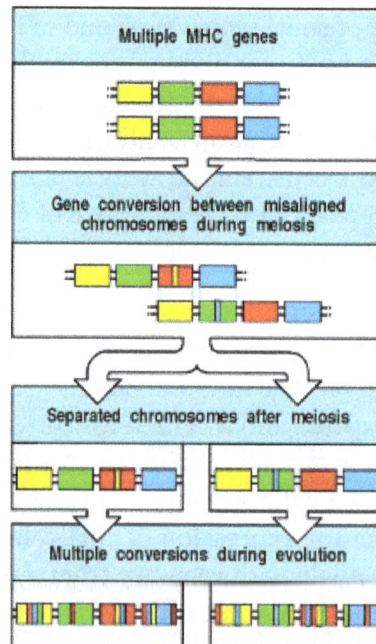

Figure shows gene conversion can create new alleles by copying sequences from one MHC gene to another. Sequences can be transferred from one gene to a similar but different gene by a process known as gene conversion. For this to happen, the two genes must become apposed during meiosis. This can occur as a consequence of the misalignment of the two paired homologous chromosomes when there are many copies of similar genes arrayed in tandem—somewhat like buttoning in the wrong buttonhole. During the process of crossing-over and DNA recombination, a DNA sequence from one chromosome is sometimes copied to the other, replacing the original sequence. In this way several nucleotide changes can be inserted all at once into a gene and can cause several simultaneous amino acid changes between the new gene sequence and the original gene. Because of the similarity of the MHC genes to each other and their close linkage, gene conversion has occurred many times in the evolution of MHC alleles.

Evidence for gene conversion comes from studies of the sequences of different MHC alleles. These reveal that some changes involve clusters of several amino acids in the MHC molecule and require multiple nucleotide changes in a contiguous stretch of the gene. Even more significantly, the sequences that have been changed frequently derive from other MHC genes on the same chromosome, which is a typical signature of gene conversion. Genetic recombination between different alleles at the same locus may, however, have been more important than gene conversion in generating MHC polymorphism. A comparison of sequences of MHC alleles shows that many different alleles could represent recombination events between a relatively small set of hypothetical ancestral alleles.

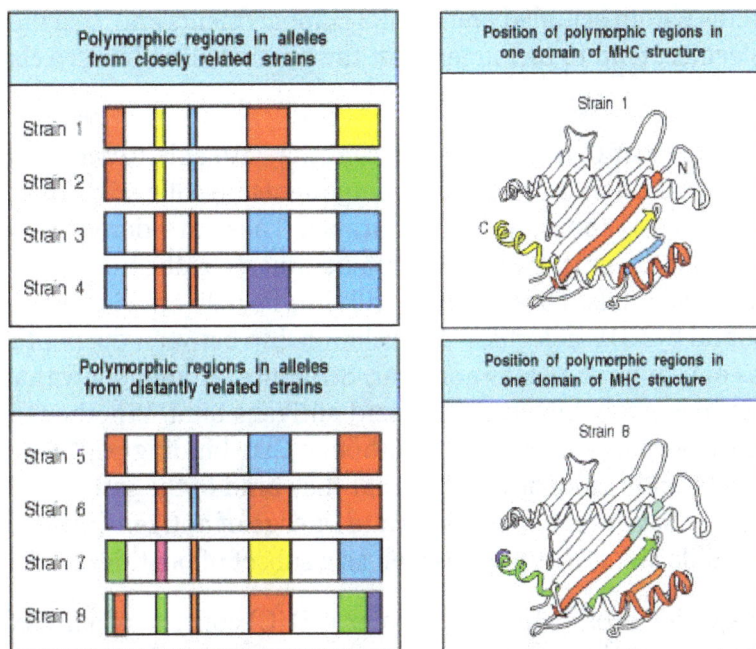

Genetic recombination can create new MHC alleles by DNA exchange between different alleles of the same gene. Conventional meiotic recombination differs from gene conversion in that DNA segments are exchanged between alleles on the two homologous chromosomes rather than, as in gene conversion, being copied in one direction only. Analysis of many MHC allele sequences has shown that the swapping of segments of DNA has occurred many times in the evolution of MHC alleles. Closely related strains of mice have MHC genes where only one or two segments have been swapped between alleles (first panel), whereas more distantly related strains show a patchwork effect that results from the accumulation of many such recombination events (second panel). The variable parts of MHC molecules correspond to segments of the structure around the peptide-binding groove, such as the β strands or parts of the α helix shown in the bottom panels.

The effects of selective pressure in favor of polymorphism can be seen clearly in the pattern of point mutations in the MHC genes. Point mutations can be classified as replacement substitutions, which change an amino acid, or silent substitutions, which simply change the codon but leave the amino acid the same. Replacement substitutions occur within the MHC at a higher frequency relative to silent substitutions than would be expected, providing evidence that polymorphism has been actively selected for in the evolution of the MHC.

10. Some peptides and lipids generated in the endocytic pathway can be bound by MHC class I-like molecules that are encoded outside the MHC. Some MHC class I-like genes map outside the MHC region. One family, called CD1, expressed on dendritic cells and monocytes as well as some thymocytes, functions in antigen presentation to T cells, but the molecules it encodes have two features that distinguish them from classical MHC class I molecules. The first is that the CD1 molecule, although similar to MHC class I molecules in its subunit organization and association with β_2-microglobulin, behaves like an MHC class II molecule. It is not retained within the endoplasmic reticulum by association with the TAP complex but is targeted to vesicles, where it binds its peptide ligand. The peptide antigens bound by CD1 are therefore derived from the breakdown of extracellular proteins within acidified endosomal compartments and, like the peptides that bind to MHC class II molecules, tend to be longer than the peptides that bind to classical MHC class I molecules.

The second unusual feature of CD1 molecules is that they are able to bind and present glycolipids, in particular the mycobacterial membrane components mycolic acid, glucose monomycolate, phosphoinositol mannosides, and lipoarabinomannan. These are derived either from internalized mycobacteria or from the uptake of lipoarabinomannans by the mannose receptor that is expressed by many phagocytic cells. These ligands will thus be delivered into the endocytic pathway, where they can be bound by CD1 molecules. The relationship between the peptide-binding and lipid-binding capacities of CD1 molecules is not clear. Structural studies show that the CD1 molecule has a deep binding groove into which the glycolipid antigens bind. Whether the peptide antigens also bind in this deep groove is not yet known; although CD1-binding peptides are predominantly hydrophobic in character, it is thought unlikely that they bind to the same site as the lipids. It appears that the CD1 genes have evolved as a separate lineage of antigen-presenting molecules able to present microbial lipids and glycolipids, as well as a subset of peptides, to T cells.

In conclusion, the major histocompatibility complex (MHC) consists of a linked set of genetic loci encoding many of the proteins involved in antigen presentation to T cells, most notably the MHC class I and class II glycoproteins (the MHC molecules) that present peptides to the T-cell receptor. The outstanding feature of the MHC molecules is their extensive polymorphism. This polymorphism is of critical importance in antigen recognition by T cells. A T cell recognizes antigen as a peptide bound by a particular allelic variant of an MHC molecule, and will not recognize the same peptide bound to other MHC molecules. This behavior of T cells is called MHC restriction. Most MHC alleles differ from one another by multiple amino acid substitutions, and these differences are focused on the peptide-binding site and adjacent regions that make direct contact with the T-cell receptor. At least three properties of MHC molecules are affected by MHC polymorphism: the range of peptides bound; the conformation of the bound peptide; and the direct interaction of the MHC molecule with the T-cell receptor. Thus the highly polymorphic nature of the MHC has functional consequences, and the evolutionary selection for this polymorphism suggests that it is critical to the role of the MHC molecules in the immune response. Powerful genetic mechanisms generate the variation that is seen among MHC alleles, and a compelling argument can be made that selective pressure to maintain a wide variety of MHC molecules in the population comes from infectious agents.

Antigen Processing

The T cell arm of the adaptive immune response has evolved to recognize the products of partial intracellular proteolysis. CD8$^+$ T cells recognize protein-derived peptides in association with Major Histocompatibility Complex (MHC) class I molecules (MHC-I) while CD4$^+$ T cells recognize peptides bound to MHC class II molecules (MHC-II). There are also T cells that recognize lipid antigens associated with CD1 molecules, but CD1 functions and the processing mechanisms that regulate their interaction with lipids will not be considered here.

All vertebrates possess an MHC, a large multigenic region with many conserved genes in addition to MHC-I and MHC-II molecules. Some of these encode products essential to MHC-I and MHC–II function. In many species the MHC encodes multiple MHC-I and MHC-II molecules, presumed to have arisen by gene duplication. For example, in mice, depending on the strain, there are two to three genes encoding 'classical' MHC-I molecules, called H2-D, -K and –L, within the H2 complex, and most strains have two MHC-II molecules, called I-A and I-E. Humans have three 'classical' MHC-I genes within the HLA complex, called HLA-A, -B, and –C, and there are three MHC-II molecules, called HLA-DR, -DQ, and –DP. In both mice and man there are other class I genes present in the MHC. These are known as class Ib genes.

Multiple structures of MHC-I and MHC-II molecules have been determined, and a schematic structure of each is presented in figure. MHC-I and MHC-II genes exhibit enormous allelic polymorphism, and amino acid sequence variation is heavily concentrated in the part of each structure that interacts with peptides, allowing different alleles to bind a different range of peptides. The peptide-binding structure consists of a membrane-distal groove formed by two anti-parallel α-helices overlaying an eight-strand β-sheet. In the case of MHC-I the groove corresponds to a contiguous amino acid sequence formed by the N-terminal region of the single MHC-encoded subunit, or heavy chain, while for MHC-II it is formed by the juxtaposition of the N-terminal regions of two MHC-encoded α- and β-chains. For both molecules the membrane-proximal region consists of two conserved domains that are homologous to Ig constant region domains. For MHC-I, one is provided by the heavy chain and the other is a separate protein, β$_2$-microglobulin (β$_2$m), a soluble product of a non-MHC-linked gene. For MHC-II one conserved domain is part of the α-subunit and the other part of the β-subunit. The MHC-I heavy chain and the MHC -II α- and β-subunits are transmembrane glycoproteins with short cytoplasmic domains. The theme that emerges is that MHC-I and -II molecules each have a structurally homologous platform capable of binding peptides with very high affinity that can engage the T cell receptor. A significant difference is that for MHC-I the peptide is confined by binding groove interactions at both the N and C-termini, while for MHC-II each end of the peptide can overhang the binding groove.

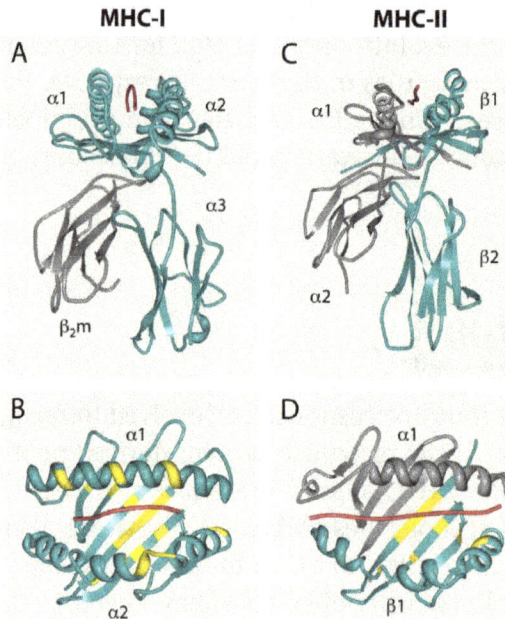

Figure shows three dimensional structures of MHC-I and MHC-II molecules with peptide ligands. A and B) Structure of the MHC-I molecule (HLA-A2 complexed with residues 58-66 of the influenza matrix protein, MHC-I heavy chain, blue; β_2m, grey; peptide, red. C and D) Structure of the MHC-II molecule (HLA-DR1 complexed with residues 306-318 of influenza haemagglutinin. MHC-II α chain, grey; MHC-II β chain, blue; peptide, red. Highly polymorphic residues of HLA-A (B) and HLA-DR (D) proximal to the peptide binding groove are highlighted in yellow. Note that polymorphism of the MHC-II alpha chains is limited, and they are essentially non-polymorphic for HLA-DR alpha chains.

Peptides are the products of proteolysis, and there are two major proteolytic systems operating within the cell that contribute to MHC-dependent T cell recognition. In the cytosol the vast majority of proteolysis is mediated by the proteasome. The proteasome (reviewed in) will not be discussed extensively, but in brief its core is a barrel-shaped 20S structure consisting of four stacked rings of seven subunits each. The outer rings are composed of α-subunits and the middle two of β-subunits, three of which, β1, β2 and β5, constitute the active proteolytic components. Variants of the active β-subunits are induced by interferon-γ (IFN-γ) and replace the constitutive versions. These were historically called LMP1, LMP2 and MECL1, and the genes encoding LMP1 and LMP2 are MHC-linked. Commonly the IFN-γ–inducible subunits are now called β1i, β2i and β5i, and proteasomes that contain them are called immunoproteasomes. The cleavage specificities of standard protaseomes and immunoproteosomes differ. The 20S core is capped at each end by an additional 19S multi-subunit complex that recognizes ubiquitin-conjugated proteins targeted for degradation. The 19S component has deubiquitinase activity and an unfoldase activity that allows the targeted proteins to enter the channel in the center of the barrel where the β-subunit active sites reside. The unfolding function, in particular, necessitates that proteolysis by the capped (26S) proteasome is ATP-dependent. There is an alternative capping structure (11S) comprised of a different set of IFN-γ-inducible proteins that allow a level of ATP-independent proteolysis of peptides but not of folded proteins. The end products of proteolysis by the 26S proteasome (20S plus 19S) form the dominant source of peptides for MHC-I binding.

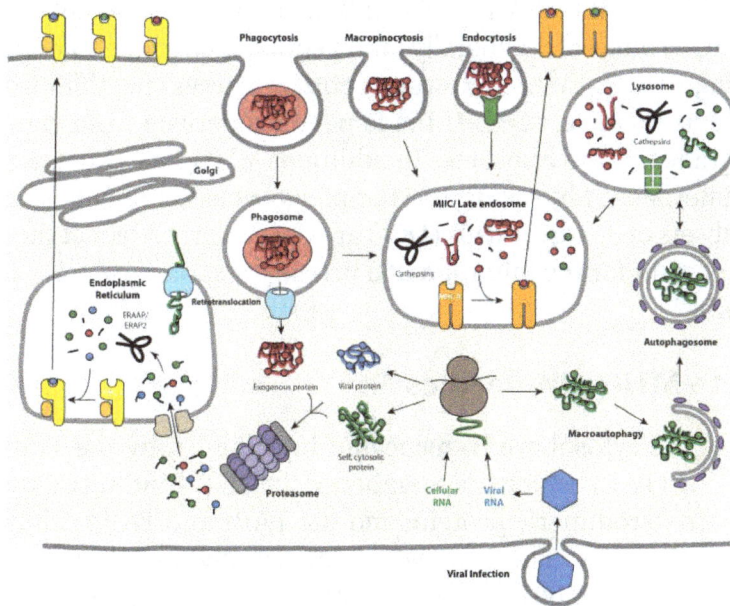

Figure shows trafficking of antigens for processing and presentation with MHC molecules: basic pathways and exceptions to the "rules". Cytosolic proteins are processed primarily by the action of the proteasome. The short peptides are then transported into the ER by TAP for subsequent assembly with MHC-I molecules. In certain antigen presenting cells, particularly dendritic cells, and exogenous proteins can also be fed into this pathway by retrotranslocation from phagosomes, a phenomenon known as cross-presentation. The retrotranslocation channels may be recruited from the ER, where they are used for ER-associated degradation, or ERAD, of misfolded trans-membrane or secretory proteins. Exogenous proteins, however, are primarily presented by MHC-II molecules. Antigens are internalized by several pathways, including phagocytosis, macropino-cytosis, and endocytosis, and eventually traffic to a mature or late endosomal compartment where they are processed and loaded onto MHC-II molecules. Cytoplasmic/nuclear antigens can also be trafficked into the endosomal network via autophagy for subsequent processing and presentation with MHC-II molecules.

Proteins that are internalized by a cell from exogenous sources are degraded by lysosomal prote-olysis. In brief, endocytosed proteins enter a vesicular pathway consisting of progressively more acidic and proteolytically active compartments classically described as early endosomes, late en-dosomes and lysosomes. Particles internalized by phagocytosis follow a similar path, terminating in phagolysosomes that are formed by the fusion of phagosomes and lysosomes. Lysosomes and phagolysosomes have a pH of 4 to 4.5, and contain a number of acid pH-optimum proteases ge-nerically called cathepsins. In highly degradative cells such as macrophages, successive cleavages by these enzymes result in very short peptides and free amino acids that are translocated into the cytosol to replenish tRNAs for new protein synthesis, but in less proteolytically active antigen presenting cells (APCs), larger intermediates form the dominant source of peptides for MHC-II binding.

The trafficking of exogenous and endogenous proteins for antigen processing and presentation are summarized in figure. In general, MHC-I molecules bind peptides generated by proteasomal pro-teolysis and they bind them in the endoplasmic reticulum (ER) after the peptides are translocated from the cytosol. Peptide binding by MHC-I is integrated into the assembly pathway of the heavy chain-β_2m dimer. MHC-II molecules generally bind peptides generated by lysosomal proteolysis in the endocytic and phagocytic pathways. However, both can access peptides from endogenous and exogenous antigens. For example, MHC-II binds peptides derived from endogenous membrane proteins that are degraded in the lysosome. In addition, MHC-I can bind peptides derived from exogenous proteins internalized by endocytosis or phagocytosis, a phenomenon called cross-presentation. Specific subsets of dendritic cells (DCs) are particularly adept at mediating this process, which is critically important for the initiation of a primary response by naïve CD8[+] T cells when it is termed cross-priming.

Peptide Binding to MHC-I Molecules

Peptides generated in the cytosol are translocated into the ER by the Transporter associated with Antigen Processing (TAP), which is a member of the ATP-Binding Cassette (ABC) family of transporters. TAP is a heterodimeric protein, and the TAP1 and TAP2 subunits are encoded by closely linked genes in the MHC. These are widely distributed in both prokaryotes and eukaryotes and transfer a variety of molecules across membranes. Biochemical evidence combined with molecular modeling suggests that each TAP subunit consist of a central core domain of 6 transmembrane α-helices, which constitute the channel that is immediately N-terminal to the Nucleotide Binding Domain (NBD). The NBD structure is known for TAP1 and it is similar to that of other ABC family members, with the classical Walker A and B motifs present in many ATPases. Cytosolic loops in the core domains that are proximal to the NBDs constitute the peptide recognition site, and ATP hydrolysis mediates the translocation event. Both subunits have additional N-terminal domains (N-domains), comprising 4 transmembrane segments for TAP1 and 3 for TAP2, which have no counterparts in other members of the ABC family of transporters.

The TAP heterodimer associates with a number of other proteins to form the Peptide Loading Complex, or PLC. The transmembrane glycoprotein tapasin, which is encoded by an MHC-linked gene, interacts within the membrane with the N- domains. Tapasin has a bridging function, recruiting MHC-I-β_2m dimers and the chaperone calreticulin (CRT) to the PLC. Recent experiments have confirmed that there are two tapasin molecules in the PLC, one associated with each TAP subunit. Tapasin in turn is stably linked via a disulfide bond to a second molecule, the protein disulfide isomerase homologue ERp57, and the structure of the lumenal region of human tapasin conjugated to ERp57 has been solved. The N-terminal domain of tapasin consists of a β barrel fused to an Ig-like domain, and, as for the MHC-I and -II proteins, the membrane proximal domain is Ig-like. ERp57 has a slightly twisted U-shaped structure and tapasin is inserted into the U in a way that results in extensive protein-protein interactions with ERp57, particularly with the a and a' domains, each of which contains a double cysteine 'CXXC' motif that constitute its two redox active sites. As predicted by earlier biochemical experiments a disulfide bond connects cysteine 95 of tapasin with cysteine 57 of ERp57, which is the N-terminal cysteine residue of the a domain CXXC motif. Normally, disulfide bonds involving cysteine 57 are transiently formed during the reduction of a disulfide-containing ERp57 substrate protein, and reduction of this enzyme-substrate bond by the second cysteine in the motif releases the substrate. The interactions of tapasin with the a domain and a' domains appear to trap the disulfide linked species, explaining the stability of the tapasin-ERp57 disulfide bond.

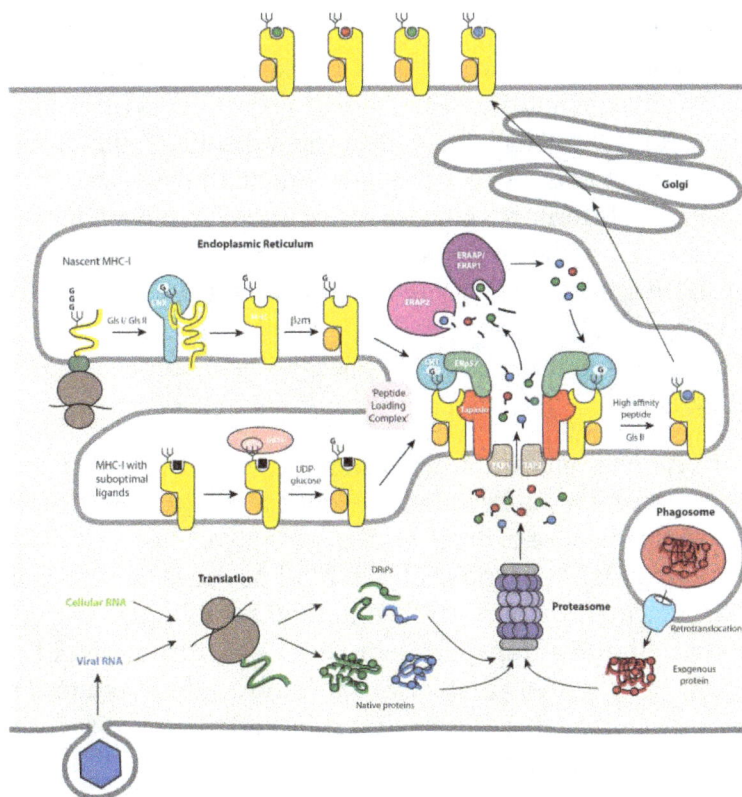

MHC-I biosynthesis and antigenic peptide binding in the ER.

In figure, trimming of the N-linked glycan by glucosidases I and II (GlsI/ GlsII) to a single terminal glucose residue ("G") permits the interaction of the MHC-I heavy chain with lectin-like chaperones at several stages during folding and assembly. The initial folding events involve the chaperone calnexin (CNX) and allow subsequent assembly with β_2m. The empty heterodimer, which is inherently unstable, is then recruited by calreticulin (CRT) via the monoglucosylated N-linked glycan to the PLC. The association of MHC-I/β_2m heterodimers with the PLC both stabilizes the empty MHC-I molecule and maintains the binding groove in a conformation that favors high affinity peptide loading. These functions are mediated by direct interactions between the MHC-I heavy chain and tapasin and are supported by coordinating interactions with CRT and ERp57 in the PLC. MHC-I molecules with suboptimal peptides are substrates for UGT1 which reglucosylates the heavy chain glycan, allowing re-entry of the MHC-I into the PLC and exchange for high affinity peptides. Peptides translocated into the ER by TAP originate primarily from the proteasomal degradation of endogenous proteins or DRiPs. These proteins may arise from the translation of either self or foreign (i.e. viral) RNA or, in the case of cross-presentation, by translocation into the cytosol from endosomes or phagosomes. Many of the peptides that are delivered into the ER are longer than the 8-10 residues preferred by MHC-I molecules and undergo trimming by ER aminopeptidases known as ERAAP/ERAP1 and ERAP2. Finally, high affinity peptides bind preferentially to MHC-I molecules in the PLC by a tapasin-mediated editing process, MHC-I-peptide complexes are released and then transit to the cell surface for T cell recognition by CD8+ T cells.

ERp57 assists the folding of newly synthesized glycoproteins in the ER by mediating disulfide bond isomerization. Its specificity for glycoproteins results from its ability to associate via its *b'* domain with CRT and a second lectin-like ER chaperone, the transmembrane CRT homologue calnexin (CNX). Both CNX and CRT are important in MHC-I assembly. CNX and CRT normally function in a quality control cycle that depends on their interactions with the N-linked glycans of the glyco-proteins. They then recruit ERp57, which mediates proper disulfide bond formation in the folding glycoprotein. Glycan binding to CNX or CRT is dependent on the precise structure of the N-linked glycan, which must bear a single terminal glucose residue and is a biosynthetic intermediate main-tained in this form by the competing actions of two enzymes. One, glucosidase II, removes the glucose and the other, UDP-glucose glycoprotein transferase-1 (UGT1), replaces the glucose only if the glycoprotein bearing the glycan is partially unfolded. This cycle does play a role in MHC-I peptide loading, but the one step that does not appear to be involved is the reduction-oxidation cycle mediated by ERp57.

Cells that lack TAP1 or TAP2 do not form MHC-I-peptide complexes because no peptides are im-ported into the ER. There are a few published exceptions to this rule, some of which lead to CD8$^+$ T cell recognition, but the only major one, in terms of quantitative effects on MHC-I assembly, is the unusual and specific ability of HLA-A2 molecules to bind peptides derived from signal sequences of certain ER-targeted molecules. Because of the inherent instability of 'empty' MHC-I molecules, and because they do not fold into a transport-competent structure in the ER, TAP-negative cells express very little surface MHC-I. Cells that lack tapasin also exhibit reduced surface MHC-I, but the defect is much less drastic than in TAP-negative cells and the magnitude of the effect depends on the individual MHC-I allele expressed. Data from tapasin knockout mice showed an essential function for tapasin in generating CD8$^+$ T cell responses, and data based on T cell recognition demonstrated that tapasin plays a 'peptide editing' role, mediating the binding of high affinity pep-tides at the expense of peptides with lower but still significant affinity, and that because of this sur-face MHC-I molecules on tapasin-negative cells are less stable than those on tapasin-positive cells. Subsequently, in vitro data produced using recombinant tapasin-ERp57 conjugates confirmed that tapasin facilitates high affinity peptide binding and further showed that its association with ERp57 is essential.

The addition of tapasin-ERp57 conjugates to extracts of human tapasin-negative cells expressing HLA-B8 was found to facilitate the binding of added high affinity peptides to HLA-B8-β_2m dimers. Lower affinity peptides were much less successful competitors for binding in the presence of the conjugate than in its absence, indicative of a peptide editing effect. The tapasin-ERp57 conjugate was also found to mediate peptide binding to purified, soluble, recombinant HLA-B8-β_2m dimers provided the HLA-B8 molecules expressed a monoglucosylated N-linked glycan. While this re-action depended on the addition of recombinant CRT, presumably to provide a bridge between MHC-I and the tapasin-associated ERp57, no other components were required. In a more simpli-fied in vitro system neither CRT nor tapasin-associated ERp57 were needed for peptide binding when the MHC-I heavy chain and tapasin were artificially coupled by the addition of leucine zip-pers to their C-termini.

ERp57-negative cells, as well as CRT-negative cells, also have reduced numbers of MHC-I mol-ecules on the cell surface. The initial identification of ERp57 in the PLC led to considerable speculation suggesting that its redox activity was important for generating stable MHC-I-pep-tide complexes. However, the structural data indicated that tapasin obstructs both of the ERp57 active sites, rendering this unlikely. In fact, when the second active site cysteine in the *a* domain and both active site cysteine residues in the a' domain were mutated to serine residues, the combined substitutions had no effect on the ability of tapasin to reconstitute MHC-I cell surface expression when it was introduced into an ERp57-deficient cell line. This triply mutated ERp57 was still disulfide-linked to tapasin. However, further analysis in both cell-free systems and intact cells using ERp57 mutated in the b' domain showed that the ability of ERp57 to bind CRT is essential for MHC-I recruitment to the PLC and normal MHC-I peptide loading. In addition to the CRT-dependent interactions with the MHC-I glycan and ERp57 that mediate MHC-I binding to the PLC, there is also a direct interaction between MHC-I and tapasin. Mutagenesis of specific tapasin residues and expression of the mutants as recombinant tapasin-ERp57 conjugates revealed a 'patch' on the surface of tapasin that binds to the MHC-I molecule, and there was a positive correlation between the relative abilities of different mutants to bind MHC-I and their efficiency in mediating peptide binding to MHC-I in vitro. In addition, a tapasin mutant that was non-functional in cell-free assays also failed to function when expressed as a full-length protein in a tapasin-negative cell.

The PLC consists of the TAP heterodimer and two tapasin-ERp57 conjugates, and up to two CRT molecules and MHCI-β_2m dimers can be recruited. The MHC class I glycan must be in the monoglucosylated form, consistent with the CRT requirement. Cellular expression of UGT1 is essential for optimal MHC-I peptide loading and, in vitro, the enzyme can discriminate between MHC-I molecules bound to high affinity peptides and those associated with lower affinity peptides. This suggests a mechanism that resembles the normal CRT/CNX quality control cycle.

A plausible model is that there are two discriminatory events that regulate peptide editing. First, after peptide-free MHC-I-β_2m dimers bearing a monoglucosylated N-linked glycan are recruited to the PLC by CRT, there is a direct interaction of the MHC-I molecule with tapasin. This interaction is sensitive to the peptide occupancy of the MHC-I molecule such that when a peptide is bound the affinity of the MHC-I interaction with tapasin is reduced, perhaps by a conformational change in the MHC-I heavy chain similar to that proposed to explain the ability of DM molecules to regulate peptide binding to MHC-II. Thus peptide binding induces dissociation of the MHC-I molecule from tapasin, and because the affinity of the CRT interaction with the monoglucosylated MHC-I glycan is low, the glucose residue becomes accessible to the enzyme glucosidase II, which removes it. If the peptide affinity is sufficiently high, the MHC-I molecule can be transported from the ER through the Golgi apparatus and ultimately to the cell surface. If the affinity of the peptide is low there are two possible scenarios for the second stage. Either the peptide dissociates and the transiently 'empty' MHC-I molecule now becomes a substrate for UGT1 and glucose is added back to the N-linked glycan, or the UGT1 can recognize that the conformation of the MHC-I-peptide complex is in some way imperfect and re-glucosylates the glycan. In either case the consequence of the addition of the glucose residue is that the MHC-I molecule re-associates with CRT, re-integrates completely into the PLC, and is subjected to further rounds of tapasin-mediated peptide binding and selection. Ultimately the MHC-I molecule will escape with a high affinity peptide, or, in common with other glycoproteins that are subject to the CRT/CNX/ERp57 quality control cycle, enzymatic removal of mannose residues from the N-linked glycan will render it unsusceptible to re-glucosylation by UGT1. This acts as a 'timer', leading to irreversible dissociation of the MHC-I from the PLC and its degradation by the ER-associated degradation (ERAD) pathway.

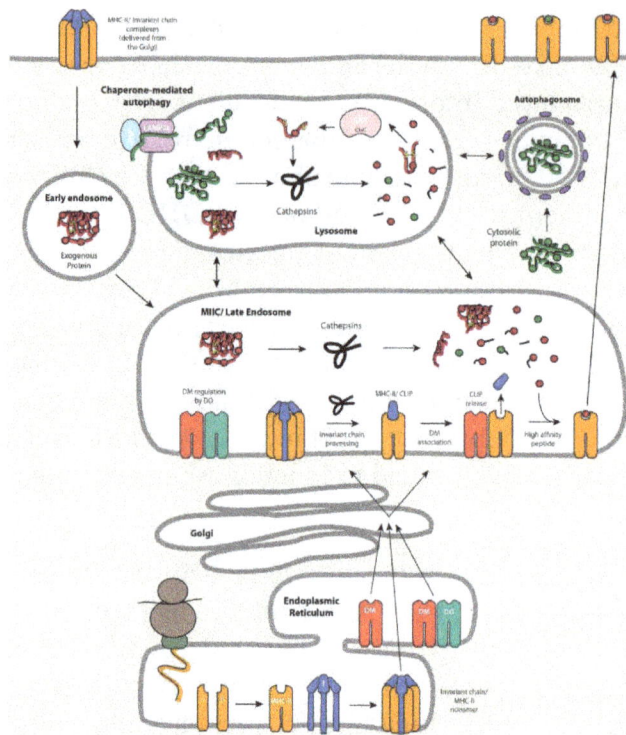

Figure shows MHC-II biosynthesis and antigenic peptide binding in the endocytic pathway. MHC-II α and β associate with I chain trimers to form nonamers. These complexes transit to mature endosomes either via the TGN or by recycling from the cell surface. Within endosomes, I chain is sequentially proteolyzed to yield the residual I chain fragment, CLIP. Displacement of CLIP from the ligand groove of MHC-II αβ is mediated by DM and blunted by DO. Expression of DO and regulation of DM function involves the assembly of DM-DO complexes in the ER and co-transport to endocytic compartments. Antigens delivered to late endosomes by phagocytosis, pinocytosis, endocytosis, and autophagy, are processed by cathepsins and the thiol oxidoreductase GILT, and acquisition of high affinity peptides by MHC-II is facilitated by DM. The MHC-II-peptide complexes are subsequently transported to the cell surface for T cell recognition by CD4+ T cells.

One other ER luminal component that is critically important for the proper generation of MHC-I-peptide complexes is an aminopeptidase, in the mouse called ER Aminopeptidase associated with Antigen Processing (ERAAP) and in humans called ER Aminopeptidase-1 (ERAP1). A second aminopeptidase, ERAP2, is present in humans but not in mice and can also play a role. Peptides associated with MHC-I are generally 8-10 amino acids in length, but TAP can translocate peptides into the ER that are significantly longer. These peptides can be amino-terminally trimmed in the ER by ERAAP/ERAP1 to yield peptides of the appropriate length for MHC-I binding. A structural change required for cleavage that can only be induced by a longer peptide prevents ERAP1 from 'overtrimming' TAP-translocated peptides to a length that would eliminate their ability to bind MHC I. Many of the peptides associated with MHC-I molecules expressed on cells derived from ERAAP knockout mice are elongated, and the MHC-I molecules are relatively unstable The absence of ERAAP results in such a severe alteration in the range of bound peptides that wildtype and knockout mice on the same background are actually histo-incompatible, with wildtype mice able to generate CD8+ T cell responses, and even antibody responses, against knockout cells. The antibodies generated recognize the MHC-I molecules complexed with elongated peptides and can block recognition of ERAAP-negative cells by the ERAAP-positive CD8+ T cells.

Peptide Binding to MHC-II Molecules

MHC-II molecules assemble within the ER, followed by functional maturation in endosomal compartments rich in antigenic peptides. Upon ER translocation MHC-II α and β subunits associate in a process facilitated by a specific chaperone, the invariant chain (I chain) or CD74. Studies using I chain-deficient cells and animals have shown that I chain promotes MHC-II αβ folding, protects the MHC-II ligand binding groove, and directs MHC-II molecules to endosomal compartments for ligand capture. I chain is a non-polymorphic, type II transmembrane glycoprotein not encoded in the MHC. Several forms of I chain exist due to alternative splicing and the use of alternate start codons. Nomenclature for the variants is based on their molecular mass, with the shortest form, p33, being most abundantly expressed. A larger splice variant p41 contains a glycosylated domain, homologous to domains present in thyrogloblulin, which can inhibit the activity of the protease cathepsin L . All forms of I chain contain a conserved di-leucine motif in the N-terminal cytoplasmic domain required for targeting I chain and associated MHC-II to late endosomal compartments. In humans an alternate upstream translational start site gives rise to two additional forms of I chain, p35 and p43, each with an N-terminal 16 amino acid extension. This extended cytoplasmic domain encodes an ER retention motif, which may facilitate ER accumulation and the folding of nascent MHC-II αβ. A limited number of I chain molecules are also modified via linkage of a chondroitin sulfate chain; these molecules reach the cell surface and facilitate cell-cell adhesion. Several other molecules involved in antigen presentation or transport have been reported to associate with I chain, including CD1, MHC-I, and the neonatal Fc gamma receptor. While I chain expression is not required for the function of CD1 or MHC-I, it may enhance antigen presentation by these molecules. I chain expression negatively regulates DC motility in vitro, but it is unknown whether this facilitates antigen presentation or if it is related to the role of I chain as a receptor for the macrophage and stem cell chemoattractant migration inhibitory factor (MIF).

Newly synthesized I chain variants form homo- or mixed trimers, involving p33, p35, p41 and p43 in humans, which accumulate in the ER. These multimers act as a nucleus for MHC-II α and β assembly giving rise to nonamers with 3 α, 3 β and 3 I chains. Distinct MHC-II alleles have different affinities and requirements for I chain binding that can influence their expression and function. In the absence of I chain, some MHC-II αβ complexes are unstable, resulting in their aggregation, retention in the ER, and failure to reach cell surface. Association of I chain with MHC-II αβ dimers prevents antigenic peptide binding, consistent with minimal peptide acquisition early in MHC-II biosynthesis. After assembly the MHC-II-I chain complexes leave the ER and are routed to the endocytic pathway by the I chain di-leucine motifs. This may occur by direct targeting from the Trans Golgi Network (TGN) or by endocytosis from the plasma membrane.

A chain release is initiated by progressive proteolysis in acidic endosomes. This culminates in a variably extended peptide of roughly 20 residues that is associated with the MHC-II binding groove. This is called CLIP, for class II-associated invariant chain peptide he structure of CLIP bound to HLA-DR3 is virtually identical to the structure of MHC-II bound to antigenic peptides indicated in. There are some MHC-II alleles with a low affinity for CLIP and they are genetically associated with the development of autoimmunity. This may reflect a role for MHC-II-CLIP complexes in regulating thymic selection, or skewing of T helper cell subset differentiation. Alternatively, premature release of CLIP from these disease-associated MHC-II alleles may favor the selection of epitopes from autoantigens or the capture of self-peptides within distinct endosomal compartments.

CLIP release from MHC-II is facilitated by another MHC-encoded heterodimeric glycoprotein, DM, which is highly homologous to conventional MHC-II. In humans DM is known as HLA-DM and in mice as H2-DM. The DM α and β subunits display limited genetic polymorphism and the assembled dimer lacks an open or accessible ligand binding groove. The cytoplasmic domain of the DM β chain contains a tyrosine motif which is responsible for sorting assembled DM molecules to late endosomes; DM may also bind I chain which may facilitate but is not required for DM assembly and stability. DM interaction with MHC-II-CLIP complexes occurs in late endosomes where DM acts to promote a conformational change that induces CLIP dissociation, analogous to the role of tapasin in MHC-1 peptide editing. This reaction can be replicated using purified MHC-II-CLIP and DM, and displays Michaelis-Menten kinetics and an acidic pH optimum. CLIP removal facilitates MHC-II loading with antigenic peptides, which influences the repertoire of CD4+ T cells selected in the thymus. DM can remove any low affinity peptides from MHC-II, and, analogous to the role of tapasin in MHC-I peptide editing, repetitive interactions with DM lead to the accumulation MHC-II complexes with high affinity peptides. While MHC-II binding to peptides derived from endocytosed antigens is inefficient in the absence of DM, there is a slow release of CLIP from MHC-II even in DM-negative APCs. As a consequence synthetic peptides bind efficiently to surface MHC-II in these cells and presentation of endogenous antigens can be detected, while in B cells BcR-mediated targeting of antigens can overcome the loss of DM, presumably by increasing the amount internalized over a critical threshold.

The function of DM is modulated by another MHC-encoded MHC-II-like αβ heterodimer, DO, and it is generally accepted that that DO inhibits DM function. DO is expressed in B cells and thymic epithelium and at low levels in select DC subsets, where there is evidence that it is regulated by Toll-like receptor (TLR) agonists. DO αβ dimers associate tightly with DM molecules, and are retained in the ER in the absence of DM, suggesting that in DO-positive cells DM and DO move in concert to endosomes. Studies using Fluorescence Resonance Energy Transfer (FRET) and mutational analysis that defined the DM/DR interface suggested that that DO and DR bind to the same region of DM. Recently the crystal structure of the DO/DM complex confirmed this, and demonstrated an apparent displacement of a segment of the DO α-chain α-helix compared with that of this α-helix in MHC-II-peptide complexes, which may reflect the conformational alteration that DM imparts to induce the dissociation of low affinity peptides.

A precise biological function for DO has been hard to define. Studies in mice deficient in DO have revealed subtle defects in MHC-II antigen presentation, although the effects observed were influenced by the genetic background of the mice and MHC-II allele examined. In vivo, over-expression of DO in dendritic cells can impair MHC-II presentation of antigenic epitopes and, presumably because of this, reduce type I diabetes development in NOD mice.

Antigen and Proteolysis in the Endocytic Pathway

Exploiting conserved pathways established for nutrient and growth factor uptake, APCs sample soluble and particulate matter from extracellular fluids. Many pathogens, including viruses, bacteria and fungi use these same pathways as conduits into cells, favoring immune recognition and antigen presentation. Pathogen driven disruption of these pathways allows immune evasion. Among these transport pathways three routes, clathrin-mediated endocytosis, phagocytosis, and macropinocytosis, efficiently promote antigen internalization and sorting to vesicular organelles for processing and presentation by MHC molecules. During clathrin-mediated endocytosis, cell surface receptor-ligand complexes, membrane proteins and soluble macromolecules are internalized. Regulated capture of particulate antigens and pathogens is mediated by phagocytosis, a process which synchronizes engulfment with delivery into a microenvironment containing reactive oxygen species (ROS), proteases, and anti-microbial agents to promote pathogen destruction. The non-selective process of macropinocytosis captures larger quantities of extracellular material, including proteins, bacteria, and viruses, via plasma membrane ruffling and folding. All of these pathways exist in DCs, macrophages and B lymphocytes, although there are variations in efficiency and regulation. For example, B cells are less efficient at fluid phase endocytosis than DCs or macrophages. However, soluble antigen uptake and MHC-II presentation by B cells can be detected in vivo using antibodies recognizing specific MHC-II-peptide complexes. Surface Ig as a component of the BcR promotes rapid and efficient internalization of antigens, enhancing the potency of antigen-specific B cells 10^3-10^4 fold as stimulators of CD4$^+$ T cells.

APCs in general display multiple cell surface receptors that can capture antigens or intact pathogens to promote internalization and processing. Enhanced antigen presentation by MHC-II has been observed following antigen uptake via several receptors that cluster in clathrin-coated domains, including the BcR, Fc receptors and the C-type lectin family receptor DEC205, as well as mannose and transferrin receptors. MHC-I cross-presentation was also increased following the internalization of ovalbumin (OVA) via the mannose receptor on DCs and macrophages. DEC205 can promote efficient antigen internalization and presentation by both MHC-I and MHC-II, and conjugation of antigens to antibodies recognizing DEC205 has been used to induce tolerance. APCs also express receptors for self and microbial heat shock proteins (HSP) such as Hsp70, Hsp90, and gp96, which promote endocytic uptake of these chaperones and associated ligands (including peptides and antigens) for MHC-I and MHC-II presentation.

Receptors on the surface of APCs promote the phagocytosis of bacteria, fungi, select viruses, and apoptotic or necrotic cells. Macrophages and DCs are well-established phagocytes but this process can also be observed in B cells, which can present phagocytosed antigens to CD4$^+$ T cells. MHC-I cross-presentation as well as MHC-II presentation of opsonized antigens is enhanced by receptor engagement upon phagocytosis, which may reflect intracellular receptor signaling rather than simply enhanced uptake of these particles. Thus, IgG-coated bacteria were effectively presented to CD8$^+$ T cells while complement C3 opsonization of bacteria facilitated phagocytosis but not antigen presentation. Signaling by receptors such as the C-type lectin family receptor DNGR-1 promotes MHC-I and MHC-II presentation of antigens from phagocytosed necrotic cells. Internalization and presentation of self-antigens associated with necrotic cells may contribute to autoimmunity or allograft rejection. Indeed, while all the above pathways promote uptake of extracellular antigens by APCs, internalization and recycling of the plasma membrane also delivers endogenous proteins for processing; peptides derived from membrane proteins, such transferrin receptor and MHC-I heavy chain, are abundantly associated with MHC-II molecules.

Endocytic Compartments in Antigen Processing and Presentation

Internalized antigens enter organelles with microenvironments favoring protein denaturation and proteolysis. While these pathways permit MHC-II access to exogenous antigens, MHC-I molecules also use these routes to acquire antigens for cross-presentation. Electron microscopy initially revealed an abundance of MHC-II molecules distributed in the endocytic pathway, concentrated in late endosomal vesicles, originally defined as MHC-II compartments, or MIICs, in contrast to only limited amounts of MHC-I . The role of this MHC-I in cross-presentation has been debated. Disrupting expression of HS-1, a modulator of endocytic invaginations, demonstrated that endocytosis delivers extracellular antigens for presentation by MHC-I as well as MHC-II in DCs. However, in DCs antigens can transit from within endosomes to the cytoplasm or the ER, raising questions as to the role of endocytosed MHC-I in antigen cross-presentation. A tyrosine motif in the cytoplasmic tail of MHC-I heavy chain facilitates recycling of low levels of these molecules from the cell surface into endosomes, but direct delivery of immature MHC-I from the ER may also occur in DCs, possibly facilitated by associated I chain.

Early endosomes mature into late endosomes and lysosomes driven in part by processes such as increased luminal acidification and fusion with TGN-derived vesicles delivering enzymes that promote antigen denaturation and proteolysis. Low temperature (18°C) can block the maturation step and disrupts the presentation of several exogenous antigens by MHC-II. However, MHC-II presentation of select antigenic epitopes processed within early endosomes can be detected. MHC-I-restricted cross-presentation via the mannose receptor was favored by its delivery of antigen into early endosomes. Whether this is due to limited antigen processing in these vesicles, favoring epitope recovery by endocytic MHC-I, or enhanced translocation of antigens into the cytoplasm for re-direction via TAP to MHC-I, is not clear. Co-localization of MHC-I in endosomes with the insulin-regulated aminopeptidase (IRAP), potentially a substitute for ERAP1, also promoted antigen cross-presentation. MHC-I presentation was also facilitated by liposome-mediated antigen delivery into early but not late endosomes, and neutralization of the acidic pH in the latter enhanced antigen presentation by MHC-I. By contrast, antigens delivered via liposomes into early or late endosomes were processed for MHC-II presentation.

Mature or late endosomal vesicles are heterogeneous in morphology and content, and include translucent and electron dense vesicles, multi-vesicular bodies (MVB) containing intra-lumenal vesicles (ILV), multi-lamellar vesicles, and pre-lysosomes. Antigen processing in these vesicles is influenced by their pH, which regulates the activity of resident proteases and other relevant enzymes, such as gamma interferon inducible lysosomal thiol reductase . Differences in the ability of distinct APCs to regulate endocytic processing have also been documented. For example, the limited protease content and higher pH of DC endocytic compartments may enhance their capacity for presenting antigens via MHC-I and MHC-II compared with macrophages. The precise steps in I chain processing vary between APC types, consistent with their differential expression of cathepsins. Studies using protease inhibitors and protease-deficient mice revealed that several enzymes including cathepsins (S, L, F) and asparaginyl endopeptidase (AEP) mediate I chain cleavage. While cathepsin S plays a key role in the late stages of I processing in DCs and B cells, in macrophages cathepsin F is required. Cathepsin L or V is necessary for terminal I chain proteolysis in cortical thymic epithelial cells. Disruptions in I chain processing can impede MHC-II binding to peptides as well as the transit of the complexes to the cell surface.

While it is well established that I chain guides MHC-II to endosomes, the regulation of MHC-II transport within and out of endosomal compartments is not well understood and may differ between APC types. Myosin II, an actin-based motor, may modulate this process in B cells, while in DCs MHC-II internalization is mediated by ubiquitination of the cytoplasmic tail of the β chain; DC maturation promotes the expression of MHC-II-peptide complexes on the cell surface. Recently down-regulation of the MIR family ubiquitin ligase MARCH-1 has been implicated in the reduction of MHC-II ubiquitination and retention of surface expression. Sub-compartments within mature endosomes may also regulate MHC-II acquisition of peptides. In MVB, the interaction of DM and DO favors their co-localization with HLA-DR in the outer or limiting membrane of these endosomes, whereas DM without DO migrates into internal vesicles which can be shed from cells as exosomes. At the cell surface MHC-II peptide presentation is greatly enhanced by the clustering in lipid raft microdomains.

Phagocytosis and Macropinocytosis and Antigen Presentation

MHC-I as well as MHC-II is detectable within phagosomes. Phagosomal antigen processing and MHC-II presentation are well established and newly formed MHC II-peptide complexes can be detected in these organelles. In contrast with endocytosed antigens, MHC-II presentation of phagocytosed antigens was impaired in DCs lacking the cytoplasmic adaptor, AP-3, due to defective transit of MHC-II-peptide complexes to the cell surface. Recent studies have revealed the importance of phagocytosis in cross-presentation, which typically leads to antigen translocation into the cytoplasm for processing and subsequent delivery for presentation by MHC-I. Processing of phagocytosed antigen by cathepsins has been observed to promote MHC-I cross-presentation, in some cases by a vacuolar peptide exchange pathway. In DCs, antigen cross-presentation by MHC-I is enhanced within newly formed phagosomes, which maintain a neutral pH by regulated delivery of NADPH oxidase to the phagosomal membrane. In contrast, phagosome maturation and acidification can facilitate MHC-II presentation of pathogen-associated antigens.

Exposure of APCs to TLR ligands and pro-inflammatory cytokines can influence the microenvironment within phagosomes by reducing protease content, controlling luminal pH, and modulating the binding of cytoplasmic regulatory proteins such as LC3 and GTPases which mediate phagosome maturation. In macrophages, phagosome maturation was found to be independent of TLR2 or TLR4 signaling, while in DCs, TLR4 activation within a specific phagosome drives maturation and MHC-II-restricted antigen presentation within the organelle. The pH is higher and the protease content lower within DC endosomes and phagosomes than in macrophages, which preserves epitopes and favors antigen presentation. Macrophages, on the other hand, are more proficient in killing engulfed pathogens, at least partly because of their higher phagosomal protease content and more acidic phagosomal pH.

Macropinocytosis does not rely on receptors, but nevertheless captures large antigens and extracellular material into vesicles termed pinosomes . These vesicles share features with early and late endosomes but are distinct, although pinosomes eventually fuse with lysosomes. TLR ligands can promote a rapid burst of macropinocytosis in DCs which then abruptly halts, stimulating preferential MHC-I and MHC-II presentation of the bolus of internalized antigen. A lack of specific inhibitors has limited analysis of macropinocytosis in APC, although studies suggest a role for this pathway in MHC-II presentation of the autoantigen type II collagen and liposome-coupled antigen presentation via MHC-I.

Autophagy and Antigen Presentation

Between 10-30% of the peptides bound to MHC-II are derived from cytoplasmic and nuclear proteins. Within APC, three routes of autophagy promote the delivery of proteins and peptides from the cytoplasm and nucleus into the endosomal network. In macroautophagy, nuclear and cytoplasmic material, including mitochondria, peroxisomes, and some intracellular bacteria, are engulfed by isolation membranes to form autophagosomes. These fuses with endosomes and lysosomes', facilitating antigen presentation by MHC-II as well as the delivery of nucleic acids to TLRs. MHC-II presentation of Epstein Barr virus nuclear antigen I as well as ectopically expressed recombinant viral and bacterial antigens, was perturbed in APCs deficient in macroautophagy. Macroautophagy is readily detected in thymic epithelial cells and disruption of Atg5, a regulator of this process, perturbed the selection of thymic CD4$^+$ but not CD8$^+$ T cells, implying an effect on MHC-II but not on MHC-I processing. The induction of macroautophagy in macrophages and DCs also enhanced MHC-II presentation of mycobacteria, likely due to more efficient phagosome maturation. In B cells, chaperone-mediated autophagy also promoted MHC-II presentation of autoantigens to CD4$^+$ T cells. In this pathway, cytoplasmic chaperones such as Hsc70 and Hsp90, together with the lysosomal transmembrane protein LAMP-2A, selectively deliver epitopes to MHC-II. Proteins may also be captured by microautophagy for delivery into endosomes via Hsc70 and the ESCRT system, although whether this contributes to antigen presentation is unclear.

APCs readily acquire and present antigens from target or dying cells for MHC-I and MHC-II, promoting graft rejection and autoimmunity as well as immune responses to pathogens. In APCs, MHC-II presentation of cytoplasmic antigens derived from target cells with diminished TAP, ERAAP, and proteasome activity was enhanced, suggesting a role for these molecules in subverting cross-presentation of cytoplasmic antigens. In addition, induction of macroautophagy in tumor or target cells can enhance their phagocytosis and MHC-I cross-presentation to CD8$^+$ T cells. By contrast in DCs, MHC-II direct presentation of membrane antigens from influenza virus required TAP and proteasome activity. A requirement for proteasomal processing of some cytoplasmic antigens and a role for ERAAP in MHC-II presentation has been documented, but the mechanisms by which these components influence the MHC-II pathway remain unclear.

Epitope Selection and Guided Antigen Processing

Proteins can contain multiple sequences capable of binding MHC molecules, but only a handful of peptides are selected for presentation to T cells. T cell responses are influenced by the diversity of the T cell repertoire but the steps in antigen processing and presentation play a major role. The concept that a hierarchy of antigenic epitopes is recognized by the immune system is well established; the strongest are called immunodominant, and there are subdominant and cryptic epitopes. Immunodominant epitopes are important for immunity to tumors and pathogens, while a shift in the hierarchy of T cell responses to subdominant epitopes is associated with autoimmune disorders. Multiple factors contribute to the process of epitope selection by MHC-I and MHC-II molecules. In the case of MHC-I, the specificity of the proteasome, ERAAP/ERAP1, tapasin, and TAP can influence epitope generation and transport to receptive MHC-I molecules. For MHC-II, antigen unfolding and proteolysis influence processing and epitope presentation. Multiple endocytic proteases have been implicated in processing antigens for MHC-II, including cathepsins B, D, L, S and AEP, and several of these enzymes also function in I chain processing. Antigen reduction facilitates protease access for processing, influencing the generation of antigenic epitopes, and GILT is the key enzyme implicated in this process. In melanoma cells, the hierarchy of epitopes presented by MHC-II is GILT dependent. GILT expression also influences autoantigen processing and the development of experimental autoimmune encephalomyelitis and tolerance development to melanocyte antigens. MHC-I and MHC-II epitopes can also be destroyed by proteases, which may result in differential epitope presentation by different APC types as well as tissue specific differences in presentation.

The open groove of MHC-II allows large fragments of antigen to bind. This led to the concept of guided antigen processing, in which MHC-II binding to epitopes within antigens shapes proteolytic cleavage. In B cells the specific interaction of antigens with the Ig component of the BcR also influences processing and presentation by MHC-II. An *in vitro* system reconstituting antigen binding to the BcR followed by digestion with the enzyme AEP favored epitope capture by proximal MHC-II. Similarly MHC-II binding to immunodominant epitopes from an intact protein was reconstituted in vitro using soluble purified components, including cathepsins to yield peptides and DM to promote editing of the resulting MHC-II-peptide complexes. Epitopes may bind MHC-II in an unstable conformation, and editing of these complexes by DM alters the hierarchy of peptides displayed to CD4+ T cells. Notably, DM-independent epitope conformations can persist, particularly when the antigen is available to APCs as a peptide rather than an intact protein, and may induce unusual CD4+ T cells (so-called Type B T cells) that can lead to autoimmunity. Far less is known about the endosomal factors that influence epitope selection for MHC-I cross-presentation, although GILT expression is required for cross-presentation of a disulfide-containing glycoprotein antigen from herpes simplex virus 1. Notably, during cross-presentation innate signaling via TLRs appears to influence antigen presentation, as suggested by a shift in the dominant CD8+ T cell epitopes during LCMV infection.

Antigen Introduction and Proteolysis in the Cytosol

Protein antigens are conventionally introduced into the cytosol by the cellular protein synthetic machinery. When a virus infects a cell the viral genes are transcribed into mRNAs and these are translated on host ribosomes to generate viral proteins. While autophagic mechanisms can give them access to the MHC-II pathway, cytosolic antigens are the prime source of MHC-I-associated peptides. Their proteolysis generates peptides that are translocated into the ER by TAP, and ultimately bind to MHC-I molecules. If they are too long they are trimmed in the ER by ERAAP/ERAP1. This process is not specific for viral proteins; host proteins are similarly degraded and generate peptides that bind to MHC-I. In fact, in the case of autoimmunity or tumor immunity MHC-I-associated, host protein-derived peptides can be recognized by CD8+ T cells. For example, CD8+ T cell-mediated killing of melanoma cells, which is exploited for immunotherapy, often involves the recognition of MHC -I-associated peptides derived from melanocyte-specific glycoproteins . These proteins are found in melanosomes, the pigment-containing organelles of melanocytes from which melanomas originate. In an infected cell viral proteins must compete with host proteins for representation in the peptide profile presented to CD8+ T cells.

Protein Sources of MHC-I-associated Peptides

Epitopes from viral glycoproteins, as well as melanosomal glycoproteins, can be recognized by CD8+ T cells. These peptides are generally derived from parts of the antigen that are luminal, not cytosolic. Nevertheless, the generation of these MHC-I-peptide complexes is virtually always TAP- and proteasome-dependent. This implies that, in spite of the presence of a signal sequence and the potential for translocation into the ER, the processing mechanisms at work are no different from those involved in the generation of peptides from exclusively cytosolic antigens. These observations have contributed to the hypothesis that intact, folded, cytosolic proteins are not the major source of peptides that bind to MHC-I. Instead the sources are proteins that are either incomplete, perhaps because of premature termination, or misfolded because cytosolic chaperones are not 100% effective in mediating the folding of newly synthesized proteins. In mammalian cells approximately 30% of total proteins are degraded extremely rapidly following synthesis. Yewdell has been a strong advocate of the hypothesis that this rapidly degraded pool is the primary source of MHC-I-associated peptides, and coined the acronym DRiP, for Defective Ribosomal Product, to describe them, and has recently reviewed the evidence supporting the hypothesis. Briefly, very early experiments showed that expression in cells of truncated proteins, which are unstable, generated MHC-I-peptide complexes as effectively as full-length proteins.

In fact, the experiments that mapped and defined the first MHC-I-restricted epitope, an influenza nucleoprotein-derived peptide that binds to H2-D^b, relied on the expression of truncated proteins. Work by Neefjes and co-workers suggested that newly synthesized proteins are the primary source of TAP-translocated peptides. They showed by FRAP (Fluorescence Recovery After Photobleaching) analysis that the lateral mobility of TAP in the ER membrane decreases when active peptide translocation is occurring, and that inhibiting protein synthesis by cycloheximide addition rapidly enhanced TAP mobility. Kinetic analysis of the synthetic rates of cytosolic antigens versus the rates at which complexes of MHC-I and peptide derived from them are generated confirmed a general principle that the accumulation of the protein lags considerably behind the acquisition of the complexes. Using the SILAC (Stable isotope labeling with aminoacids in cell culture) technique, in which cellular proteins, and the peptides derived from them, are labeled with specific isotopic variants of amino acids upon synthesis and identified by mass spectrometry, it has been observed that there is no clear relationship between the abundance of MHC-I-bound peptides and the abundance of the proteins from which they derive. In fact, some MHC-I-associated peptides are derived from proteins that are undetectable in the cell.

Exactly what the mechanisms are that drive DRiP formation are still not entirely clear, although there are increasing suggestions that one component may involve modifications to normal translational processes. Work by Fahraeus and co-workers adapted the phenomenon of nonsense mediated decay, in which mRNA with a premature stop codon is degraded after only a single round of translation, to show that an epitope encoded by such an mRNA is produced with high efficiency for T cell recognition. More recently, Granados et al. used the SILAC method to analyze MHC-I-associated peptides in human EBV-transformed B cell lines and made the intriguing observations that, first, many of the peptides were derived from proteins associated with B cell differentiation rather than more abundant house-keeping proteins, and second, that the peptides were preferentially derived from proteins encoded by transcripts that were the targets of microRNAs (miRNAs), which are known to regulate transcript stability. Analysis of literature data covering multiple epitopes and their sources determined that this is a general phenomenon, not specific for transformed B cell lines. The precise mechanistic connection between mRNA instability and the generation of MHC-I-associated peptides remains unknown.

Chaperones and Cytosolic Peptide Generation

While DRiPs are a significant, perhaps major, source, MHC-I-associated peptides can be derived from intact proteins. Proteins introduced directly into the cytosol of a cell, for example proteins such as listeriolysin and other proteins secreted by *Listeria monocytogenes* after its internalization by macrophages, can be processed and recognized by CD8⁺ T cells. What then are the intracellular processing steps that proteins, or DRiPs, follow before they degenerate into the peptides that are translocated into the ER by TAP? Shastri and co-workers developed exceptionally clever techniques to identify the cytosolic precursors of MHC-I binding peptides and have shown that they are associated with cytosolic chaperones. The approach draws on the ability of exogenous MHC-I-binding peptides to sensitize cells for recognition by CD8⁺ T cells.

In the most refined version of the method, the epitope, derived from OVA, is flanked with lysine residues and embedded in a protein that is then expressed in cells. The precise epitope (SIINFEHL, a modification of the classical H2-K^b-associated SIINFEKL epitope with histidine substituted for the normal internal lysine residue) is released from any cytosolic precursor of the peptide by digestion with trypsin, which produces the correct N-terminal amino acid, and carboxypeptidase B, which removes the C-terminal lysine. The exceptional sensitivity of a T cell hybridoma recognizing this epitope allowed the identification of precursors which co-immunoprecipitated with anti-chaperone antibodies, as saying the proteolytically released epitope by sensitization of an H2-K^b-positive target cell. Large intermediate degradation fragments of the protein were found in association with the chaperone Hsp90α. shRNA-mediated knockdown of Hsp90α inhibited accumulation of the fragments and processing of the antigen, as well as its recognition by CD8⁺ T cells, as did knockdown of a co-chaperone, CHIP, which ubiquitinates Hsp70 or Hsp90α-associated proteins and delivers them to proteasomes for degradation. This suggests that these fragments are pre-proteasomal. Consistent with this, the addition of a proteasome inhibitor to the cell increased the amounts of the fragments, and they were extended at the C-terminus beyond the actual epitope; the C-terminal residue of peptides translocated by TAP and associated with MHC-I is generally generated by proteasomal cleavage. Other fragments were associated with another chaperone, the Tailless Complex Polypeptide-1 (TCP-1) Ring Complex or TRiC. These fragments were N-terminally extended but not C-terminally extended, i.e. all of them ended with the precise epitope sequence that was originally embedded in the protein. This indicates that they are post-proteasomal. Thus the pathway that has emerged is that a cytosolic protein, usually a recently synthesized or somehow defective one (a DRiP), associates with Hsp90α, is ubiquitinated by CHIP, and is degraded by the proteasome to yield truncated fragments which then associate with TRiC. Cytosolic aminoterminal trimming, for example by leucine aminopeptidase, can then reduce them to an appropriate size for TAP mediated transport into the ER. For individual epitopes, cytosolic peptidases, including leucine aminopeptidase and tripeptidyl peptidase II, may facilitate or inhibit their generation.

Nonconventional Sources of MHC-I-associated Peptides

The extraordinary sensitivity of T cell recognition is well established. Very low numbers of MHC-I peptide complexes are required; even a single complex may be sufficient to trigger a T cell. Possibly because of this some MHC-I-associated peptides have origins that do not depend on conventional translation. There are examples of antigenic peptides that are out of frame with regard to their proteins of origin and others derived from sequences embedded in introns. There are peptides that derive from translation initiated at codons other that the conventional methionine codon, ATG. Shastri and co-workers have identified a novel translational mechanism that involves leucine-tRNA-mediated initiation of translation at a CUG codon and suggest that other codons may be functional. These experiments constitute recent examples of a historically common phenomenon; immunological studies often enhance our understanding of molecular biological processes.

There are also examples of peptide epitopes derived from non-contiguous sequences in proteins. Many of these have derived from studies of human epitopes recognized by patient-derived tumor specific CD8$^+$ T cells. Vigneron et al. described an HLA-A32-associated epitope derived from the melanosomal glycoprotein gp100 (or pmel17) that was a nonamer but was derived from a 13 amino acid precursor by removal of four internal residues. They showed that this excision/splicing event was mediated by the proteasome and involved a mechanism in which the hydrolysis of a bond between the peptide and a threonine residue in the active site of the proteasome β-subunit, normally the final step of proteolysis, is replaced by reaction with the N-terminal amino group of a second peptide instead of water. A number of other examples of this have been described, including one peptide in which the N-terminal sequence of the peptide is actually C-terminal to the N-terminal peptide sequence in the intact protein.

Another example of an epitope that does not represent the primary sequence of a protein also involves a melanosomal glycoprotein. In this case, an asparagine residue present in the melanosomal enzyme tyrosinase was replaced by an aspartic acid residue in a tyrosinase-derived HLA-A2.1-associated nonameric peptide. This occurs because the peptide is generated from the protein after its signal sequence-mediated entry into the ER and subsequent degradation following retrotranslocation into the cytosol. This is the conventional mechanism for disposal of misfolded proteins and glycoproteins and is known as ER-associated degradation, or ERAD. The proteasome is the normal destination for such retrotranslocated proteins. A component of the pathway for glycoproteins involves their cytosolic deglysosylation by an N-glycanase that converts the glycan-bearing asparagine residue to an aspartic acid; the epitope encompassed a glycosylated sequence in tyrosinase that was deglycosylated in the cytosol.

Implications of ERAD for Cross-presentation

A pathway in which proteins that enter the ER are retrotranslocated into the cytosol and generate peptides that are potentially available for MHC-I-restricted T cell recognition has a clear parallel to the dominant mechanism involved in cross-presentation. Here the compartment is an endosome or phagosome rather than the ER, but the underlying principle is the same. A luminal protein internalized by a DC must enter the cytosol and be degraded by the proteasome to generate the relevant peptide, in principle the same peptide that would be generated by a normal cell expressing the protein as an endogenously translated protein. Thus a CD8$^+$ T cell induced by cross-presentation of a viral protein would recognize the epitope generated in the infected cell, allowing its destruction. The seductive logic of this argument has led to a considerable body of work suggesting, although not without controversy, that the mechanisms responsible for cross-presentation are an adaptation of ERAD. This was first suggested by the work of Desjardin and coworkers, who identified ER-derived proteins in phagosomes purified from a macrophage cell line, with the implication that the ERAD retrotranslocation machinery could be recruited to phagosomes from the ER. Experimental evidence supporting this rapidly followed. DCs and DC-like cell lines were found to be capable of transferring proteins into the cytosol from endosomes or phagosomes, including enzymes such as luciferases, as well as cytochrome C. The addition of cytochrome C to DCs and its entry into the cytosol caused apoptosis, mimicking the effect of cytochrome C released from mitochondria in conventionally induced apoptosis. Processing and presentation of soluble, exogenous OVA by H2-K^b expressed in a human DC-like cell line, KG-1, could be blocked by a cytosolically expressed dominant-negative, ATPase-defective, mutant version of the AAA-ATPase p97, which normally mediates the extraction of proteins from the ER during ERAD.

In addition, phagosomes derived from KG-1 were capable of extruding luciferases that were internalized along with the phagocytic substrate, a latex bead, into the external milieu, topologically equivalent to the cytosol. This was ATP-dependent, could be enhanced by recombinant p97, and inhibited by recombinant dominant-negative p97, all of which is consistent with an ERAD-like mechanism. TAP and other PLC components were also identified in purified phagosomes, and they were capable of internalizing peptides via TAP and assembling them with MHC-I molecules present in the phagosome. This led to the concept that phagosomes in DCs are compartments specialized for MHC-I-restricted antigen processing, later extended to endosomes. This is an interesting but not essential element of a coherent hypothesis involving ER recruitment to phagosomes. The critical step is the role of ERAD in mediating cytosolic access; after that proteolytic degradation and TAP-mediated transport of peptides into the ER would be sufficient. However, as mentioned earlier the ERAP1-like aminopeptidase IRAP is present in DC phagosomes and can facilitate cross-presentation, which is consistent with the idea that they may be dedicated cross-presenting organelles.

Vesicular fusion events in cells are regulated by the interactions of SNARE proteins present on the vesicles involved. Recently it has been shown that recruitment of ER resident proteins to the phagosome, and cross-presentation, in DCs is dependent on Sec22b, a SNARE localized to the ER-Golgi intermediate compartment (ERGIC), that interacts with a partner SNARE, syntaxin 4, normally present on the plasma membrane but present on phagosomes in DCs. This appears to have resolved some of the controversies surrounding the connection of ERAD and cross-presentation, although the nature of the channel that mediates the translocation of internalized antigens into the cytosol of the cross-presenting cell remains unknown.

In conclusion, the study of antigen processing is now over three decades old, yet novel findings continue to surprise and delight those of us working in the field. For MHC-I the mechanisms of cross-presentation and the precise mechanisms that regulate DRiP formation and the cytosolic generation of peptides are areas in need of clarification. For MHC-II the mechanisms that regulate the formation of the peptide complexes recognized by Type A and Type B CD4$^+$ T cells, in particular the role of DM in the process, and the precise function of DO remain to be uncovered. In addition, recent demonstrations of phagocytosis in B cells underlines the need for additional work to determine how this modulates MHC-I and -II functions in these cells, given the clear differences in the process between B cells, DCs and macrophages. Applications of mechanistic insights to vaccine development are likely to be important.

Antigen Presentation

Major histocompatibility complexes (MHC) class I and class II proteins play a pivotal role in the adaptive branch of the immune system. Both classes of proteins share the task of presenting peptides on the cell surface for recognition by T cells. Immunogenic peptide–MHC class I (pMHCI) complexes are presented on nucleated cells and are recognized by cytotoxic CD8+ T cells. The presentation of pMHCII by antigen-presenting cells [e.g., dendritic cells (DCs), macrophages, or B cells], on the other hand, can activate CD4+ T cells, leading to the coordination and regulation of effector cells. In all cases, it is a clonotypic T cell receptor that interacts with a given pMHC complex, potentially leading to sustained cell:cell contact formation and T cell activation.

Major histocompatibility complex class I and class II share an overall similar fold. The binding platform is composed of two domains, originating from a single heavy α-chain (HC) in the case of MHC class I and from two chains in the case of MHC class II (α-chain and β-chain). The two domains evolved to form a slightly curved β-sheet as a base and two α-helices on top, which are far enough apart to accommodate a peptide chain in-between. Two membrane-proximal immunoglobulin (Ig) domains support the peptide-binding unit. One Ig domain is present in each chain of MHC class II, while the second Ig-type domain of MHC class I is provided by non-covalent association of the invariant light chain beta-2 microglobulin (β_2m) with the HC. Transmembrane helices anchor the HC of MHC class I and both chains of MHC class II in the membrane.

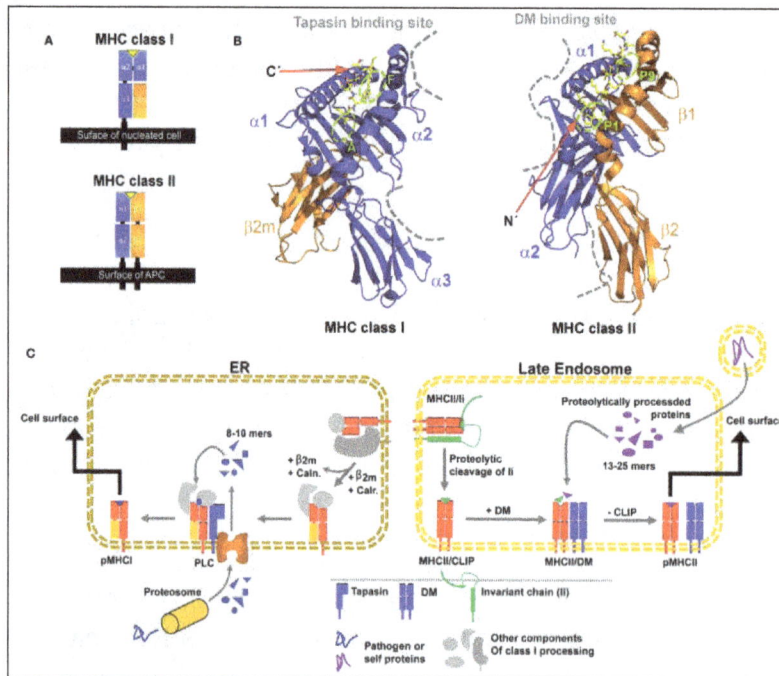

Figure shows structural characteristics of major histocompatibility complex (MHC) class I and MHC class II proteins and their compartment-dependent loading with processed peptides. (A) Domain topology of a pMHC class I and pMHC class II complex. (B) Structure of HLA-A68 in complex with an HIV-derived peptide (PDB: 4HWZ, left) and HLA-DR1 in complex with a hemagglutinin-derived peptide (1DLH, right). Indicated are the supposed interaction sites of MHC class I with tapasin and of MHC class II with DM as dashed gray lines. The peptide is shown in yellow with its N and C-terminus marked and relevant pockets are labeled green (C) Simplified illustration of MHC class I (left) and II (right) processing and peptide-editing pathways. CLIP, class II-associated invariant chain peptide; Caln., calnexin; Calr., calreticulin; ER, endoplasmic reticulum; PLC, peptide loading complex.

The groove in-between the two helices accommodates peptides based on (i) the formation of a set of conserved hydrogen bonds between the side-chains of the MHC molecule and the backbone of the peptide and (ii) the occupation of defined pockets by peptide side chains (anchor residues P2 or P5/6 and PΩ in MHC class I and P1, P4, P6, and P9 in MHC class II. The type of interactions of individual peptide side-chains with the MHC depend on the geometry, charge distribution, and hydrophobicity of the binding groove. Predicting the affinity of these distinct MHC–antigen interactions for individual allotypes has been a long-standing goal in the community. While good progress has been made in developing and optimizing bioinformatic algorithms to estimate peptide binding to MHC proteins, these *in silico* predictions, however, still yield false positives, and often fail in predicting immunodominance. We argue that understanding the relevance of transient or energetically excited protein conformations that are visited during the equilibrium fluctuations of the molecular structure is important for making good predictions.

In MHC class I, the binding groove is closed at both ends by conserved tyrosine residues leading to a size restriction of the bound peptides to usually 8–10 residues with its C-terminal end docking into the F-pocket. In contrast, MHC class II proteins usually accommodate peptides of 13–25 residues in length in their open binding groove, with the peptide N-terminus usually extruding from the P1 pocket. It has been reported that the interactions at the F pocket region in MHC class I and the P1 region (including the P2 site) in MHC class II appear to have a dominant effect on the presentation of stable pMHC complexes and on the immunodominance of certain peptidic epitopes. Interestingly, these pockets are located at opposite ends of the binding groove of the respective MHC class I and MHC class II structures.

The most polymorphic human MHC class I and class II proteins (human leukocyte antigens, HLAs) are each expressed from three gene regions (MHC class I: HLA-A, -B, -C; MHC class II: HLA-DR, -DP, -DQ), which are all highly polymorphic. This allelic variation mainly affects the nature and composition of the peptide-binding groove and thus modulates the peptide repertoire that is presented on the surface by MHC class I or MHC class II proteins for CD8+ or CD4+ T cell recognition, respectively. A good match of the peptide and the MHC binding groove is an important, but certainly not the sole determinant of its presentation. In fact, the formation of a pMHC complex depends on its peptide-loading pathway, in which the selection of peptides is influenced by several factors, such as antigen availability, protease activity, or the availability of chaperones. In addition, for each MHC class, a "catalyst" is available to enhance peptide exchange for certain peptides: tapasin for MHC class I and HLA-DM for MHC class II. These molecules edit the presented peptide repertoire and bias the exchange reaction toward the presentation of thermodynamically stable complexes. Tapasin and HLA-DM thus act similar to typical enzymes by reducing the energy barrier for peptide exchange. However, in the case of HLA-DM and tapasin, no covalent bonds are formed or cleaved during the exchange reaction.

The MHC class I HC folds and assembles with β_2m in the lumen of the endoplasmic reticulum (ER). The partially folded heterodimer is then incorporated into the peptide-loading complex (PLC) for peptide binding and exchange. In the PLC, tapasin is a protein that catalyzes, together with other chaperones, the loading of high-affinity peptides derived from proteolysis of endogenously ex-pressed proteins. In the absence of tapasin, some class I allotypes (such as HLA-B*44:02) are retained in the ER (tapasin-dependent), whereas other class I proteins (tapasin-independent, such as HLA-B*44:05 and HLA-B 27:09) can bind peptides and travel to the cell surface. There is no crystal structure of the MHC class I/tapasin complex, but several structural models and mutational studies suggested that tapasin binds two regions in the HC of MHC class I, a loop in the α_3 domain (residues 222–229), and a region of the α_2 domain (residues 128–137) adjacent to the F-pocket.

Major histocompatibility complex class II proteins fold in the ER in complex with a protein called invariant chain (Ii) and are then transported to late endosomal compartments (also coined MHC class II compartment, MIIC). There, Ii is cleaved by cathepsin proteases and a short fragment remains bound to the peptide-binding groove of MHC class II proteins, termed class II-associat-ed invariant chain peptide (CLIP). This placeholder peptide is then normally exchanged against higher affinity peptides, which are derived from proteolytically degraded proteins available in en-docytic compartments. HLA-DM accelerates peptide exchange, with different allelic variants being more or less susceptible to catalysis. HLA-DM has a highly similar structural fold compared to classical MHC class II proteins, but its closed-up binding groove prevents peptide binding. Crystal structures of HLA-DM in complex with the MHC class II protein HLA-DR1 and in complex with the competitive inhibitor HLA-DO revealed that HLA-DM mainly contacts the α_1-domain of MHC class II proteins close to the P1 pocket and additionally the membrane-proximal β2-domain, in line with previous mutational analyses.

Despite the structural differences between tapasin and HLA-DM as well as their presumably oppo-site sides of interaction with regard to the orientation of the binding groove, a similar mode of ac-tion has been suggested, hinting at a possible convergent evolution of the two exchange catalysts. A common feature seems to be that both catalysts target regions in the vicinity of those pockets in the peptide-binding groove that are of great relevance for the stability of the respective pMHC com-plex . Furthermore, in both cases, the binding of a high-affinity peptide is able to release the in-teraction with tapasin/DM and allows for transport of stable pMHC complexes to the cell surface.

While the general hallmarks of antigen processing and editing have been established, the discus-sion is now moving toward the dynamics of the system, both at the cellular and molecular level. The mechanistic questions relate to a description of how exactly peptides are selected for presen-tation and how tapasin and HLA-DM catalyze this reaction in an allele-specific manner.

Structural variations in MHC Complexes

Many allelic variants of MHC class I and MHC class II bound to individual peptide antigens dis-play different biochemical features, but surprisingly, their "ground-state," i.e., thermodynamical-ly most stable conformations reported by the many available pMHC X-ray structures are very similar. In contrast, increasing experimental and computational evidence of wild type (WT) and mutant MHC complexes over the past years incontestably revealed that changes in conformational dynamics in MHC proteins have to accompany peptide loading and exchange.

To highlight possible dynamic regions within ground-state crystal structures of human MHC class I and class II proteins bound to a peptide, we performed a global B-factor analysis of all available X-ray crystal structures of human MHC complexes in the absence of any other binding partner.

In each structure, we normalized the B-factor values of each alpha carbon (CA) atom to the global mean. Then the variance of all the normalized B-factor values for each CA atom, in 297 human pMHC class I and 41 human pMHC class II structures, was calculated and depicted with a blue to red color spectrum, respectively (heat map on structures of HLA-A 0201 and HLA-DR1. Overall in the binding groove of class I (class II), the α-helix in the α2 (β1) domain displays higher B-factor variation values than the α-helix in the α1 (α1) domain and the β-strands from both domains. Among the pMHCI structures, although B-factor variation values in the N-terminus-proximal helical segments indicate the existence of a certain degree of dynamics, the α2-helical region around the peptide C-terminus displays the highest variation in B-factors. Among the class II structures, high B-factor variation values are found especially in β-strands 2 and 4 of the α-chain, the 3_{10} helical regions and almost the entire β-chain α-helix. Our analysis is corroborated by a previous comparison of 91 different pMHC class II crystal structures. In this analysis, conformational heterogeneities were observed in three regions: the 3_{10}-helical region (α45–54), the kink region in the β1-helix (β62–71), and the β2-domain (β105–112).

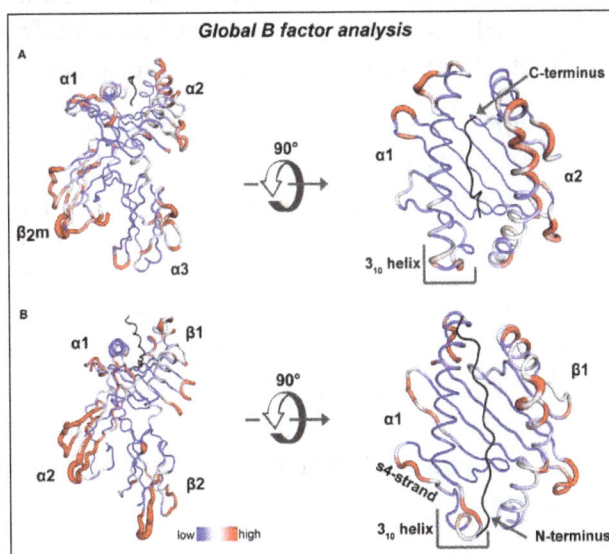

Global B-factor analysis of X-ray crystal structures of MHC class I and MHC class II.

In figure, shown is the variance of the normalized residual B factor values of CA atoms (A) derived from 297 human pMHC class I structures is plotted as blue to red spectrum on a HLA-A*0201/peptide complex (PDB: 5HHN) and (B) from 41 human pMHC class II structures is plotted on a DR1/peptide complex (PDB: 4X5W).

It is known that, to some extent, structural variations can be introduced by variable peptide-binding modes. In this context, peptides longer than 8–10 residues have been reported to bind to the MHC class I binding groove. To accommodate the increase in length, the peptides have to bulge out, leaving the central residues (between p2 and pΩ) exposed to solvent. This is usually achieved by a kink in the backbone in the middle part of the peptide. Recently, two crystal structures of HLA-A2 bound to 15-mer peptides have been solved. The two peptides follow a binding mode similar to that of the canonical peptides with two anchor residues in the B and F pockets. While one of the peptides showed a mobile central conformation similar to another reported long peptide, the other peptide adopted an unusual rigid β-hairpin secondary structure. Although the binding of the N- and C-termini at both ends of the binding groove is conserved in almost all the MHC class

I complexes, some exceptions have been reported. For example, in the F pocket of HLA-A2, the C terminal residue of the peptide extends by ~1Å leading to a significant rearrangement of the pocket with only one of the standard hydrogen bonds (at Thr143) preserved. Another example is seen in the HLA-B35 protein, the short N-terminus of the 8-mer peptide does not reach the A pocket. Instead, the hydrogen bonds between the amino group of P1 residue and residue 45 of MHC class I are mediated by a water molecule.

Since, in the case of MHC class II proteins, the peptide ligand within the binding groove usually adopts a pseudosymmetrical PPII helix-like conformation, bidirectional binding is theoretically possible. An interesting case represents a crystal structure of a DR1/CLIP complex, in which the peptide binds in a very unusual, inverted orientation (C-terminus close to the P1 pocket). The driving force for this peptide inversion is the formation of three additional H-bonds of P1-close residues and the backbone of the peptide's C-terminus. Biological and biochemical evidence for the existence of other pMHC class II isomers have been described in the context of autoimmunity. Since MHC class II proteins have open binding grooves, peptides can protrude outwards and even bind in different registers. In this regard, an insulin B chain-derived peptide ($InsB_{9-23}$) was suggested to induce type 1 diabetes (T1D) in a thermodynamically less favored, low-affinity binding register.

Apart from variable peptide binding, catalyst binding can induce more significant conformational variation, as seen in DM-bound DR. By designing a P1-anchor-free pMHC class II complex, Pos et al. could increase the affinity for the pMHC class II to DM and solve the crystal structure for the covalently tethered DR1/HA/DM complex. In this MHC class II/DM complex, the interaction interface is primarily composed by the α-subunits of DM and DR1 (~65% of the entire interaction surface, Figure. DM binding to DR stabilizes a rearranged conformation in the vicinity of the P1 pocket of DR1 resulting from the absence of critical peptide-MHC class II interactions in this region. The extended region in the DR1α-chain (α52–55) and the 3_{10}-helix adopt an α-helical fold. Compared to other parts of the pMHC class II structure, it was shown that this site indeed represents a conformationally labile region. In addition, the C-terminal part of the β1-α-helix (β86–91) becomes slightly less structured.

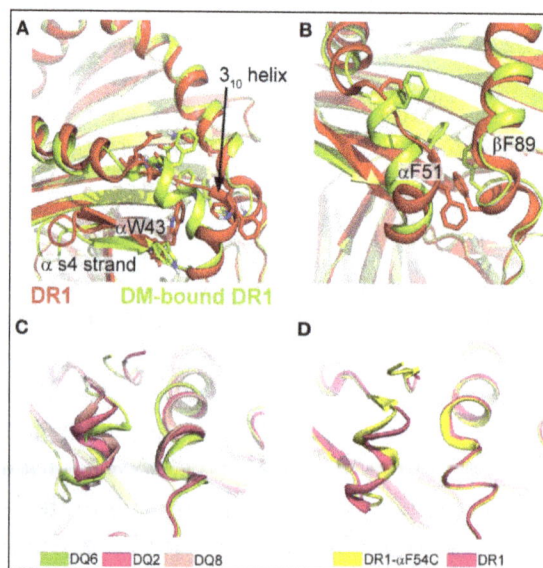

Conformational rearrangements upon DM binding and structural variations in type 1 diabetes-susceptible DQ complexes.

In figure, (A) Structural rearrangement in the α1-S4 strand and 3_{10}-helical region seen in DR1 when bound to DM (limon cartoon) compared to DR1 unbound DM (red). (B) DM-induced rearrangements in the P1-pocket and the surrounding helical segments. PDBs used in (A,B) 1DLH and 4FQX. (C) Overlay of DQ2/ag (PDB: 1S9V), DQ6/hyp$_{1-13}$ (PDB: 1UVQ) and DQ8/InsB$_{9-23}$ (PDB: 1JK8) showing the structural variations of the 3_{10} helix and the P1-proximal β1-helix. Interdomain communication as exemplarily indicated by the hydrogen bond between αR52 and βE86/βT89 in the DQ8 allele variant is thought to increase the stability of these regions and was previously discussed to be linked to a lowered DM-susceptibility. ag, αI-gliadin; hyp, hypocretin peptide 1–13; InsB, insulin B chain 9–23. (D) Structural alignment of DR1/CLIP (PDB: 3QXA) and DR1-αF54C/CLIP (PDB: 3QXD), a mutant that shows an altered conformation in the 3_{10} helix and an increased DM susceptibility.

A feature, which is also present in DM-bound DO, is the intermolecular H-bonds between two conserved residues (DRα W43 and DMα N125). The formation of these critical bonds (as well as other interactions) likely depends on the "flipping out" movement of αW43 from the P1 pocket of DR1 toward DMα. This movement of DR1 αW43 was suggested to be triggered by partial dissociation of the peptide's N-terminus or by transient destabilization of contacts of the peptide N-terminus when bound to MHC class II. As a consequence, the P1 site is stabilized by a repositioning of two phenylalanine sidechains (DRα F51 and DRβ F89), thereby compensating for the loss of peptide anchors and αW43 from this region. Incoming peptides have to compete with these repositioned Phe residues for the P1/P2 site in order to be selected for display. Interestingly, structural characteristics of T1D-conferring HLA-DQ alleles were indeed discussed to be linked to decreased DM-sensitivity. The analysis of several DQ variants indicated structural differences of the T1D-risk variants DQ2 and DQ8 when compared to DQ1, DQ 6, or DR variants. The decrease in DM-susceptibility of these two proteins was explained by a stabilization of the 3_{10} helical regions. However, the exact relationship between structural variations in the 3_{10} helixes and DM-susceptibility are not clear, as highly DM-susceptible DR complexes can display a different conformational mode, compared to DM-susceptible DQ alleles.

The observed changes lead to the question as to how much structural plasticity in these regions preexists in the peptide-loaded form and provide a prerequisite for catalyzed as well as for spontaneous peptide exchange. For example, do pMHC complexes sample conformations observed in simulations of empty proteins or in complex with the catalyst? How would allelic variation affect the distribution of MHC proteins within the conformational space and thereby influence the presented peptide repertoire? Could variation in protein plasticity also account for the association of specific MHC alleles with immune diseases? Since the polymorphic peptide-binding groove of MHC proteins defines its affinity for a certain peptide, substitutions of even a single amino acid may lead to significantly different affinities for individual peptides. In general, the critical factors defining whether a peptide is presented or not are determined at the different levels of antigen processing and presentation such as uptake route, amount, and folding state of the antigenic protein, amenability to proteolytic degradation, and catalysis of the complex, etc. However, at the molecular level, it has been shown that certain polymorphisms shape individual pockets in the peptide-binding groove to optimally present an auto-immunogenic self-peptide. In other cases, the functional impact of disease-associated polymorphisms remained enigmatic and suggests that dynamics might account for the observed differences.

Dynamics of Peptide-free MHC Proteins

While simulations and experimental studies vary in the features ascribed to peptide-free MHC proteins, they certainly agree in attributing a substantial degree of dynamics to the peptide-binding groove. Thus, binding of peptides to MHC proteins is of utmost importance for the stabilization of the known MHC fold. The lack of a crystal or an NMR structure of peptide-free MHC protein hinders an accurate description of the structural changes upon peptide binding and this is probably due to the ensemble character of the peptide-free conformers. This ensemble character, however, has been probed by computational techniques.

MHC Class I

Most of the conformational dynamics information on the peptide-free class I have been revealed by molecular dynamics (MD) simulations. In such simulations, peptide-free class I protein is modeled from the crystal structure by deleting the atoms of the bound peptide. In the absence of peptide, an increased conformational flexibility of the F pocket region was observed for several allelic variants (HLA-A 02:01, HLA-B 44:02, HLA-B 44:05, HLA-B 27:05, HLA-B*27:09, H-2D^b, and H-2K^b). Longer simulations of chicken and human class I allotypes showed increased global motion in the peptide-free form when compared to the peptide-bound proteins. By combining molecular docking and MD simulations, a conformational transition of the 3_{10} helical segment of H-2L^d between the peptide-bound and peptide-free class I was observed. Thus, a conformational reorganization close to the A and B pockets upon peptide binding was proposed.

Experimentally, circular dichorism (CD) was used to measure the thermal denaturation temperature (T_m) of the peptide-free HLA-B 07:02 (B7/β2m). By increasing the temperature, a gradual loss of the structure-specific signal of B7/β_2m in the CD spectrum of peptide-free class I was detected, indicating a more heterogeneous conformational population. Furthermore, in the absence of peptide, the binding groove of B7/β_2m was more sensitive to enzymatic proteolysis when compared to the peptide-bound form. Saini et al. studied the unfolding of H-2K^b by measuring the intrinsic tryptophan florescence. The results pointed to a folding intermediate of peptide-free class I proteins that are more structured than a molten globule. This was in line with a previous study arguing for a native-like conformation of *in vitro* refolded empty murine class I proteins.

Structural studies using NMR indicated a loss of the binding-groove fold in the peptide-free form of a HLA-C allotype. In particular, NMR spectra of these peptide-free MHC class I protein show the loss of selected methionine NH resonances of the β-sheet floor of the peptide-binding groove, which indicated unfolding or conformational exchange of this part of the protein. This is consistent with previous reports indicating that especially the binding groove is undergoing conformational exchange in the absence of the bound peptide.

A work that focused on complexes with a partly filled MHC class I binding groove pointed to a requirement of the stabilization of the F pocket region. By using a refolded H-2D^b in the presence of a pentamer peptide (NYPAL), which binds to the C to F pockets in the binding groove, a X-ray crystal structure of the pMHCI complex could be solved. Thus, peptide/class I interactions at the F pocket region seem to be sufficient to keep class I in a folded state. In agreement, short dipeptides mimicking the peptide C-terminus of high-affinity ligands support the folding of HLA-A*0201, displaying high peptide-receptivity. To stabilize peptide-free class I in a folded form independently from the peptide, the Springer group created a novel variant by introducing a disulfide bond to restrain the high flexibility of the F pocket region. The disulfide mutant showed an increased peptide and β_2m affinity and bypassed the cellular quality control.

MHC Class II

Physiologically, the question if peptide-free MHC class II proteins play a role in adaptive immunity is posed by studies indicating that unloaded MHC class II proteins are abundantly present on the surface of immature DCs. There, they are able to bind ligands from the extracellular milieu and activate T cells. Two isomers of peptide-unloaded MHC proteins seem to exist, each displaying different kinetic properties. While the peptide-receptive empty isomer of DR1 binds peptide rapidly, the conversion to the non-receptive isomer within less than 5 min dramatically reduces the peptide-binding capacity of human DR. Studies using circular dichroism and size exclusion chromatography predicted a conformational change of peptide-free MHC class II upon peptide binding, and an increase in the overall stability. Peptide-free MHC class II proteins thus show a lower degree of helicity and an increased hydrodynamic radius compared to peptide-loaded MHC class II.

Carven and Stern studied ligand-induced conformational changes by selective chemical side-chain modification of peptide-free DR1 followed by mass spectroscopy analysis. The results of this study were inconsistent with a partly unfolded state of DR1 in the absence of ligand, but rather indicated a more localized conformational change induced upon peptide binding. However, empty MHC class II proteins harbor the hallmarks of partially unstructured peptide-binding domains when studied spectroscopically. NMR-spectra of the α-chain of such peptide-free MHC class II proteins barely display any signals for residues corresponding to the folded peptide-binding groove, indicating that the binding groove undergoes conformational exchange. Taken together, it appears likely that the empty binding groove dynamically samples different native-like conformations. Interestingly, similar to MHC class I, certain small molecules and dipeptides increase peptide-receptivity of peptide-free MHC class II proteins, presumably by preventing a "closure" of the binding groove. In similar to the F pocket of MHCI, the predicted site of interaction is the most dominant pocket of the binding groove (P1).

In a MD simulation study combined with peptide-binding assays, it was shown that a well-conserved residue, βN82, which also contributes disproportionally to pMHCII stability, is participating in the control of peptide receptivity. The authors suggested that the "non-receptive" state of peptide-free DR1 is induced by a molecular lock through the formation of a hydrogen-bond between DRβ N82A and DRα Q9. The observed narrowing of parts of the binding groove-flanking α-helices likely represents the trigger for such a clamped conformation. Using MD simulations, another investigation suggested a movement of the α51–59 region into the P1–P4 site of the binding groove in the empty state. In this state, the α51–59 region adopted a ligand-like conformation. In addition, an increased flexibility of the β2 domain as well as the β50–70 helical region was observed. A higher flexibility of the β58–69 helical region was also seen in MD simulations of the HLA-DR3 protein upon *in silico* peptide removal. Interestingly, this helical segment is also recognized by monoclonal antibodies designed to bind to the peptide-free conformation.

Table: Computational studies on MHC class I and II dynamics.

MHC	Molecular dynamics parameters	Outcome
MHC class I		
HLA-B*2705, HLA-B*2709	GROMACS, OPLS-AA/L, TIP4P, 310K	Polymorphism of major histocompatibility class I (MHC class I) influences the dynamics of the binding groove and the bound peptide
HLA-A*02:01, HLA-B*44:02, HLA-B*44:05	Amber, parm03, TIP3P, 300K	Peptide-free MHC class I shows a varying flexibility at the F pocket region
HLA-A2:01, H-2K^b	Amber, parm03, TIP3P, 300K	Prominent role of peptide C-terminus in long-range stabilization of MHC class I binding groove
HLA-B*44:02, HLA-B*44:05, H-2K^b, HLA-B*2705, HLA-B*2709	(Amber, parm03, TIP3P, 300K) (GROMACS, Amber99SB-ILDN, TIP3P, 300K)	Dynamics of the F pocket region is important for MHC stability and modulates MHC class I tapasin dependance
BF2*15:01, BF2*19:01, HLA-B*44:02, HLA-B*44:05	GROMACS, Amber99SB-ILDN, TIP3, 300K	MHC intrinsic plasticity determines the bound peptide and can be modulated allosterically by tapasin
HLA-A2:01, HLA-B*3501, HLA-B*3508	(GROMACS, GROMOS43a1, SPC, 300 K) (NAMD, CHARMM22, TIP3P, 300K)	Peptide-MHC dynamics determine the T cell receptor (TCR) binding mode
HLA-B*2705, HLA-B*2709, H-2D^b	(GROMACS, OPLS-AA/L, TIP4, 310 K) (Amber, parm03, TIP3P, 350K)	Peptide-MHC interactions at the A pocket region modulate TCR recognition
H-2L^d	NAMD, CHARMM27, TIP3P, 310K	Peptide-receptive MHC class I shows a varying flexibility at the A pocket region
HLA-A2:01	(Normal mode analysis) (Modified Amber force fields, 300K)	Anti-correlative motion of residues in the binding groove is important for peptide binding "dynamic fit"
MHC class II		
HLA-DR1, HLA-DR1	GROMACS, GROMOS9643a1, SPC, 298 K, GROMACS, GROMOS (ffG43a1), SPC, 310 K	Peptide-free MHC class II show a large conformational flexibility around the P1 pocket
HLA-DR1 (1DLH)	GROMACS, GROMOS, 310 K	Occupation of P1 with an amino acid side chains prevents the "closure" of the empty peptide binding site into the non-receptive state
HLA-DR3, HLA-DR1	(Amber, parm03, TIP3, 300K) (GROMACS, GROMOS, SPC3, 310K)	Prominent role of peptide N–terminus in long-range stabilization of MHC class II binding groove
I-Au, HLA-DR1 HLA-DR4	GROMACS, GROMOS, SPC3, 310K	Peptide-MHC dynamics influences T cells costimulation
HLA-DR4	GROMACS, GROMOS96, SPC, 310K	Different dynamics of soluble and membrane anchored pMHC
		The membrane anchored is more conformationally and energetically stable
HLA-DR1	NAMD, CHARMM22, explicit water model, 298K	Conformational entropy of peptide binding to DR1 correlates with the DM-susceptibility
HLA-DR1	ACEMD, ff99SB, TIP3P, 310K	β-chain around peptide N-terminus and αW43 sample DM-bound-like conformations

HLA-DR1	(Normal mode analysis) (Modified Amber force fields, 300K)	Anti-correlative motions in the binding groove is important for binding of long peptides "dynamic fit"
HLA-DR1	(Normal mode analysis) (Modified Amber force fields, 300K)	The membrane-proximal domains of ~MHC class II modulate the dynamics of P1 pocket and have a greater influence on the binding groove than those of MHC class I
MHC I, major histocompatibility class I.		

Finally, it has to be noted that the timescale of the experimental descriptions of empty MHC molecules differs vastly from the theoretical studies. While the latter describe the initial events of conformational changes accompanying peptide removal, the experimental investigations observe the properties of the empty MHC species at or near equilibrium.

Dynamic Features of Peptide-bound MHC Complexes

While the study of empty MHC proteins is of theoretical and conceptual interest, nature has engineered the antigen-presenting system in a way that prevents the accumulation of isolated, non-peptide-bound MHC molecules. Endogenous peptides derived from the proteasome in case of class I or from the invariant chain in the case of class II first bind and eventually are replaced by antigenic peptide. This inherently dynamic process is enabled by intrinsic features of the MHC molecules and several studies suggest that pMHC complexes sample different and transient conformations dependent on the bound peptide and the allelic variant under investigation.

MHC Class I

Changes in conformational dynamics in MHC class I are heterogeneously distributed along its peptide-binding groove, as suggested by both computational and experimental studies. For example, MD simulations showed a subtype-dependent conformational flexibility of the F pocket region. Residues 114 and 116 of the HC, at the bottom of the F pocket, and residues 74 and 77 from the α_1-helix, engaging the peptide's C-terminus, show an altered mobility in different MHC class I allotypes . Consistently, it was shown that the dynamics of the MHC class I binding groove was most profoundly affected by C-terminal residues of the peptide. In longer MD simulations, in addition to varying protein plasticity in the F pocket region, an enhanced sampling of conformations in the α_3-domain upon peptide binding was observed.

Experimental observations at the atomistic level, derived from NMR-based relaxation-dispersion experiments, have elucidated the peptide dependency of minor states on the stability of pMHCI complexes. Conformational fluctuations of different HLA-B*35:01 complexes were localized to the peptide-binding groove, including residues of the B, E, and F-pocket, but not in the IgG-like domains. Interestingly, the presence of minor conformations in pMHCI complexes (ranging from approximately >1 to 4.5%) could be positively correlated to the thermostability and surface presentation of the pMHCI complex under investigation, implying that a minor conformation considerably contributes to pMHCI stability. Similar, investigations of HLA-A*02:01 loaded with different peptides by HD exchange/MS and fluorescence anisotropy revealed that fluctuations within the binding groove depend on the ligand bound to MHC class I. Despite these ligand-sensitive changes in dynamics, the α_2-helix showed a general higher flexibility than the α_1-helix. The authors concluded that the observed variations in dynamics throughout the peptide-binding site could influence receptor engagement, entropic penalties during receptor binding, and the population of binding-competent states.

Table: Experimental studies on major histocompatibility complex (MHC) class I and II dynamics.

MHC	Method	Outcome
MHC class I		
HLA-B*2705, HLA-B*2709	IR spectroscopy, crystallography	The heavy α-chain (HC) of B27:05 shows a higher flexibility than that of B27:09
HLA-B*2705, HLA-B*2709	1H-15N-HSQC (NMR)	HLA-B27 polymorphism influences the β_2m plasticity at the HC/β_2m interface
HLA-Cw*07:02	1H-15N-HSQC (NMR)	Peptide binding domains are "unstructured" in the peptide-free form
HLA-B*2709	T1/T2 and HetNOE measurements	Regions of β_2m remain flexible upon HC binding
HLA-A2	HDX/MS combined with fluorescence anisotropy	Fluctuations within the binding groove depend on the ligand bound to MHC class I
HLA-B*35:01	NMR (relaxation-dispersion)	Stability of pMHC class I is determined by peptide-dependent fluctuations defining minor states
MHC class II		
HLA-DR1	HDX combined with mass spectroscopy	3_{10} helix shows a conformational lability
		DM-susceptible conformations show weakened interactions around the P1-pocket
HLA-DR1	NMR combined with crystallography	Peptides can bind in an bidirectional mode to DR1
HLA-DR1	SACS, NMR, crystallograpy	Susceptibility to HLA-DM depends on a dynamic conformation of pMHC class II
HLA-DR1	NMR detected HDX, HSQC spectra	Dynamics in helical segments and and αS2/S4 strand of binding groove
		Peptide binding domains are "unstructured" in the peptide-free form

HDX, hydrogen/deuterium (H/D) exchange; HSQC, heteronuclear Single Quantum Coherence; SAXS, small-angle X-ray scattering.

Another study also showed that β_2m seems to sense allelic as well as peptide-induced conformational variations and accommodates to them, showing a high degree of plasticity within the inter-domain interface with the HC domains. NMR-chemical-shift changes of complexes were most pronounced in the region close to the F-pocket. By comparing the dynamics in the ns–ms timescale of HC-bound and free β_2m, Hee et al. demonstrated that most residues gain rigidity upon HC binding. Nevertheless, three sites (region around His31, site around Asp53 and Lys58, and region around Ser88) remained flexible in the mature complex. Interestingly, His31 and Ser88 are located underneath the F-pocket, which stability is known to be important for tapasin function. Moreover, Lys58 and Ser88 are also known to interact with several other proteins, including the natural killer cell receptors Ly49A CD8 and LIR1. Conformational sampling of these regions could thus be critical for the interaction with these receptors.

MHC Class II

A similarly heterogeneous picture in regards to altered binding groove dynamics can be observed for MHCII: by dissecting the thermodynamics of peptide MHC class II interactions, Ferrante et al. conclusively demonstrated how dynamics of pMHCII complexes are linked to peptide affinity and DM-susceptibility. Using different biophysical techniques and MD simulations, the authors showed that peptide binding events can be driven by a considerable proportion of conformational entropy (if enthalpic interactions are less favored). MD simulations suggest that peptide-dependent conformational fluctuations involve alterations of α-chain residues DR1α-43–54 and β-chain residues 63–68 and 79–90. Wieczorek et al. performed H/D-exchange measurements in combination with NMR spectroscopy to obtain residue-specific experimental information about the stability of individual secondary structure elements. Several regions undergoing conformational fluctuation even in highly stable pMHCII complexes were thus revealed. These fluctuations are confirmed by extensive (~100 μs) MD simulations and Markov model analyses that reveal transient conformations with obvious relevance for the peptide-exchange pathway. In particular, the highest lability was seen in DRα 46–62, in parts of β-strands s2–s4 sitting underneath the N-terminal part of the α_1 helix, β65–93 and several loops connecting the β-strands of the peptide-binding site. Interestingly, this experimental piece of evidence is also in line with the global B-factor analysis presented here; a certain degree of dynamics thus seems to already be encoded even in the context of a high affinity pMHC complex. Earlier on, it was shown by HD-exchange/MS measurements that conserved peptide–MHC class II contacts (H–bonds) are strong at the P1 pocket-proximal site of the peptide (especially position βN82) in highly stable immunodominant complexes, which is in agreement with previous biochemical studies. However, local destabilization induced by a point mutation in the DR1 complex and the use of a different ligand (DR1-αF54C/CLIP) strongly enhanced fluctuations of the peptide and especially weakened contacts around the P1 site. This implies that weakening interactions by substitutions in the peptide or MHC (allelic variation) would have an influence on conformational fluctuations that correlate with DM-susceptibility.

MHC Dynamics during Peptide Exchange

While the studies described in the above topic unambiguously demonstrate the dynamic features of pMHC complexes; the question arises naturally in how far these properties translate into peptide exchange. For pMHCII complexes experimental progress has been made in identifying intermediate or transient conformations of pMHCII with regard to catalyzed or intrinsic peptide exchange. For pMHCI molecules the atomistic description of structural changes during peptide exchange mostly relies on MD simulation studies, supported by mutational analysis and circumstantial biophysical evidence.

MHC Class I

Within cells, tapasin is a key protein that mediates the binding of high-affinity peptides to most class I proteins. To date, there is no crystal structure of the tapasin/MHC class I complex. Based on mutational studies, however, two regions have been shown to be essential for tapasin interaction with the HC of MHC class I: a loop in the α_3 domain (residues 222–229) and a part of the α_2 domain (residues 128–137). Two major functions have been proposed for tapasin: (i) a chaperone-like stabilization of empty class I proteins and (ii) a peptide-editing function through peptide-exchange catalysis. Several computational models have been published to describe the mechanism of action of tapasin on MHC class. Most researchers agree on the importance of the F-pocket region for peptide exchange. However, the association of F-pocket dynamics and the peptide-exchange mechanism remain a matter of debate. So far, dynamics in the F-pocket region in the presence of peptide have not revealed any significant conformational exchange phenomena in most MD simulations. Recently, longer MD simulations (microsecond timescale) of tapasin/pMHCI complexes indicated that binding of tapasin to HLA-B*44:02 accelerates the dissociation of low-affinity peptides. Using a computational systems model, it was shown that peptide exchange seems to depend on the opening and closing rate of the binding groove in the presence of peptide. According to this study, the pMHCI opening rate is peptide-dependent, but pMHCI closing is allele-dependent. Consequently, a low-affinity peptide complex would display fast opening rates, but only if the MHC allele variant has an F-pocket signature (more plasticity) that allows for fast closing in the presence of a high-affinity peptide (as B44:05), it would lead to efficient peptide exchange in the absence of catalyst. Allele variants with a rigid F-pocket conformation (as B44:02) in contrast depend on tapasin to sample the necessary conformational states to close the binding groove quickly.

It has to be considered that as a default, tapasin is present in the cell and that it may also provide the necessary function as a chaperone to prevent the collapse of empty MHC class I molecules into a non-receptive state as it is experimentally measured in tapasin-deficient cells. However, in the absence of a crystal structure of the tapasin/MHC class I complex, it is difficult to rationalize the dynamics with regard to tapasin binding and exchange.

MHC Class II

Two seminal studies made it unambiguously clear that HLA-DM recognizes complexes showing a P1-destabilized conformation. However, since DM-susceptible structures rarely show any of the changes present in the DM-bound structure (e.g., folding of α-46–55 into an α-helix and unfolding of C-terminal β-helix), the question of the conformational prerequisites for DM binding arises. As mentioned previously, an important study indeed demonstrated that HLA-DM attacks pMHC class II complexes at a site of conformational lability, the 3_{10}-helical region. This segment, together with a neighboring unstructured segment (α52–55) folds into an α-helix when bound to DM. Interestingly, increased fluctuations of this region could be observed by other computational and experimental studies, implying the existence of higher conformational entropy within this region. Noteworthy, the α-helix in the region β86–β91 opens up to a certain degree in the DM-bound structure of DR1. However, a considerable influence of P1-remote sites on conformational dynamics and DM-dependence was recently demonstrated. In this study, alteration of P9-pocket/peptide interactions influenced dynamics of the pMHCII, likely in regions relevant for DM binding. The authors concluded that the key determinants for HLA-DM recognition are conformational dynamics present in HLA-DR1. Similarly, Ferrante et al. explained the relationship between entropic penalties and DM binding in a thermodynamic context. According to their experimental and computational results, higher conformational entropy of pMHCII complexes correlates with DM susceptibility.

A recent study by our group in the MHC class II field explored internal motions of pMHC class II molecules along the conformational peptide-exchange pathway in a more conceptual model. Using NMR/HDX (hydrogen deuterium exchange) and MD simulations of over 200 μs in total, followed by Markov State model (MSM) analysis , we have identified transient conformations relevant for the DM-catalyzed and non-catalyzed (spontaneous) peptide-editing process. In agreement with the general view, the catalyzed pathway depends on the particular destabilization of the region surrounding the P1 pocket, sharing in part features of MHC class II bound to DM. More specifically, it has been suggested for MHC class II that pMHC complexes have to sample P1-pocket-destabilized conformations to allow for HLA-DM binding.

The non-catalyzed pathway, however, was correlated to the ground state of the pMHCII complex and, therefore, is directly correlated with thermodynamic stability. Indeed, it was shown that, removal of two hydrogen bonds between β82N of the MHC class II and the backbone of the peptide in the mutant DR1βN82A drastically reduces stability and, at the same time, dramatically enhances non-catalyzed peptide exchange. Nevertheless, binding to HLA-DM is also enhanced for the βN82A mutant, leading to the somewhat paradoxical finding that an MHCII molecule might bind tightly to a catalyst that it does not need for exchanging peptide. This can be best conceptualized when assuming that the βN82A mutant of HLA-DR1 in addition to increased spontaneous exchange more frequently samples a rare conformation along the pathway of catalyzed exchange. MD simulations in conjunction with MSM analysis indeed show that an excited state structurally correlated with features of the HLA-DM bound conformation. This excited state was seen to be significantly more frequently sampled in the mutant compared to WT HLA-DR1.

However, a similar intermediate state can be defined for the very stable WT protein, where peptide release from the pockets was not mandatory for the observation of the early intermediates. Thus, if the pMHCII forms a stable complex, the peptide editing depends on the population of rare conformations that can be selected by the catalyst DM for binding. This study demonstrated the critical importance of residues 80–93 of the β1 helix for catalyzed exchange, suggesting that β1 helical unfolding is critical for the rearrangement of this segment as it is observed in the DR1-DM structure. As the study shows, mutations in the β1 helix (e.g., βE87P) designed to specifically destabilize the C-terminal part of the β1 helix without disrupting H-bonds to the peptide, are able to over-proportionally shift the dynamics toward the HLA-DM-dependent pathway.

In conclusion, this model helps to reconcile discrepancies in the hypothesized correlations of peptide affinity, pMHC stability, DM susceptibility, and catalytic effect.

Chapter 3

T Cells and B Cells

The lymphocytes which develop in the thymus gland and are vital for the immune response in organisms are known as T cells. B cells refer to a type of white blood cells which belong to the subtype lymphocyte. This chapter closely examines the key concepts of B cells and T cells such as their development and activation to provide an extensive understanding of the subject.

T Cells

T cells are part of the immune system and develop from stem cells in the bone marrow. T cells are like soldiers who seek and destroy invaders and support other immune cells for a combined response to threats. T cells are also known as T lymphocytes, with the "T" standing for "thymus", the organ in which these cells develop, and because they mature from thymocytes (hematopoietic progenitor cells present in the thymus), though a few also mature in the tonsils.

Types of T Cells

The majority of human T cells are part of the adaptive immune system. T cells have a number of variants that perform differing roles within the immune system.

1. Effector: These are relatively short-lived activated cells that defend the body during the immune response. The category of effector T cells is a broad one that includes various T cell types, which carry out cell-mediated responses and actively respond to stimulus, such as co-stimulation. This category includes helper, killer, regulatory, and potentially other T cell types as well as B cells.

2. Helper: The helper T cells support other white blood cells with immunologic processes, including the maturation of B cells into plasma cells and memory B cells along with the activation of cytotoxic T cells and macrophages. These cells are also called CD4+ T cells because they express the CD4 glycoprotein on their surfaces.

Helper T cells become activated by certain antigens on the surface of antigen-presenting cells (APCs), which include macrophages, dendritic cells, langerhans cells, and B cells. T cells detect fragments of protein antigens that have been partly degraded inside the APC. These peptide fragments are carried to the surface of the APC on special molecules called MHC proteins, which then allow the T cells to detect them and become activated.

Once they are activated, they divide quickly and secrete protein signals known as cytokines, which regulate and support the immune response. These cells can differentiate into one of several subtypes (TH1, TH2, TH3, TH17, TH9, or TFH), which secrete different cytokines for different kinds of immune responses. The signalling from the APC determines what subtype a helper T cell becomes.

3. Cytotoxic T Cell: These cells are also known as CD8+ T cells, since they express the CD8 glycoprotein at their surfaces, but are more commonly called the killer T cells. These cells are designed to seek and destroy pathogens, including viruses and bacterial invaders, and tumors. Killer T cells detect these threats by sensing antigens (toxins or other foreign substances) when encountering a threat.

Once the T cells have located a threat, such as an influenza virus for example, they have three weapons in their arsenal to use.

The first is the secretion of cytokines, in particular the cytokines TNF-α and IFN-γ, which have antitumor, antiviral, and antimicrobial effects.

The second is the production and release of cytotoxic granules known as granzymes. These granzymes are also found in natural killer cells and contain two families of proteins, perforin, and granzymes. Perforin forms a pore in the membrane of the target cell, allowing the granzymes to enter the target cell. The granzymes then cleave the proteins inside the cell, shutting down the production of viral proteins and ultimately resulting in apoptosis (cellular death).

The third is using Fas/FasL interactions. Activated killer T cells express FasL on the cell surface, which binds to its receptor, Fas, on the surface of a target cell. The binding causes the Fas molecules on the surface of the target cell to trigger the caspase cascade, which also results in apoptosis of the target cell. Importantly, killer T cells also express both molecules, making Fas/FasL interactions a mechanism by which killer T cells can destroy each other – a process called "fratricide" – to remove themselves at the end of an immune response.

4. Memory: Memory T cells are a type of antigen-specific T cell that remains long after an infection has resolved. When they encounter an antigen associated with a pathogen they encountered in the past, they quickly expand to large numbers of effector T cells capable to destroy the pathogen. This provides the immune system with a "memory" against past infections and allows a faster response to attack. For example, if you had an illness such as chickenpox or the mumps as a child, you are much better able to fight off any future occurrences, as your immune "memory" can identify them faster.

5. Regulatory: These T cells are crucial for the upkeep of immunological tolerance, ensuring that there is no immune response to self-antigens and for suppressing excessive immune responses damaging to the host. Their main role is to shut down T cell-mediated immunity towards the end of an immune reaction and to suppress autoreactive T cells that escape the process of negative selection in the thymus.

Regulatory T cells can develop either in the thymus, making them thymic Treg cells, or they can also be induced peripherally, making them peripherally derived Treg cells.

6. Natural killer T cell: Natural killer T cells (NKT cells) are different from natural killer cells of the innate immune system, as they link the adaptive immune system and the innate immune system. Similar to regular T cells, which recognize certain antigens, these cells detect a different set of antigens (glycolipid antigens); once activated, they can function in a double capacity, as if they were T helper and T killer cells combined into one.

This means that NKTs can release cytokines to support the active immune response and use the cytotoxic weapons available to regular T cells.

7. Others: There are some other types of T cells, such as mucosal associated invariant T cells and gamma delta T cells (part of the innate immune system), but these are only present in very small numbers and are beyond the scope of this general introduction.

T Cell Receptor

Initial descriptions of T cell receptors were made 30 years ago primarily through similarity with immunoglobulin DNA sequences. From this beginning, a clearer picture of TCRs as a pair of clone-specific, heterodimeric polypeptide chains consisting of both constant and variable regions has developed. In humans, the majority of T cells express a TCR composed of alpha (α) and beta (β) chains (95%), and a smaller subset of T cells express a TCR with gamma (γ) and delta (δ) chains.

The TCR, through its CDRs, endows the T cell with the ability to recognize and respond to foreign or "non self" material. Antigen presenting cells (APCs) digest pathogens and display their fragments on major histocompatibility complex (MHC) molecules. This MHC/antigen complex binds to the TCR while other co-stimulatory molecules (e.g. CD28) are activated leading to T cell activation, proliferation, differentiation, apoptosis, or cytokine release. MHC/antigen complexes are, however, not the only molecules capable of interaction with TCRs. Non-peptide antigens such as lipids can interact with TCRs via some of the five isoforms of CD1 (a-e), and several studies describe TCRs binding to metabolic intermediates bound to the MHC like molecule MR1.

TCRs have been described as the most intricate receptor structures of the mammalian immune system. In the following sections, we describe how these unique structures are developed, the mechanisms used to drive immune responses via TCR signaling, the effects of their dysfunction and their exploitation as therapeutics.

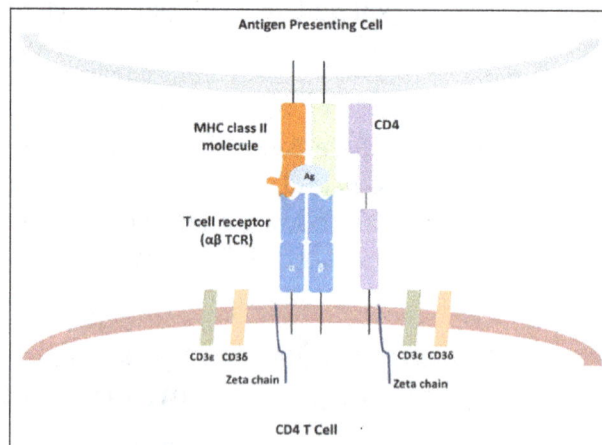

Diagram of TCR engagement with the peptide antigen MHC complex using the CD4 T cell as an example.

TCR Development and Diversity

The TCR is a disulfide-linked membrane bound heterodimeric protein normally consisting of the highly variable α and β chains expressed as part of a complex with the invariant CD3 chain molecules. T cells expressing these two chains are referred to as α:β (or $\alpha\beta$) T cells, though a minority of T cells express an alternate receptor, formed by variable γ and σ chains, referred as γσ T cells. TCR development occurs through a lymphocyte specific process of gene recombination, which assembles a final sequence from a large number of potential segments. This genetic recombination of TCR gene segments in somatic T cells occurs during the early stages of development in the thymus. The TCRα gene locus contains variable (V) and joining (J) gene segments (Vβ and Jβ), whereas the TCRβ locus contains a D gene segment in addition to Vα and Jα segments. Accordingly, the α chain is generated from VJ recombination and the β chain is involved in VDJ recombination. This is similar for the development of γδ TCRs, in which the TCRγ chain is involved in VJ recombination and the TCRδ gene is generated from VDJ recombination. Recombination is temporally regulated by the access of recombinant activating gene (RAG) 1 and RAG2 to recognizable sequences. TCR recombination occurs at two stages during the process of T cell development. First, the β chain gene undergoes Dβ – Jβ rearrangement before Vβ – DJβ recombination in the double negative cells of the thymus. Rearrangement of the α chain gene takes place in double positive thymocytes. RAG1/2 bind to and introduce double strand breaks at recombination signal sequences (RSS), which flank all TCR gene segments. DNA repair machinery completes the recombination reaction. RAG1/2 are expressed by all lymphoid progenitors and immature T and B cells.

The TCR α chain gene locus consists of 46 variable segments, 8 joining segments and the constant region. The TCR β chain gene locus consists of 48 variable segments followed by two diversity segments, 12 joining segments and two constant regions. The D and J segments are located within a relatively short 50 kb region while the variable genes are spread over a large region of 1.5 mega bases (TCRα) or 0.67 megabases (TCRβ). Therefore, the process of VDJ recombination requires contraction of the entire locus by looping. In precursor cells, the gene loci are localized at the periphery of the nucleus where gene transcription is less active. However the proximity allows for D-J recombination at this stage. As differentiation progresses the gene locus moves to a more central nuclear position which likely promotes chromatin opening. As the cells commit to a particular lineage, the variable (V) gene loci undergo a contraction that places usually distant V genes next to the already arranged D-J segments. The contraction produces a looping that allows the different V genes access to the already combined DJ segment with similar frequency.

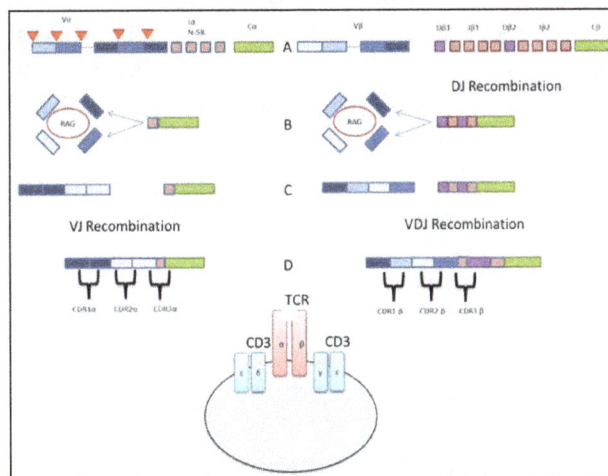

Simplified overview of VJ & V(D)J recombination of alpha and beta chains of TCRs:

- A: TCR gene locus showing the (V) variable, (J) joining and (C) constant regions. Red triangles denote the RSS at the edge of each gene segment. DJ recombination of the beta chain occurs.

- B: Following DJ recombination in the precursor cells. The locus has moved to a more central location. The V gene segments undergo the looping allowing each at chance at combination with the DJ segments.

- C: Combination of the selected V regions with DJ segment.

- D: Mature TCR transcripts showing the approximate location of complementary determining regions (CDRs).

The ultimate goal of the recombination process is diversity among the CDRs. CDRs are the antigen binding sections of TCRs and a diverse recognition capability leads to efficient protection against pathogens and the generation of optimal immune responses. VDJ recombination, along with the addition or deletion of nucleotides at the junctions between gene segments helps to generate an astounding amount of TCR diversity. The diversity generated by VDJ recombination is estimated to exceed 10^{15} TCRs. CDRs can be re-edited in the periphery, in a process called TCR revision. This results in a change in the antigen specificity of the TCR, and is initiated by reactivation of recombinases that initiate gene recombination. TCR revision is a carefully regulated process that induces tolerance to self-antigens, while still inducing protection against invading pathogens.

In addition to the diversity of TCRs, their cross-reactivity also contributes to host defense. Cross-reactivity of TCRs means giving a single T cell host the ability to react to multiple peptide ligands. This is achieved by a degree of flexibility in TCR-MHC/peptide binding. This means fewer T cells are required to detect foreign material. Additionally antigen may be detected by several T cells leading to a polyclonal response, which will make pathogen escape more difficult. This wide ranging cross-reactivity is not without its problems as the concept of T cells being activated by antigen and then cross-reacting to self-ligands is possible. This is known as molecular mimicry and it represents one theory of the root cause of auto-immunity.

TCR Activation and Signaling

The function of T cells is controlled by TCR activation and signaling. Stimulation of T cell function is initiated upon interaction of the TCR with short peptides presented by MHC class I or II molecules (MHC 1 for CD8 T cells and MHC II for CD4 T cells). However, the TCR heterodimer by itself is incapable of activating downstream pathways to initiate T cell activation. Initiation of TCR signaling requires co-receptors such as CD4 for helper T cells and CD8 for cytotoxic T cells. These co-receptors act as cellular adhesion molecules that bind their respective MHC molecules and stabilize the interaction of T cells and antigen presenting cells.

The TCR is also located in close proximity to a complex of signaling molecules, which help to mediate T cell activation. These include the CD3 family of proteins (CD3δ, CD3ε, and CD3γ) as well as a TCR zeta (ζ) chain. Once the TCR is properly engaged with the peptide-MHC complex, conformational changes in the associated CD3 chains are induced, which leads to their phosphorylation and association with downstream proteins. The TCR ζ chain is also phosphorylated upon TCR engagement. These molecules are phosphorylated via their c-terminal immunoreceptor tyrosine-based activation motifs (ITAMs) by the Src kinases leukocyte-specific tyrosine kinase (LCK) and Fyn.

Phosphorylated CD3 ITAMs then recruit and activate the Syk family kinase zeta-activated protein 70 kDa (ZAP70) via Src-homology-2 (SH2)-domain interactions. ZAP70 then phosphorylates a membrane associated scaffolding protein called linker for activation of T cells (LAT). LAT in turn recruits a second molecular scaffold, SH2-domain containing leukocyte protein of 76 kDa (Slp-76). Slp-76 is then phosphorylated by ZAP70 and the resulting LAT-Slp-76 complex acts as a scaffold for the recruitment of signaling effector molecules (Koretzky et al. 2006). Interleukin-2 inducible tyrosine kinase (ITK) then interacts with the LAT-Slp-76 complex and becomes activated by autophosphorylation. This promotes phosphorylation of the effector molecule phospholipase C gamma 1 (PLC-γ1). PLC-γ1 transduces TCR signals by cleaving phosphatidylinositol triphosphate (PIP2) in the plasma membrane to generate the second messengers' diacylglycerol (DAG) and inositol trisphosphate (IP3).

DAG, a membrane associated lipid, activates a number of downstream proteins, including various isoforms of protein kinase C (PKC) and RAS guanyl nucleotide-releasing protein (RasGRP). Upon activation by DAG, PKC-theta participates in activating the NF-κB pathway, whereas RasGRP is a crucial activator of MAPK signaling pathways. IP3, on the other hand, stimulates the efflux of Ca^{2+} from the endoplasmic reticulum to the cytoplasm. Elevated Ca^{2+} levels induce activation of the protein phosphatase, calcineurin, which then dephosphorylates the T cell transcription factor nuclear factors of activated T cells (NFAT). Dephosphorylated NFAT then migrates to the nucleus to join other transcription factors in inducing the transcription of specific genes.

In general, the signaling events described ultimately lead to cytoskeletal changes and transcription of relevant T cell genes. However, signaling solely through the TCR is not sufficient for T cell activation, and can result in induction of an anergic state in which T cells fail to respond to antigen stimulation and cannot be restimulated. Therefore, a central tenet of T cell activation is the requirement of co-stimulation through ligation of the TCR with other cell surface receptors which provide additional signals to promote productive T cell activation. Several co-stimulatory molecules have been identified, including CD28, CD2, CD5, CD30, 4-1BB, OX40, LFA-1 and inducible costimulatory (ICOS). CD28-deficient mice demonstrate dampened immune responses to a number of infectious agents. However, not all immune responses are severely impacted by loss of CD28, indicating the dual role of other co-stimulatory molecules in T cell activation.

TCR signaling is still an active area of research and future studies will undoubtedly reveal new interactions between current proteins involved in TCR signaling as well as identify new proteins and interactions.

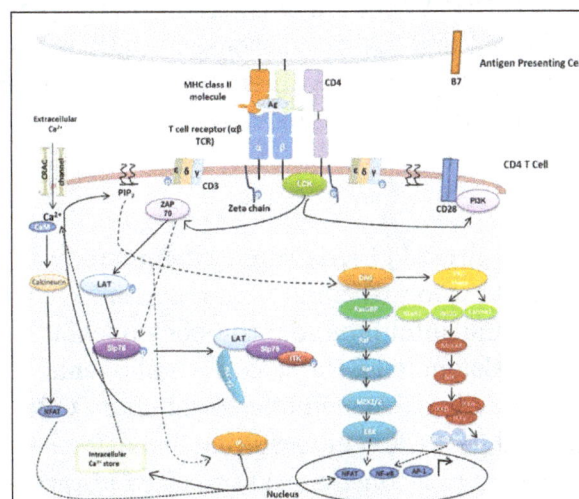

Overview of TCR signaling.

In figure, TCR signaling is activated upon interaction of the TCR with cognate peptide antigen bound to a major histocompatibility complex (MHC) molecule, and co-stimulation by co-receptor molecules such as CD28. AP-1, activator protein 1; Bcl10, B cell lymphoma 10; Ca^{2+}, calcium; CaM, calmodulin; Carma1, caspase recruitment domain membrane-associated guanylate kinase protein 1; CRAC, calcium release-activated Ca^{2+}; DAG, diacylglycerol; IP3, inositol trisphosphate; IKK, I kappa B kinase; ITK, interleukin-2 inducible tyrosine kinase; LAT, linker activation of T cells; LCK, leukocyte-specific tyrosine kinase; Malt 1, mucosa-associated lymphoid tissue protein 1; NFAT, nuclear factors of activated T cells; NF-κB, nuclear factor kappa B; NIK, NF-kappa-B-inducing kinase, PI3K, phosphatidylinositol-3 kinase; PIP2, phosphatidylinositol bisphosphate; PKC-theta, protein kinase C-theta; PLC-γ1, phospholipase C gamma 1; RasGRP, RAS guanyl nucleotide releasing protein; Slp76, SH2-domain containing leukocyte protein of 76 kDa; ZAP70, zeta-activated protein 70 kDa.

Clinical Manifestations of Aberrant TCR Signaling

Genetic defects in critical TCR signaling proteins have been shown to result in distinct clinical and immunological phenotypes. Mutations in ZAP70, LCK and ITK genes have been identified in patients demonstrating various immune pathologies. Below we describe the reported studies of the clinical manifestations of these defects in humans.

Effect of Defects in ZAP70 Function

It was in the early 1990s that scientists first discovered that mutations in the ZAP70 gene were directly associated with a rare primary immunodeficiency called CD8. CD8 deficiency was first characterized as a lack of circulating CD8+ T cells, with the presence of non-functional CD4+ T cells. Studies investigating the mechanism of immune dysregulation associated with ZAP70 defects in humans have shown that CD4+ cells from ZAP-70 deficient patients have an altered T cell repertoire. These cells express a phenotype consistent with autoimmunity, which includes reduced levels of CTLA4, IL-10 and TGFβ gene transcripts and decreased sensitivity to FAS-mediated apoptosis

A study by Katamura et al. described a patient with CD8 deficiency, with a unique subset of CD4 T cells. The patient presented with infiltrative cutaneous erythematous lesions and accumulation of activated CD4+ CD25+ CD45RO+ DR+ T cells and eosinophils in the perivascular area of the skin. Another more recent study showed that ZAP70 missense mutations resulted in a clinical phenotype characterized by immune dysregulation, with wheezing, generalized erythroderma, lymphadenopathy, eosinophilia and elevated serum IgE levels.

Effects of LCK Deficiency

The first report of molecularly-confirmed LCK deficiency in humans was published in 2012. Hauck et al. described the case of a child who presented with recurrent respiratory infections, nodular skin lesions, arthritis, vasculitis and autoimmune thrombocytopenia. In addition to these clinical manifestations, the researchers also noted CD4+ T cell lymphopenia, including reduced T-regulatory (Treg) cells, and an increase in exhausted effector memory CD8+ T cells. Genetic analyses identified a missense mutation in the LCK gene, resulting in a defective protein lacking kinase activity. Associated with this defect in LCK function was impaired intracellular signaling in response to TCR/CD3 stimulation. It is likely that the abnormal TCR signaling as well as the low number of

Treg cells may have contributed to the induction and perpetuation of the clinical manifestations of immune dysregulation observed.

Effects of ITK Deficiency

ITK is critical to TCR signaling and subsequently T cell activation as it promotes PLC-γ1 activation and Ca²⁺ influx in response to TCR stimulation. ITK is also necessary for maintaining peripheral immune homeostasis. Accordingly, ITK deficiency or impaired function results in severe immune pathology in humans. In recent years, several patients with autosomal recessive ITK deficiency have been reported. Their clinical phenotype includes infections, primarily due to herpesviruses, autoimmune cytopenias, lymphadenopathy, hepatosplenomegaly and lymphoproliferative disease, particularly of the lungs. Molecular studies have also demonstrated naïve CD4⁺ T cell lymphopenia, increased proportion of activated T cells, defective proliferation to CD3 stimulation, deficiency of NKT cells and progressive hypogammaglobulinemia in patients with ITK deficiency.

In addition to the described consequences of mutated or non-functional ZAP70, LCK and ITK, other examples of altered T cell signaling associated with defects in critical proteins have been described in mice. Identification of these conditions could lead to the development of novel therapeutics to treat autoimmune diseases.

T Cell Mediated Therapies

T cell immunotherapies are beginning to emerge as potential breakthrough in cancer therapeutics with initial clinical trials reporting high levels of remission. There are several types of existing T cell based immunotherapies.

Adoptive cell therapy (ACT), a technique pioneered by Philip Greenberg, MD, and a team at the Hutchinson Center in the early 1990s is perhaps the most basic and the foundation of other techniques. In this treatment, a patient's white blood cells are collected in a process called leukapheresis. Isolation of the specific T cells with the most cancer-fighting potency is followed by *in vitro* culture of the cells. This hugely expanded T cell population is then reinfused into the patient to work against the cancer.

A further twist on the adoptive cell therapy is the Chimeric Antigen Receptor (CARs) based therapy. CARs are engineered receptors, which graft an arbitrary specificity onto an immune effector cell. Typically, these receptors are used to graft the specificity of a monoclonal antibody onto a T cell, with transfer of their coding sequence facilitated by retroviral vectors. The receptors are called chimeric because they are composed of parts from different sources. First generation CARs typically had the intracellular domain from the CD3 ζ- chain, which is the primary transmitter of signals from endogenous TCRs. Second generation CARs add intracellular signaling domains from various costimulatory protein receptors (e.g., CD28, 41BB, ICOS) to the cytoplasmic tail of the CAR to provide additional signals to the T cell. Cell based therapies are not without challenges; particularly their ability to induce large scale damaging and non-specific immune responses.

Soluble T cell receptor therapy represents a potential alternative to cell based immunotherapies. Bispecific T cell engaging TCR can recognize tumor peptides on the cell surface. This engagement can be used to target therapeutics to this cell or engage further T cell responses.

T Cell Development

The thymus is the site of T cell development, providing a microenvironment that supports and guides the generation of a diverse T cell repertoire, which is self- restricted and self-tolerant. Thymic seeding progenitor cells (TSPs), or early thymic progenitor cells (ETPs), arrive from the adult bone marrow (BM), enter the thymus at the cortico medullary junction, and undergo T-lineage specification, followed by a series of well-characterized developmental check- points. These cells lack the expression of CD4 and CD8 and are termed double-negative (DN) cells [or triple negative if it is not already presumed that these cells are also CD3/TCR negative]. They are subdivided by the expression of the cell surface markers CD44 and CD25. DN1 cells (CD44$^+$CD25$^-$) are heterogeneous and have the potential to give rise to $\alpha\beta$ T cells, $\gamma\delta$ T cells, NK cells, dendritic cells, macrophages, and B cells. Further characterization of the DN1 subpopulation into five subsets based on CD117 and CD24 expression (DN1a–e) revealed that the DN1a and DN1b subsets, which express CD117, are the most potent at giving rise to T-lineage cells. Figure provides an overview of T cell development.

After specification to the T cell lineage, DN2 cells (CD44$^+$ CD25$^+$) migrate through the cortex and begin TCR-β, TCR-γ, and TCR-δ gene segment rearrangements, which are mediated by RAG1 and RAG2. Full commitment to the T cell lineage occurs following the transition from the DN2 to the DN3 stage of development. DN3 cells (CD44$^-$CD25$^+$) that have successfully rearranged their TCR b-chain associate with an invariant pre-TCR a-chain and CD3 signaling molecules to form the pre-TCR complex, which enforces b-selection, rescuing cells from apoptosis, mediating allelic exclusion at the TCR b-chain locus, and initiating cellular proliferation, permitting passage along the $\alpha\beta$ lineage. In the subcapsular region, b-selection also leads to CD25 downregulation, producing an apparent and transient DN4 population (CD44$^-$CD25$^-$) that upregulates expression of CD4 and CD8 to yield double-positive (DP) cells, which usually progress through an immature cycling CD8$^+$ intermediate SP pop- ulation , and initiates TCR-α gene rearrangements. DP cells that have successfully rearranged their TCR a-chain, to produce an $\alpha\beta$-TCR, undergo positive and negative selection in the cortex, as well as further negative selection in the medulla, and typically become MHC class I or MHC class II restricted. During positive selection, thymocytes bearing "useful" TCRs undergo differentiation to the CD4$^+$ helper or CD8$^+$ cytotoxic lineage, and mature CD4$^+$ or CD8$^+$ single- positive (SP) cells exit the thymus and circulate in the periphery. $\gamma\delta$ T cells do not undergo a selection checkpoint in the same manner as $\alpha\beta$ T cells, but they adopt this lineage from the strength of the $\gamma\delta$ TCR signal. Other nonclassical lineages that develop in the thymus include innate NKT cells and natural T regulatory cells.

The Notch-signaling Pathway

The Notch-signaling pathway is critical for the specification, commitment, and development of thymocytes . Notch is a heterodimeric receptor (in mammals Notch1–4) that binds to two families of Notch ligands: the Delta family (in mammals, Delta-like [Dll]–1, Dll3, and Dll4) and the Serrate family (in mammals, Jagged [Jag]-1 and Jag2). Upon ligand– receptor interactions, the Notch receptor undergoes two proteolytic cleavage events, the first mediated by ADAM metal- loproteases and the second mediated by g-secretase activity; this causes the release of the intracellular portion of Notch, which translocates into the nucleus and, in cooperation with coactivators, induces target gene transcription.

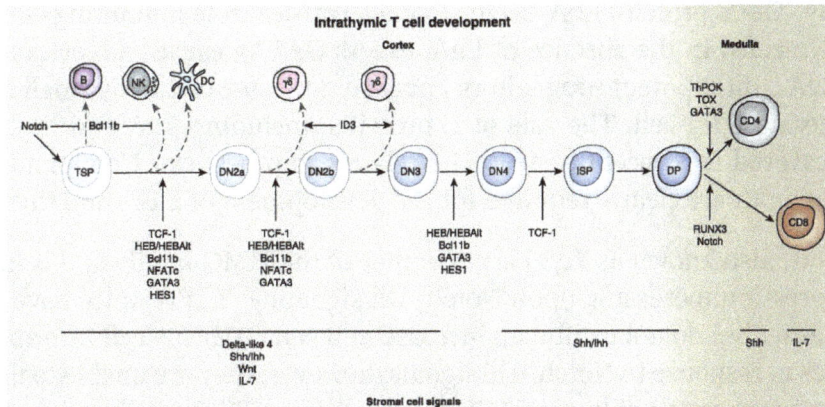

Overview of thymocyte development, highlighting role of key transcription factors and signaling molecules at specific developmental points.

In figure, the main stages of thymocyte development are depicted, with transcription factors marked with arrows and signals provided by thymic stromal cells, including receptor– ligand interactions, shown at the bottom. Notch–Dll4 signaling is required for specification of TSPs to the T cell lineage and for instructing transcription factors to adopt and commit to the T cell pathway at specific stages during differentiation. Thymic epithelial signals, such as those from the Hh- (Shh and Ihh), Wnt-, and IL-7–signaling pathways, aid in the commitment to the T cell lineage and continued proliferation and survival of developing thymocytes.

Unlike other hematopoietic lineages, there is no set master regulator that instructs cells to adopt the T cell lineage; rather, cells that enter the thymus lose the potential to give rise to other lineages and sequentially acquire the ability to choose their ultimate T cell fate through the expression of T-lineage genes (specification and commitment). Notch comes close to encompassing and enforcing all of these outcomes; however, other transcriptional regulators are required for Notch to instruct T-lineage adoption.

TSP to DN2 Stages

Several transcription factors have been identified recently as critical regulators of T cell specification, some of which are thought to act in concert with Notch signaling to promote T cell specification and limit other alternative fates. Notch signaling activates multiple transcription factors in thymocytes, including *Gata3*, *Tcf7*, and *Hes1*.

GATA3 is a zinc-finger transcription factor that has long been known to play a role at various stages of T cell development. GATA3 expression increases from the ETP to DN3 stages of T cell development. GATA3 hypomorphic mutant embryos, adoptive transfer of GATA3-null hematopoietic stem cells (HSC) and mice conditionally deleted for GATA3, conclusively showed that GATA3 is required for the development of functional ETPs. Recent work confirmed the requirement for GATA3 at the transition from DN1 to DN2 and its essential role in promoting a Notch-induced T cell program. *Gata3*−/− progenitors cultured on OP9-DL cells did not progress beyond the DN2 stage, although molecular analysis confirmed the T cell identity of these cells. There was also an increase in the production of CD19+ B cells, suggesting a role for GATA3 in inhibiting latent B cell potential. Beyond the specification stage, recent evidence showed that the positive and negative effects of GATA3 levels must be balanced at the DN2 stage to allow for further differentiation along the T cell pathway. The E protein, E2A, seems to play a critical role in limiting GATA3 expression specifically in DN2 cells. In the absence of E2A, excess GATA3 causes a block in T cell development, whereas E2A$^{-/-}$ multipotent progenitors knocked down for *Gata3* by small interfering RNA were able to generate DN3 cell. The role of E proteins, including E2A and E2-2, in thymocyte development is covered in a recent review. The relationship between Notch and Gata3 remains complex; however, both are clearly required for the development of ETPs and thymocytes.

TCF-1 (T cell factor, also known as *Tcf7*) is a member of the HMG family and is highly expressed in ETPs, with expression increasing upon Notch–Dll signaling. TCF1$^{-/-}$ mice have a severe reduction in the ETP subset but do not exhibit an increase in B cells. TCF-1$^{-/-}$ cells are able to upregulate Notch target genes in response to Notch–Dll signals; however, they are unable to upregulate T-lineage genes. Ectopic expression of human TCF-1 in progenitor TCF1$^{-/-}$ cells rescued T cell development, even in the absence of Notch–Dll signals, and it specifically upregulated T-lineage– specific genes (*Bcl11b* and *Gata3*), TCR genes, including *Tcf7* itself, as well as Notch1 target genes (*Deltex1* and *Ptcra*). Notch binds the *Tcf7* gene locus, and ectopic expression of Notch1 leads to transcriptional upregulation of *Tcf7*, indicating that Notch signaling is upstream of *Tcf7*.

HES1, a bHLH transcriptional repressor, is a major component of Notch1-induced signaling during T-lineage commitment and is important for constraining myeloid cell fate outcomes. ETPs and DN cells have high *Hes1* expression, whereas *Cebpa* is reduced in ETPs and absent from DN2 and DN3 cells. Ectopic expression of HES1 in BM Lin$^-$ Sca1$^+$ ckit$^+$ progenitors resulted in downregulation of *Cebpa*, and HES1 is suggested to directly regulate the *Cebpa* promoter, because it has several putative Hes1 binding sites. When cultured on OP9-DL4, *Hes1*$^{-/-}$ cells gave rise to myeloid cells, whereas *Hes1*$^{-/-}$ cells deleted for *Cebpa* re-stored T cell development, indicating an important role for HES1 in inhibiting *Cebpa* expression.

Cre-mediated deletion of *Hes1* in BM cells results in a reduction in the DN and DP cell compartments in competitive situations, and intrathymic transfer of these cells gave rise to T cells; however, there was an increase in the DN1 compartment, which was composed of immature B cells. The investigators hypothesized that this was a consequence of HSCs receiving weak Notch signals, because *Hes1*-deleted HSCs receiving suboptimal Notch signals were unable to adopt the T cell lineage, indicating that *Hes1* is essential to induce a Notch1-dependent genetic program for efficient T cell commitment.

NF-AT proteins are transcription factors that are activated by pre-TCR signaling. NF-ATc1 was recently shown to have an indispensible role during early thymocyte development, before *b* selection. NF-ATc1 activation increases as DN1 cells differentiate into DN3 thymocytes, and NF-ATc1 cooperates with STAT5 in response to IL-7 signals to contribute to the survival of early DN thymocytes. Conditional deletion of NF-ATc1 results in reduced cellularity; although these cells expressed key genes, such as *Notch1* and *Tcf7*, an arrest at the DN1 stage was observed.

DN2a/b to DN3 Stages

The DN2 population recently has been subdivided, based on the expression of CD117, into DN2a (CD44$^+$ CD25$^+$ CD117^{hi}) and DN2b (CD44$^-$ CD25$^+$ CD117^{lo}) subsets. Gene expression, cell-proliferation profiles, and dependency on Notch–Dll signals show that the DN2b population is more committed to the T cell lineage than is the preceding DN2a subset, but it is not as fully locked-in as

DN3 cells. High, continuous Notch signals are required to promote and support early thymocyte populations and inhibit NK cell development, whereas low Notch signals are sufficient to in- hibit the development of B cells.

Several articles recently highlighted the role of the tumor suppressor Bcl11b in the commitment of progenitors to the T cell lineage. Bcl11b is required to suppress the NK cell lineage, by repressing NK-promoting genes (*Id2* and *Il2rβ* [CD122]). Thymocytes conditionally deleted for Bcl11b and cocultured on OP9-DL1 cells give rise to Nkp46+ CD3- NK-lineage cells and exhibit decreased expression of T- lineage genes (*Notch1, Hes1, Gata3, Tcf7*) and increased levels of genes normally associated with NK cells (*Id2, Il2rb, Zfp105*). Bcl11b is also a downstream target of both TCF-1 and Notch signaling, where it is directly upregulated upon Notch– Dll interactions.

αβ and γδ Lineages

The γδ lineage is less sensitive to Notch signals, and Id3 has been suggested to play a role in commitment and differentiation to the γδ T cell lineage by integrating Notch and TCR signals. Strong TCR signals promote the γδ lineage, whereas weak pre-TCR signals, in collaboration with Notch, cause the repression of the E protein, E47, and promote the αβ lineage. Notch signaling is absolutely required at the *b*-selection checkpoint for its functional outcomes, including survival, proliferation, and differentiation, by regulating cellular metabolism, involving the PI3K/Akt pathway. Notch signals mediate these trophic effects through HES1, PTEN, and cMyc. Notch signaling withdrawal from Rag2-/- DN3 cells resulted in decreased *Hes1* transcription and an increase in *Pten* expression, whereas cells transduced with dominant-negative Hes1, or knockdown for Hes1, showed an in- crease in PTEN protein levels, indicating that HES1 represses PTEN. In the absence of Notch signals, Pten conditionally deleted DN3 cells are able to differentiate to the DP stage, but they fail to undergo proliferation unless they overexpress cMyc. Thus, HES1 and PTEN are responsible for supporting differentiation, survival, and metabolism of pre-T cells at the *b*-selection checkpoint by bridging Notch signals to the activation of the PI3K/Akt pathway through PTEN, whereas cMyc drives proliferation of *b*-selected cells that reach the DP stage. In support of its mitogenic role at this stage, a recent global transcriptome analysis of the entire αβ T cell pathway revealed that cMyc has a steady expression pattern in DN cells, which decreases abruptly in DP thymocytes. cMyc protein levels increased after *b* selection but were absent by the DP stage. Ectopic expression of cMyc in DP cells resulted in a decrease in small DP cell maturation, indicating that cMyc regulation may be a key molecular event that drives maturation to the small DP cell.

HEB proteins are bHLH family transcription factors implicated in several stages of thymocyte differentiation: β-selection, TCRβ and TCRα gene rearrangements, regulation of pre-TCRα, and CD4 expression. Separate transcriptional start sites in HEB give rise to canonical and shorter alternate (HEBAlt) forms. A developmental block in HEB-/- cells observed at the *b*-selection checkpoint can be partially restored with transgenic expression of HEBAlt, bypassing *b*-selection, to the DP stage, thus implicating HEBAlt as a critical regulator of early T-lineage genes. In addition, HEBAlt limits myeloid cell outcomes by collaborating with intracellular Notch. Furthermore, HEB-/- cells that have compromised Notch1 activity retain lineage plasticity, producing a DN1-like phenotype that could be induced to develop into NK cells and expresses *Gata3* and *Id2* but had lower levels of *Bcl11b*, a putative Notch target gene, suggesting that the canonical form of HEB is important for inhibiting NK cell fate.

RUNX1 is a transcription factor that is highly expressed at the DN stage and downregulated by the DP stage; however, until recently, the significance of this downregulation had not been resolved. Runx deficiency leads to severe defects in DN thymocyte differentiation; whereas overexpression of the distal isoform of RUNX1 has an inhibitory effect that results in a smaller thymus and a reduction in DP cells due to decreased proliferation of the DN4 population.

GATA3—important for the CD4 lineage choice, and RUNX3 is required for the development of the CD8 lineage. The role of Notch signaling in the CD4/CD8 lineage decision is controversial, with Cre-mediated deletion of Notch1 under the CD4 promoter not affecting CD4 or CD8 SP T cell development, in contrast to a previous report that suggested a role for Notch signaling. Recent data showed that the Notch pathway and TCR signaling may work together to influence positive selection and CD4/CD8 T cell development, as evidenced in mice conditionally deleted for Presenilin1/2 and within vitro–generated CD8 T cells. A decrease in CD8 SP cells developing from MHC class I–restricted TCR Tg$^+$ DP cells was observed when cocultured in the presence of the Notch-signaling inhibitor, indicating that Notch signaling is required for the positive se- lection of CD8 SP cells.

Thymic Microenvironment

Reciprocal interactions between thymocytes and thymic epithelial cells (TECs) are essential for the development of T cells and the maturation of the thymic epithelium itself. The thymus is organized into distinct cortical and medullary regions, and the development and differentiation of the TECs depend on the transcription factor FoxN1. Several chemokines, cytokines, and ligands are produced or expressed by the thymic epithelium, which interact with the developing progenitors. Below we describe some recent advances in this field and concentrate on Notch–Dll interactions.

Recruitment and homing of TSPs to the thymus involve adhesion molecules, such as P-selectin, which signals to PSGL1, and chemokines, such as CCL25 and CXCL12, and their receptors, CCR9 and CXCR4, respectively, which have been implicated in the migration of progenitors from the corticomedullary junction to the outer cortex . Mice deficient in CCL25 or CCR9, exhibit normal T cell development, whereas mice deficient in CXCR4 or CXCL12 have a reduced number of DP cells. CXCR4, along with the pre-TCR, functions to mediate survival and proliferation at the b-selection transition. Positive se- lection of DP cells mediates downregulation of CXCR4 and upregulation of CCR7, which is required for SP cell entry into the medulla.

Adult mice lacking both CCR7 and CCR9 have a largely normal thymus but exhibit a decrease in the proportion of ETPs, suggesting an additional role for CCR7 in settling of progenitors in the thymus. Thymocyte development is not completely abolished in CCR9$^{-/-}$ CXCR4$^{-/-}$ mice, but it is severely reduced in combination with CCR7 deficiency because of the lack of chemotactic effects regulating the distribution of progenitor cells in and around the thymic anlage. When CXCL12, CCL25, stem cell factor (cKit ligand), and Dll4 are reintroduced into FoxN1-deficient thymic epithelium, there is an accumulation of CD45$^+$ T-lineage cells in and around the thymic anlage. Surprisingly, only CXCL12 and Dll4 are required for the production of DP cell, in keeping with what was shown using simple in vitro systems; where CXCR4:CXCL12, together with Notch signals , were required for DN3 cells to transit through the b-selection checkpoint to the DP stage.

IL-7 is produced by TECs and is needed to promote proliferation, survival, and differentiation of DN thymocytes Cells are refractory to IL-7 signaling during the preselection DP stage and at the CD4 lineage–commitment stage; however, postselected DP cells restore cytokine responsiveness and induce upregulation of IL-7Ra and downregulation of SOCS1. IL-7 signaling is required to express the transcription factor RUNX3, for specifying the CD8 lineage choice, and, in combination with IL-15, for the development of CD8 cells. Mice conditionally deleted for IL-7Ra in preselected DP cells fail to induce a RUNX3- dependent cytotoxic lineage gene-expression profile. IL- 7Ra is also needed for the development and proliferation of Tregs, as well as for proliferation and maturation of innate NKT cells.

Hh-signaling Pathway

The role of Hh signaling during thymocyte development remains controversial. Data for the differentiation, proliferation, and survival of the earliest DN thymocyte subsets, the transition from DN to DP, as a negative regulator of pre- TCR–induced thymocyte expansion, the transition from DP to SP, for TCR repertoire selection, at the CD4/CD8 lineage decision, and negative selection all support a role for Hh signaling in T cell development. In contrast, other work showed that the Hh signal transducer Gli1 is not needed to mediate the effects of Hh signaling at early stages of thymocyte differentiation, and gain- and loss-of-function genetic models of Smoothened show that it is not required for adult BM HSC self-renewal or differentiation or for thymocyte development. Although previous results for Ptc deletion in hematopoietic cells suggested a role in T cell development, subsequent experiments showed that it is dispensable for T cell development; the previously observed developmental block, resulting in a reduced number of ETPs, could be due to a defect in thymic-homing progenitors.

Wnt-signaling Pathway

Like Hh, the role of Wnt signaling in thymocyte development is controversial. Wnt signaling is important for proliferation and survival. Pre-TCR signals are important in in- ducing b-catenin/ TCF activity for b-selection, and b-catenin can be induced in response to $\alpha\beta$-TCR signaling and can affect DP thymocyte selection and survival. Surprisingly, conditional deletion of b-catenin does not per- turb the hematopoietic compartment or reduces thymocyte development, and this was not due to redundancy with g-catenin. The effects observed in TCF1$^{-/-}$ mice point to it acting through a Wnt-independent pathway.

Notch and Notch Ligands in T Cell Development

Although developing thymocytes express Notch receptors, recent work found Notch3 to be dispensable for T cell development, indicating that Notch1 is the key player during T cell development.

In vivo, Dll1, Dll4, Jag1, and Jag2 are expressed in the embryonic and adult thymus. FoxN1 seems to regulate the expression of Dll1, Dll4, and Jag2 expression in TEC. Conditional deletion of Dll4 in TECs revealed that it is the relevant physiological ligand for T cell development, be- cause these mice were unable to support T cell development, in contrast with conditional deletion of Dll1, which did not Jag2, Dll1, and Dll4 in vitro, but Dll4 is uniquely better suited to support T cell development in vitro compared with Dll1 when ectopically expressed in OP9 cells at levels similar to those seen in TECs.

Notch Ligand Endocytosis

Endocytosis of the Notch ligands is thought to be important for initiating cleavage of the receptor to release the intracellular domain of Notch, which is necessary for the induction of target gene transcription and could explain some of the above differences. Two models have been proposed to explain the purpose of Notch ligand endocytosis. The Recycling Model suggests that Notch ligands, present in an "inactive" state on the signal-sending cell, undergo endocytosis and unknown posttranslational modifications to become "activated" and are recycled back to the cell surface and are better able to interact with Notch receptors. The Mechanotransduction Model proposes that, upon ligand–receptor interactions, the "pulling" force generated by endocytosis of the Notch ligand into the signal-sending cell exposes the ADAM cleavage site and allows for Notch receptor cleavage and activation in the signal- receiving cell. The extracellular portion of the Notch receptor is "transendocytosed" into the signal-sending cell.

Notch Ligand Endocytosis and T Cell Development

The intracellular domain (ICD) of the Notch ligands is the target for the E3 ubiquitin ligases Mindbomb (Mib) and Neuralized, which induce their endocytosis and subsequent activation of the Notch-signaling pathway. Through the generation of constructs that modified or deleted the ICD of Dll4 and Dll1, it was shown that this domain is necessary for efficient development of T cells in vitro and highlighted some unique features of Dll4 function. Absence of the ICD caused a reduction in T cell development and Notch target gene induction, presumably as a result of reduced binding of Notch1-Fc, and it decreased internalization/recycling of Dll4. Furthermore, when Dll1 is mutated at all of its po- tential lysine residues (Dll1K17) and overexpressed in OP9 cells, it is unable to support T cell development to the DP stage or *trans*endocytose the Notch extracellular domain, indicating that ubiquitination is a requirement for ligand endocytosis and Notch activation for progenitors to adopt the T cell lineage. We and other investigators showed that Dll1 and Dll4 have strong Mib1 inter- actions; although all E3 ubiquitin ligases (Mib1, Mib2, Neur1, and Neur2) are expressed in both the stromal and hematopoietic compartments, only Mib1 is necessary for T cell development and, therefore, is the relevant physiological E3 ubiquitin ligase in the thymus. Conditional deletion of Mib1 led to the abrogation of T cell development in these mice, and knockdown of Mib1 in OP9-DL1 cells caused a block in development at the DN1 stage, indicating that Mib1 can interact with Dll1. Because Dll4 is the physiological ligand, and Mib1 seems to be the functional E3 ubiquitin ligase in the thymus, it would be interesting to in-vestigate the role of Mib1 on Dll4; presumably, Mib1 interacts with and ubiquitinates Dll4 in vivo, but this remains to be in- vestigated.

In conclusion, a critical step in thymocyte development is specification and commitment to the T cell lineage. Recent advances in trying to identify a master regulator of thymocyte development revealed that no one factor is responsible; rather, it is their interplay and cooperative actions that specify the T cell fate, and proliferative and survival signals from other molecules, provided by the thymic epithelium or the developing thymocytes themselves, support and aid in their continued development. Notch Dll signaling remains critical in instructing cells to adopt the T cell lineage at the expense of other lineages and induces the expression of many key regulators of T cell develop-ment. In addition, recent evidence has shed some light on how activation of the Notch-signaling pathway via its ligands can also influence T cell development.

T Cell Activation

Costimulatory Proteins on Antigen-presenting Cells Help Activate T Cells

To activate a cytotoxic or helper T cell to proliferate and differentiate into an effector cell, an antigen-presenting cell provides two kinds of signals. Signal 1 is provided by a foreign peptide bound to an MHC protein on the surface of the presenting cell. This peptide-MHC complex signals through the T cell receptor and its associated proteins. Signal 2 is provided by costimulatory proteins, especially the B7 proteins (CD80 and CD86), which are recognized by the co-receptor protein CD28 on the surface of the T cell. The expression of B7 proteins on an antigen-presenting cell is induced by pathogens during the innate response to an infection. Effector T cells act back to promote the expression of B7 proteins on antigen-presenting cells, creating a positive feedback loop that amplifies the T cell response.

Signal 2 is thought to amplify the intracellular signaling process triggered by signal 1. If a T cell receives signal 1 without signal 2, it may undergo apoptosis or become altered so that it can no longer be activated, even if it later receives both signals. This is one mechanism by which a T cell can become tolerant to self-antigens.

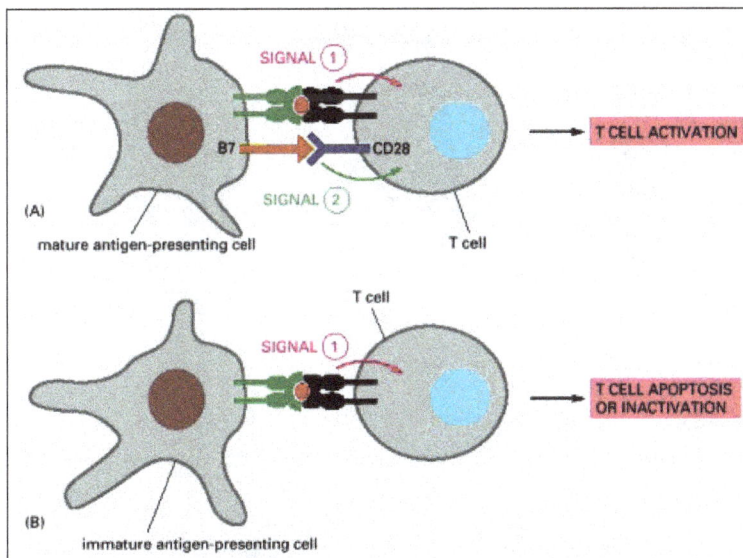

The two signals that activate a helper T cell.

In figure, (A) A mature antigen-presenting cell can deliver both signal 1 and 2 and thereby activate the T cell. (B) An immature antigen-presenting cell delivers signal 1 without signal 2, which can kill or inactivate the T cell; this is one mechanism for immunological tolerance to self-antigens. One model for the role of signal 2 is that it induces the active transport of signaling proteins in the T cell plasma membrane to the site of contact between the T cell and the antigen-presenting cell. The accumulation of signaling proteins around the T cell receptor is thought to greatly enhance the intensity and duration of the signaling process activated by signal 1. In this way, "immunological synapses" form in the contact zone, with the T cell receptors (and their associated proteins) and co-receptors in the center and cell-cell adhesion proteins forming a peripheral ring.

The T cell receptor does not act on its own to transmit signal 1 into the cell. It is associated with a complex of invariant transmembrane proteins called CD3, which transduces the binding of the peptide-MHC complex into intracellular signals. In addition, the CD4 and CD8 co-receptors play important parts in the signaling process, as illustrated in figure.

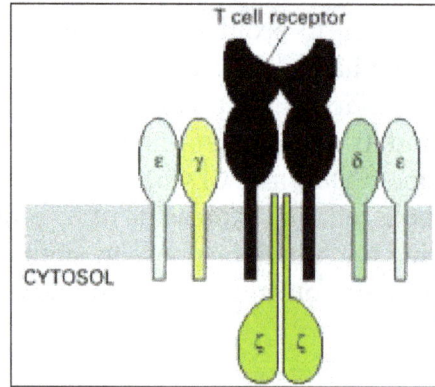

The T cell receptor and its associated CD3 complex. All of the CD3 polypeptide chains (shown in green), except for the ζ (zeta) chains, have extracellular Ig-like domains and are therefore members of the Ig superfamily.

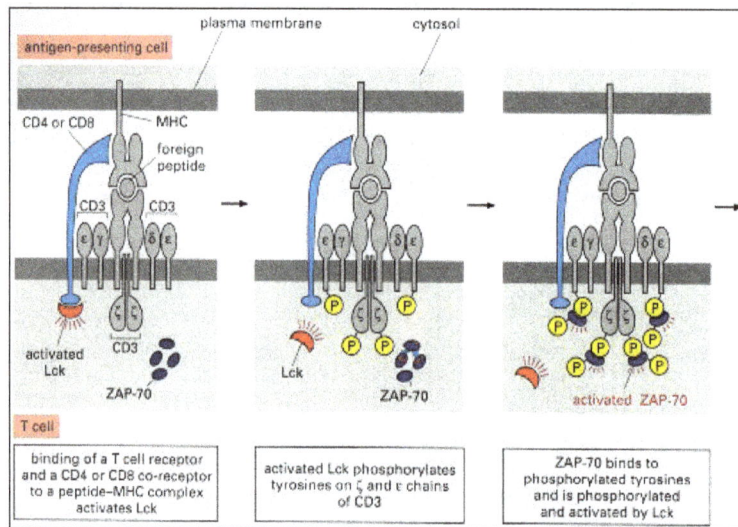

Figure shows the signaling events initiated by the binding of peptide-MHC complexes to T cell receptors (signal 1). When T cell receptors are clustered by binding to peptide-MHC complexes on an antigen-presenting cell, CD4 molecules on helper cells or CD8 molecules on cytotoxic T cells are clustered with them, binding to invariant parts of the same class II or class I MHC proteins, respectively, on the presenting cell. This brings the Src-like cytoplasmic tyrosine kinase Lck into the signaling complex and activates it. Once activated, Lck phosphorylates tyrosines on the ζ and ε chains of the CD3 complex, which now serve as docking sites for yet another cytoplasmic tyrosine kinase called ZAP-70. Lck phosphorylates, and thereby activates, ZAP-70. Although not shown, ZAP-70 then phosphorylates tyrosines on the tail of another transmembrane protein, which then serve as docking sites for a variety of adaptor proteins and enzymes. These proteins then help relay the signal to the nucleus and other parts of the cell by activating the inositol phospholipid and MAP kinase signaling pathways, as well as a Rho family GTPase that regulates the actin cytoskeleton.

The combined actions of signal 1 and signal 2 stimulate the T cell to proliferate and begin to differentiate into an effector cell by a curiously indirect mechanism. In culture, they cause the T cells to stimulate their own proliferation and differentiation by inducing the cells to secrete a cytokine called interleukin-2 (IL-2) and simultaneously to synthesize high affinity cell-surface receptors that bind it. The binding of IL-2 to the IL-2 receptors activates intracellular signaling pathways that turn on genes that help the T cells to proliferate and differentiate into effector cells; there are advantages to such an autocrine mechanism. It helps ensure that T cells differentiate into effector cells only when substantial numbers of them respond to antigen simultaneously in the same location, such as in a lymph node during an infection. Only then do IL-2 levels raise high enough to be effective.

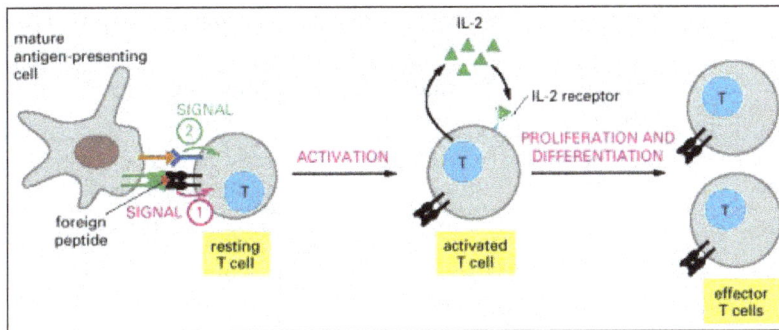

The stimulation of T cells by IL-2 in culture.

In figure, signals 1 and 2 activate T cells to make high affinity IL-2 receptors and to secrete IL-2. The binding of IL-2 to its receptors helps stimulate the cell to proliferate and differentiate into effector cells. Although some T cells do not make IL-2, as long as they have been activated by their antigen and therefore express IL-2 receptors, they can be helped to proliferate and differentiate by IL-2 made by neighboring T cells.

Once bound to the surface of an antigen-presenting cell, a T cell increases the strength of the binding by activating an integrin adhesion protein called lymphocyte-function-associated protein 1 (LFA-1). Activated LFA-1 now binds more strongly to its Ig-like ligand, intracellular adhesion molecule 1 (ICAM-1), on the surface of the presenting cell. This increased adhesion enables the T cell to remain bound to the antigen-presenting cell long enough for the T cell to become activated.

The activation of a T cell is controlled by negative feedback. During the activation process, the cell starts to express another cell-surface protein called CTLA-4, which acts to inhibit intracellular signaling. It resembles CD28, but it binds to B7 proteins on the surface of the antigen-presenting cell with much higher affinity than does CD28, and, when it does, it holds the activation process in check. Mice with a disrupted CTLA-4 gene die from a massive accumulation of activated T cells.

Most of the T (and B) effector cells produced during an immune response must be eliminated after they have done their job. As antigen levels fall and the response subsides, effector cells are deprived of the antigen and cytokine stimulation that they need to survive, and the majority die by apoptosis. Only memory cells and some long-lived effector cells survive.

Table summarizes some of the co-receptors and other accessory proteins found on the surface of T cells.

Table: Some Accessory Proteins on the Surface of T Cells.

Protein	Superfamily	Expressed on	Ligand on target cell	Functions
CD3 complex	Ig (except for ζ)	All T cells	—	Helps transduce signal when antigen-MHC complexes bind to T cell receptors; helps transport T cell receptors to cell surface
CD4	Ig	Helper T cells	Class II MHC	Promotes adhesion to antigen-presenting cells and to target cells; signals T cell
CD8	Ig	Cytotoxic T cells	Class I MHC	Promotes adhesion to antigen-presenting cells and infected target cells; signals T cell
CD28	Ig	Most T cells	B7 proteins (CD80 and CD86)	Provides signal 2 to some T cells
CTLA	Ig	Activated T cells	B7 proteins (CD80 and CD86)	Inhibits T cell activation
CD40 ligand	Fas ligand family	Effector helper T cells	CD40	Costimulatory protein that helps activate macrophages and B cells
LFA-1	Integrin	Most white blood cells, including all T cells	ICAM-1	Promotes cell-cell adhesion

CD stands for cluster of differentiation, as each of the CD proteins was originally defined as a blood cell "differentiation antigen" recognized by multiple monoclonal antibodies. Their identification depended on large-scale collaborative studies in which hundreds of such antibodies, generated in many laboratories, were compared and found to consist of relatively few groups (or "clusters"), each recognizing a single cell-surface protein. Since these initial studies, however, more than 150 CD proteins have been identified.

Before considering how effector helper T cells help activates macrophages and B cells, we need to discuss the two functionally distinct subclasses of effector helper T cells, T_H1 and T_H2 cells, and how they are generated.

Helper T Cell Determines Nature of Adaptive Immune

When a an antigen-presenting cell activates a naïve helper T cell in a peripheral lymphoid tissue, the T cell can differentiate into either a T_H1 or T_H2 effector helper cell. These two types of functionally distinct subclasses of effector helper T cells can be distinguished by the cytokines they secrete. If the cell differentiates into a T_H1 cell, it will secrete interferon-γ (IFN-γ) and tumor necrosis factor-α (TNF-α) and will activate macrophages to kill microbes located within the macrophages' phagosomes. It will also activate cytotoxic T cells to kill infected cells. Although, in these ways, T_H1 cells mainly defend an animal against intracellular pathogens, they may also stimulate B cells to secrete specific subclasses of IgG antibodies that can coat extracellular microbes and activate complement.

If the naïve T helper cell differentiates into a T_H2 cell, by contrast, it will secrete interleukins 4, 5, 10, and 13 (IL-4, IL-5, IL-10, and IL-13) and will mainly defend the animal against extracellular pathogens. A T_H2 cell can stimulate B cells to make most classes of antibodies, including IgE and some subclasses of IgG antibodies that bind to mast cells, basophils, and eosinophils. These cells release local mediators that cause sneezing, coughing, or diarrhea and help expel extracellular microbes and larger parasites from epithelial surfaces of the body.

Thus, the decision of naïve helper T cells to differentiate into T_H1 or T_H2 effector cells influences the type of adaptive immune response that will be mounted against the pathogen—whether it will be dominated by macrophage activation or by antibody production. The specific cytokines present during the process of helper T cell activation influence the type of effector cell produced. Microbes at a site of infection not only stimulate dendritic cells to make cell-surface B7 costimulatory proteins; they also stimulate them to produce cytokines. The dendritic cells then migrate to a peripheral lymphoid organ and activate naïve helper T cells to differentiate into either T_H1 or T_H2 effector cells, depending on the cytokines the dendritic cells produce. Some intracellular bacteria, for example, stimulate dendritic cells to produce IL-12, which encourages T_H1 development, and thereby macrophage activation. As expected, mice that are deficient in either IL-12 or its receptor are much more susceptible to these bacterial infections than are normal mice. Many parasitic protozoa and worms, by contrast, stimulate the production of cytokines that encourage T_H2 development, and thereby antibody production and eosinophil activation, leading to parasite expulsion.

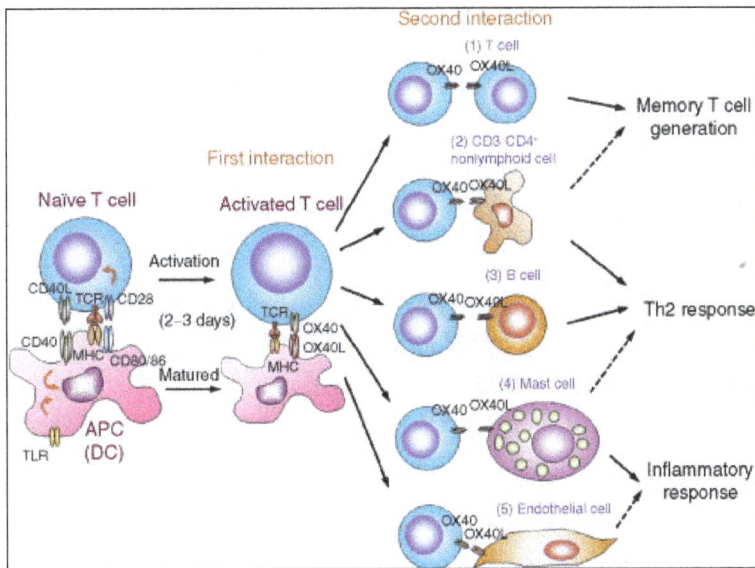

Figure shows the activation of T_H1 and T_H2 cells. The differentiation of helper T cells into either T_H1 or T_H2 effector cells determines the nature of the subsequent adaptive immune responses that the effector cells activate. Whether a naïve helper T cell becomes a T_H1 or T_H2 cell depends mainly on the cytokines present when the helper T cell is activated by a mature dendritic cell in a peripheral lymphoid organ. The types of cytokines produced depend on the local environment and the nature of the microbe or parasite that activated the immature dendritic cell at the site of infection. IL-12 produced by mature dendritic cells promotes T_H1 cell development. The cytokine(s) produced by dendritic cells that promotes T_H2 cell development (cytokine X) is not known, although IL-4 produced by T cells can serve this function. In this figure, the effector T_H1 cell produced in the peripheral lymphoid organ migrates to the site of infection and helps a macrophage kill the microbes it has phagocytosed. The effector T_H2 cell remains in the lymphoid organ and helps activate a B cell to produce antibodies against the parasite. The antibodies arm mast cells, basophils, and eosinophils, which then can help expel the parasite from the gut.

Once a T_H1 or T_H2 effector cell develops, it inhibits the differentiation of the other type of helper T cell. IFN-γ produced by T_H1 cells inhibits the development of T_H2 cells, while IL-4 and IL-10 produced by T_H2 cells inhibit the development of TH1 cells. Thus, the initial choice of response is reinforced as the response proceeds.

The importance of the T_H1/T_H2 decision is illustrated by individuals infected with Mycobacterium leprae, the bacterium that causes leprosy. The bacterium replicates mainly within macrophages and causes either of two forms of disease, depending mainly on the genetic make-up of the infected individual. In some patients, the tuberculoid form of the disease occurs. T_H1 cells develop and stimulate the infected macrophages to kill the bacteria. This produces a local inflammatory response, which damages skin and nerves. The result is a chronic disease that progresses slowly but does not kill the host. In other patients, by contrast, the lepromatous form of the disease occurs. T_H2 cells develop and stimulate the production of antibodies. As the antibodies cannot get through the plasma membrane to attack the intracellular bacteria, the bacteria proliferate unchecked and eventually kill the host.

T_H1 Cells Help Activate Macrophages at Sites of Infection

T_H1 cells are preferentially induced by antigen-presenting cells that harbor microbes in intracellular vesicles. The bacteria that cause tuberculosis for example, replicate mainly in phagosomes inside macrophages, where they are protected from antibodies. They are also not readily attacked by cytotoxic T cells, which mainly recognize foreign antigens that are produced in the cytosol . The bacteria can survive in phagosomes because they inhibit both the fusion of the phagosomes with lysosomes and the acidification of the phagosomes that is necessary to activate lysosomal hydrolases. Infected dendritic cells recruit helper T cells to assist in the killing of such microbes. The dendritic cells migrate to peripheral lymphoid organs, where they stimulate the production of T_H1 cells, which then migrate to sites of infection to help activate infected macrophages to kill the microbes harboring in their phagosomes.

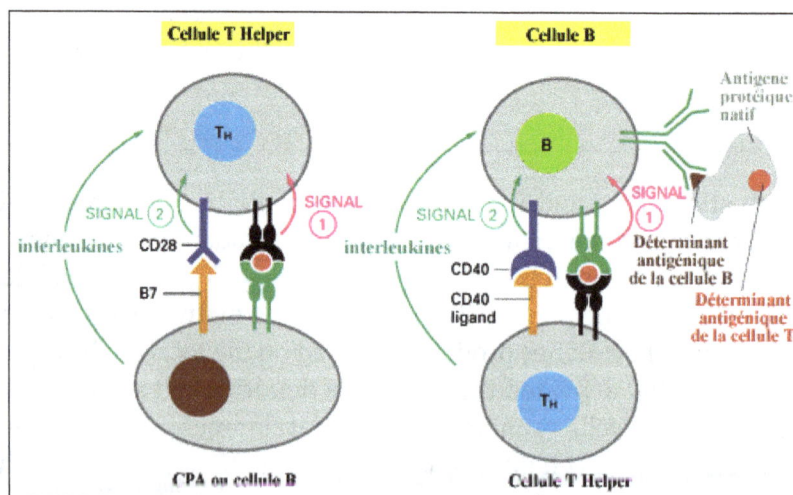

The differentiation of T_H1 cells and their activation of macrophages.

In figure, (A) An infected dendritic cell that has migrated from a site of infection to a peripheral lymphoid organ activates a naïve helper T cell to differentiate into a T_H1 effector cell, using both cell-surface B7 and secreted IL-12. (B) A T_H1 effector cell that has migrated from the peripheral lymphoid organ to an infected site helps activate macrophages to kill the bacteria harboring within the macrophages' phagosomes. The T cell activates the macrophage by means of CD40 ligand on its surface and secreted interferon-γ.

T_H1 effector cells use two signals to activate a macrophage. They secrete IFN-γ, which binds to IFN-γ receptors on the macrophage surface, and they display the costimulatory protein CD40 ligand, which binds to CD40 on the macrophage. (We see later that CD40 ligand is also used by helper T cells to activate B cells.) Once activated, the macrophage can kill the microbes it contains: lysosomes can now fuse more readily with the phagosomes, unleashing a hydrolytic attack, and the activated macrophage makes oxygen radicals and nitric oxide, both of which are highly toxic to the microbes. Because dendritic cells also express CD40, the T_H1 cells at sites of infection can also help activate them. As a result, the dendritic cells increase their production of class II MHC proteins, B7 costimulatory proteins, and various cytokines, especially IL-12. This makes them more effective at stimulating helper T cells to differentiate into T_H1 effector cells in peripheral lymphoid organs, providing a positive feedback loop that increases the production of T_H1 cells and, thereby, the activation of macrophages.

T_H1 effector cells stimulate an inflammatory response by recruiting more phagocytic cells into the infected site. They do so in three ways:

1. They secrete cytokines that act on the bone marrow to increase the production of monocytes (macrophage precursors that circulate in the blood) and neutrophils.

2. They secrete other cytokines that activate endothelial cells lining local blood vessels to express cell adhesion molecules that cause monocytes and neutrophils in the blood to adhere there.

3. They secrete chemokines that direct the migration of the adherent monocytes and neutrophils out of the bloodstream into the site of infection.

T_H1 cells can also help activate cytotoxic T cells in peripheral lymphoid organs by stimulating dendritic cells to produce more costimulatory proteins. In addition, they can help effector cytotoxic T cells kill virus-infected target cells, by secreting IFN-γ, which increases the efficiency with which target cells process viral antigens for presentation to cytotoxic T cells. An effector T_H1 cell can also directly kill some cells itself, including effector lymphocytes: by expressing Fas ligand on its surface, it can induce effector T or B cells that express cell-surface Fas to undergo apoptosis.

Both T_H1 and T_H2 cells can help stimulate B cells to proliferate and differentiate into either antibody-secreting effector cells or memory cells. They can also stimulate B cells to switch the class of antibody they make, from IgM (and IgD) to one of the secondary classes of antibody. Before considering how helper T cells do this, we need to discuss the role of the B cell antigen receptor in the activation of B cells.

Antigen Binding Provides Signal 1 to B Cells

Like T cells, B cells require two types of extracellular signals to become activated. Signal 1 is provided by antigen binding to the antigen receptor, which is a membrane-bound antibody molecule.

Signal 2 is usually provided by a helper T cell. Like a T cell, if a B cell receives the first signal only, it is usually eliminated or functionally inactivated, which is one way in which B cells become tolerant to self-antigens.

Signaling through the B cell antigen receptor works in much the same way as signaling through the T cell receptor. The receptor is associated with two invariant protein chains, Igα and Igβ, which help convert antigen binding to the receptor into intracellular signals. When antigen cross-links its receptors on the surface of a B cell, it causes the receptors and its associated invariant chains to cluster into small aggregates. This aggregation leads to the assembly of an intracellular signaling complex at the site of the clustered receptors and to the initiation of a phosphorylation cascade.

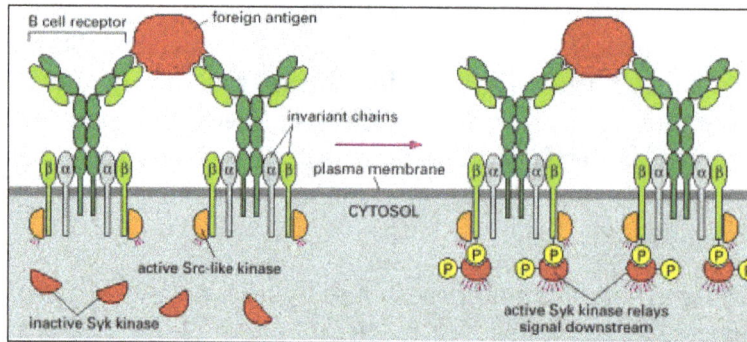

Figure shows signaling events activated by the binding of antigen to B cell receptors (signal I). The antigen cross-links adjacent receptor proteins, which are transmembrane antibody molecules, causing the receptors and their associated invariant chains (Igα and Igβ) to cluster. The Src-like tyrosine kinase associated with the cytosolic tail of Igβ joins the cluster and phosphorylates Igα and Igβ (for simplicity, only the phosphorylation on Igβ is shown). The resulting phosphotyrosines on Igα and Igβ serve as docking sites for another Src-like tyrosine kinase called Syk, which is homologous to ZAP-70 in T cells. Like ZAP-70, Syk becomes phosphorylated and relays the signal downstream.

Just as the CD4 and CD8 co-receptors on T cells enhance the efficiency of signaling through the T cell receptor, so a co-receptor complex that binds complement proteins greatly enhances the efficiency of signaling through the B cell antigen receptor and its associated invariant chains. If a microbe activates the complement system , complement proteins are often deposited on the microbe surface, greatly increasing the B cell response to the microbe. Now, when the microbe clusters antigen receptors on a B cell, the complement-binding co-receptor complexes are brought into the cluster, increasing the strength of signaling. As expected, antibody responses are greatly reduced in mice lacking either one of the required complement components or complement receptors on B cells.

Later in the immune response, by contrast, when IgG antibodies decorate the surface of the microbe, a different co-receptor comes into play to dampen down the B cell response. These are Fc receptors, which bind the tails of the IgG antibodies. They recruit phosphatase enzymes into the signaling complex that decrease the strength of signaling. In this way the Fc receptors on B cells act as inhibitory co-receptors, just as the CTLA-4 proteins do on T cells. Thus, the co-receptors on a T cell or B cell allow the cell to gain additional information about the antigen bound to its receptors and thereby make a more informed decision as to how to respond.

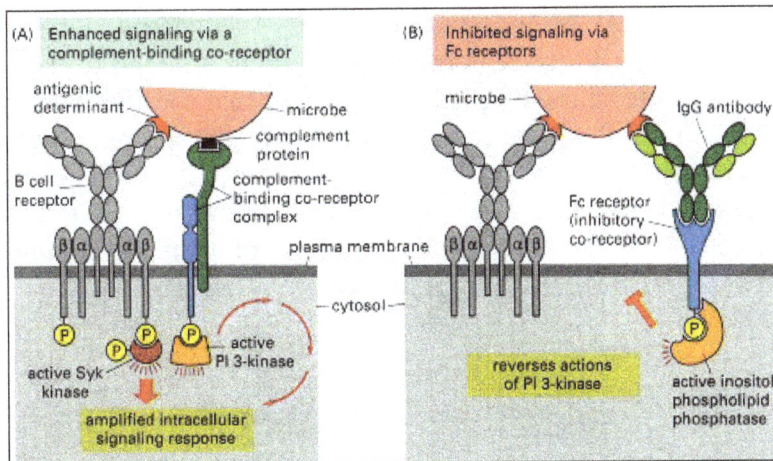

Figure shows the influence of B cell co-receptors on the effectiveness of signal I. (A) The binding of microbe-complement complexes to a B cell cross-links the antigen receptors to complement-binding, co-receptor complexes. The cytosolic tail of one component of the co-receptor complex becomes phosphorylated on tyrosines, which then serve as docking sites for PI 3-kinase. PI 3-kinase is activated to generate inositol phospholipid docking sites in the plasma membrane, which recruit intracellular signaling proteins (not shown). These signaling proteins act together with the signals generated by the Syk kinase to amplify the response. (B) When IgG antibodies become bound to foreign antigen, usually late in a response, the Fc regions of the antibodies bind to Fc receptors on the B cell surface and are thus recruited into the signaling complex. The Fc receptors become phosphorylated on tyrosines, which then serve as docking sites for an inositol phospholipid phosphatase. The phosphatase dephosphorylates the inositol phopholipid docking sites in the plamsa membrane generated by PI 3-kinase, thereby reversing the activating effects of PI 3-kinase. The Fc receptors also inhibit signaling by recruiting protein tyrosine phosphatases into the signaling complex.

Unlike T cell receptors, the antigen receptors on B cells do more than just bind antigen and transmit signal 1. They deliver the antigen to an endosomal compartment where the antigen is degraded to peptides, which are returned to the B cell surface bound to class II MHC proteins. The peptide-class-II-MHC complexes are then recognized by effector helper T cells, which can now deliver signal 2. Signal 1 prepares the B cell for its interaction with a helper T cell by increasing the expression of both class II MHC proteins and receptors for signal 2.

Helper T Cells Provide Signal 2 to B Cells

Where as antigen-presenting cells such as dendritic cells and macrophages are omnivorous and ingest and present antigens non-specifically, a B cell generally presents only an antigen that it specifically recognizes. In a primary antibody response, naïve helper T cells are activated in a peripheral lymphoid organ by binding to a foreign peptide bound to a class II MHC protein on the surface of a dendritic cell. Once activated, the effector helper T cell can then activate a B cell that specifically displays the same complex of foreign peptide and class II MHC protein on its surface.

The display of antigen on the B cell surface reflects the selectivity with which it takes up foreign proteins from the extracellular fluid. These foreign proteins are selected by the antigen receptors on the surface of the B cell and are ingested by receptor-mediated endocytosis. They are then degraded and recycled to the cell surface in the form of peptides bound to class II MHC proteins. Thus, the helper T cell activates those B cells with receptors that specifically recognize the antigen that initially activated the T cell, although the T and B cells usually recognize distinct antigenic determinants on the antigen. In secondary antibody responses, memory B cells themselves can act as antigen-presenting cells and activate helper T cells, as well as being the subsequent targets of the effector helper T cells. The mutually reinforcing actions of helper T cells and B cells lead to an immune response that is both intense and highly specific.

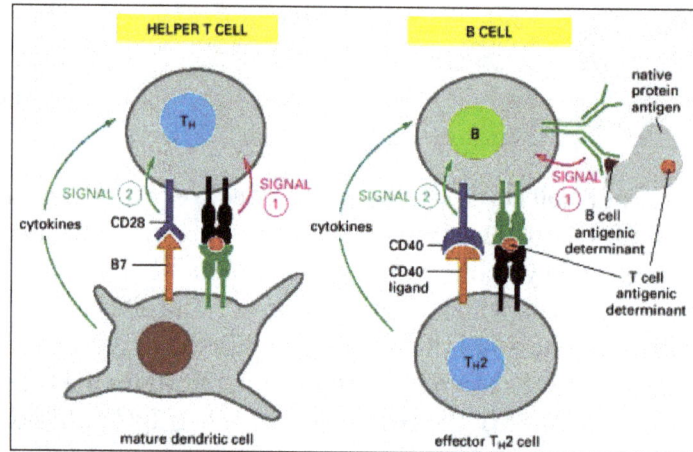

Comparison of the signals required to activate a helper T cell and a B cell.

In figure, note that in both cases secreted and membrane-bound molecules can cooperate to provide signal 2. Although not shown, CD40 is also expressed on the surface of mature dendritic cells and helps maintain helper T cells in an active state. The native protein antigen is endocytosed by both the dendritic cell and the B cell and is degraded in endosomes (not shown). The T cell antigenic determinant is presented on the surface of both the dendritic cell and the B cell as a peptide fragment bound to a class II MHC protein. By contrast, the B cell recognizes an antigenic determinant on the surface of the folded protein.

Once a helper T cell has been activated to become an effector cell and contacts a B cell, the contact initiates an internal rearrangement of the helper cell cytoplasm. The T cell orients its centrosome and Golgi apparatus toward the B cell, as described previously for an effector cytotoxic T cell contacting its target cell. In this case, however, the orientation is thought to enable the effector helper T cell to provide signal 2 by directing both membrane-bound and secreted signal molecules onto the B cell surface. The membrane-bound signal molecule is the transmembrane protein CD40 ligand, which we encountered earlier and is expressed on the surface of effector helper T cell, but not on nonactivated naïve or memory helper T cells. It is recognized by the CD40 protein on the B cell surface. The interaction between CD40 ligand and CD40 is required for helper T cells to activate B cells to proliferate and differentiate into memory or antibody-secreting effector cells. Individuals that lack CD40 ligand are severely immunodeficient. They are susceptible to the same infections that affect AIDS patients, whose helper T cells have been destroyed.

Secreted signals from helper T cells also help B cells to proliferate and differentiate and, in some cases, to switch the class of antibody they produce. Interleukin-4 (IL-4) is one such signal. Produced by T_H2 cells, it collaborates with CD40 ligand in stimulating B cell proliferation and differentiation, and it promotes switching to IgE antibody production. Mice deficient in IL-4 production are severely impaired in their ability to make IgE.

The signals required for T and B cell activation are compared in figure, and some of the cytokines discussed here are listed in table.

Table: Properties of Some Interleukins.

Cytokine	Some sources	Some targets	Some actions
IL-2	All helper T cells; some cytotoxic T cells; activated mast cells	All activated T cells and B cells	Stimulates proliferation and differentiation
IL-4	T_H2 cells and mast cells	B cells and T_H cells	Stimulates B cell proliferation, maturation, and class switching to ige and igg1; inhibits T_H1 cell development
IL-5	T_H2 cells and mast cells	B cells, eosinophils	Promotes proliferation and maturation
IL-10	T_H2 cells, macrophages, and dendritic cells	Macrophages and T_H1 cells	Inhibits macrophages and T_H1 cell development
IL-12	B cells, macrophages, and dendritic cells	naïve T cells	Induces T_H2 cell development and inhibits T_H1 cell development
IFN-γ	T_H1 cells	B cells, macrophages, endothelial cells	Activates various MHC genes and macrophages; increases MHC expression in many cell types
TNF-α	T_H1 cells and macrophages	Endothelial cells	Activates

Some antigens can stimulate B cells to proliferate and differentiate into antibody-secreting effector cells without help from T cells. Most of these T cell-independent antigens are microbial polysaccharides that do not activate helper T cells. Some activate B cells directly by providing both signal 1 and signal 2. Others are large polymers with repeating, identical antigenic determinants; their multipoint binding to B cell antigen receptors can generate a strong enough signal 1 to activate the B cell directly, without signal 2. Because T cell-independent antigens do not activate helper T cells, they fail to induce B cell memory, affinity maturation, or class switching, all of which require help from T cells. They therefore mainly stimulate the production of low-affinity (but high-avidity) IgM antibodies. Most B cells that make antibodies without T cell help belong to a distinct B cell lineage. They are called B1 cells to distinguish them from B2 cells, which require T cell help. B1 cells seem to be especially important in defense against intestinal pathogens.

Immune Recognition Molecules belong to an Ancient Superfamily

Most of the proteins that mediate cell-cell recognition or antigen recognition in the immune system contain Ig or Ig-like domains, suggesting that they have a common evolutionary history. Included in this Ig superfamily are antibodies, T cell receptors, MHC proteins, the CD4, CD8, and CD28 co-receptors, and most of the invariant polypeptide chains associated with B and T cell receptors, as well as the various Fc receptors on lymphocytes and other white blood cells. All of these proteins contain one or more Ig or Ig-like domains. In fact, about 40% of the 150 or so polypeptides that have been characterized on the surface of white blood cells belong to this superfamily. Many of these molecules are dimers or higher oligomers in which Ig or Ig-like domains of one chain interact with those in another.

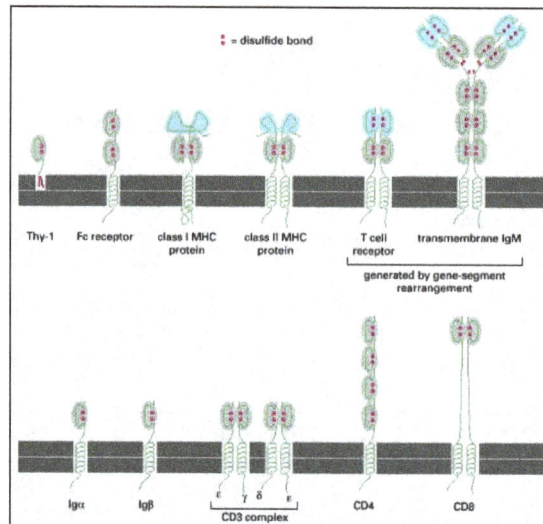

Figure shows some of the membrane proteins belonging to the Ig superfamily. The Ig and Ig-like domains are shaded in gray, except for the antigen-binding domains (not all of which are Ig domains), which are shaded in blue. The function of Thy-1 is unknown, but it is widely used to idenitfy T cells in mice. The Ig superfamily also includes many cell-surface proteins involved in cell-cell interactions outside the immune system, such as the neural cell-adhesion molecule (N-CAM). There are about 765 members of the Ig superfamily in humans.

The amino acids in each Ig-like domain are usually encoded by a separate exon. It seems likely that the entire gene superfamily evolved from a gene coding for a single Ig-like domain—similar to that encoding β_2-microglobulin or the Thy-1 protein—that may have mediated cell-cell interactions. There is evidence that such a primordial gene arose before vertebrates diverged from their invertebrate ancestors about 400 million years ago. New family members presumably arose by exon and gene duplications.

The multiple gene segments that encode antibodies and T cell receptors may have arisen when a transposable element, or transposon, inserted into an exon of a gene encoding an Ig family member in an ancestral lymphocyte-like cell. The transposon may have contained the ancestors of the rag genes, which, encode the proteins that initiate V(D)J joining; the finding that the RAG proteins can act as transposons in a test tube strongly supports this view. Once the transposon had inserted into the exon, the gene could be expressed only if the transposon was excised by the RAG proteins and the two ends of the exon were rejoined, much as occurs when the the V and J gene segments of an Ig light chain gene are assembled. A second insertion of the transposon into the same exon may then have divided the gene into three segments, equivalent to the present-day V, D, and J gene segments. Subsequent duplication of either the individual gene segments or the entire split gene may have generated the arrangements of gene segments that characterize the adaptive immune systems of present-day vertebrates.

Adaptive immune systems evolved to defend vertebrates against infection by pathogens. Pathogens, however, evolve more quickly, and they have acquired remarkably sophisticated strategies to counter these defenses.

In conclusion, naïve T cells require at least two signals for activation. Both are provided by an antigen-presenting cell, which is usually a dendritic cell: signal 1 is provided by MHC-peptide complexes binding to T cell receptors, while signal 2 is mainly provided by B7 costimulatory proteins binding to CD28 on the T cell surface. If the T cell receives only signal 1, it is usually deleted or inactivated. When helper T cells are initially activated on a dendritic cell, they can differentiate into either T_H1 or T_H2 effector cells, depending on the cytokines in their environment: T_H1 cells activate macrophages, cytotoxic T cells, and B cells, while T_H2 cells mainly activate B cells. In both cases, the effector helper T cells recognize the same complex of foreign peptide and class II MHC protein on the target cell surface as they initially recognized on the dendritic cell that activated them. They activate their target cells by a combination of membrane-bound and secreted signal proteins. The membrane-bound signal is CD40 ligand. Like T cells, B cells require two simultaneous signals for activation. Antigen binding to the B cell antigen receptors provides signal 1, while effector helper T cells provide signal 2 in the form of CD40 ligand and various cytokines.

Most of the proteins involved in cell-cell recognition and antigen recognition in the immune system, including antibodies, T cell receptors, and MHC proteins, as well as the various co-receptors discussed in this chapter, belong to the ancient Ig superfamily. This superfamily is thought to have evolved from a primordial gene encoding a single Ig-like domain.

B Cells

B cells are at the centre of the adaptive humoral immune system and are responsible for mediating the production of antigen-specific immunoglobulin (Ig) directed against invasive pathogens (typically known as antibodies). The function of B cells was discovered in the 1960s by Max Cooper who demonstrated that antibody production was completely abrogated in irradiated chickens after surgical removal of the Bursa of Fabricius (the primary site of B cell development in birds) from which the notation 'B' cell was derived. Several distinct B cell subsets have been defined that possess distinct functions in both adaptive and innate humoral immune responses.

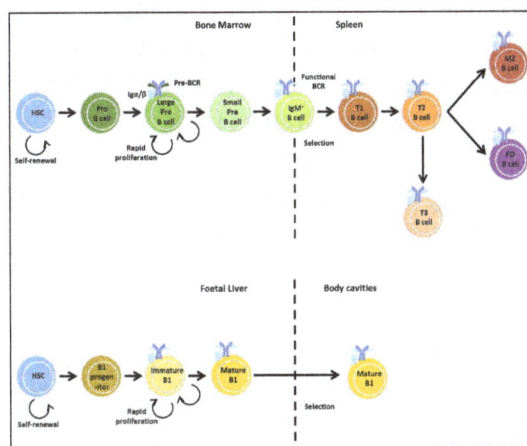

B cell development and B cell subsets.

B Cell Responses to Antigen

Mature FO B cells recirculate between secondary lymphoid organs in search of antigen. Following cognate Ag encounter, B cells receiving T cell help can enter a couple of different developmental possibilities. Firstly the cells can undergo plasmacytic differentiation, form extrafollicular plasmablasts and form IgM secreting plasma cells. These cells do not have somatically mutated Ig genes and are short lived, but provide a rapid initial response to antigen. The second developmental possibility is the establishment of a germinal centre, a specialised structure within which B cells undergo rounds of proliferation accompanied by affinity maturation: an iterative process of Ig gene mutation and selection resulting in a B cell pool which can bind to Ag with the highest affinity. The cells also undergo class switch recombination. Memory B cells and plasma cells expressing somatically mutated and generally high affinity BCRs of switched isotypes exit the GC.

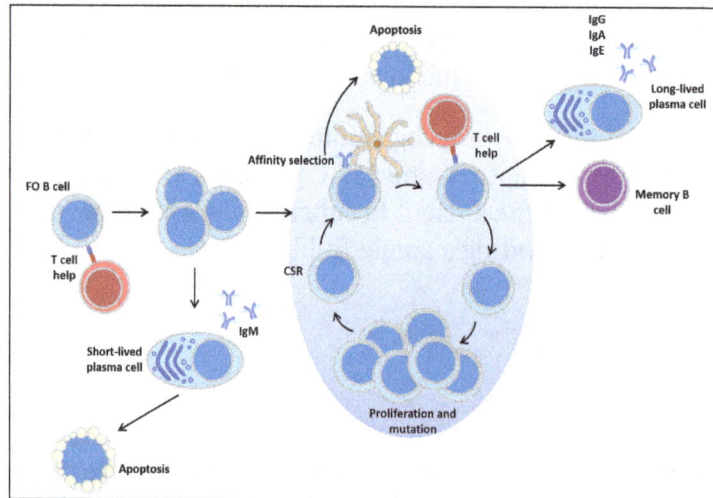

B cell responses to antigen.

Regulatory B Cells

B cells have a positive role in priming adaptive CD4+ T cells, but not CD8+ T cells. The magnitude of CD4+ T cell responses is reduced upon pathogen challenge in B cell deficient or -depleted mice. B cells are also able to dampen T cell driven immune responses, giving rise to the concept of regulatory B cells (Breg). Interleukin (IL-) 10-secreting B cells with suppressive functions are referred to as B10 Bregs. B10 Bregs reduce disease severity in animal models, e.g. during experimental autoimmune encephalomyelitis (EAE), the secretion of IL-10 in mice has the effect of countering this T cell-mediated autoimmune disease of the central nervous system. Bregs secreting IL10 or transforming growth factor β (TGFβ) have been identified in other animal models of auto-immunity, cancer and infection, supporting the concept that these cells have an important role in maintaining peripheral tolerance.

B Cell Development

B Cell Maturation and Subset Development

B cells outside the marrow are morphologically homogenous, but their cell surface phenotypes, anatomic localization, and functional properties reveal still-unfolding complexities. Immature B cells exiting the marrow acquire cell surface IgD as well as CD21 and CD22, with functionally important density changes in other receptors. Immature B cells are also referred to as "transitional" (T1 and T2) based on their phenotypes and ontogeny, and have been characterized primarily in the mouse. Immature B cells respond to T cell–independent type 1 antigen such as lipopolysaccharides, which elicit rapid antibody responses in the absence of MHC class II–restricted T cell help. The majority of mature B cells outside of the GALT reside within lymphoid follicles of the spleen and lymph nodes, where they encounter and respond to T cell–dependent foreign antigens bound to follicular dendritic cells (DCs), proliferate, and either differentiate into plasma cells or enter GC reactions.

GCs containing rapidly proliferating cells (ie, centroblasts) were first described in 1884, but were identified as the main site for high-affinity antibody-secreting plasma cell and memory B cell generation a century later. It is within GCs where SHM and purifying selection produce the higher affinity B cell clones that form the memory compartments of humoral immunity. Significantly, affinity maturation in GCs does not represent an intrinsic requirement for BCR signal strength but rather a local, Darwinian competition. The dynamics of lymphocyte entry into follicles and their selection for migration into and within GCs represents a complex ballet of molecular interactions orchestrated by chemotactic gradients and BCR engagement that is only now being elucidated.

B cell subsets with individualized functions such as B-1 and marginal zone (MZ) B cells have also been identified. First described in 1983 by Lee Herzenberg, murine B-1 cells are a unique CD5$^+$ B cell subpopulation (Hayakawa et al) distinguished from conventional B (B-2) cells by their phenotype, anatomic localization, self-renewing capacity, and production of natural antibodies. Peritoneal B-1 cells are further subdivided into the B-1a (CD5$^+$) and B-1b (CD5$^-$) subsets. Their origins, and whether they derive from the same or distinct progenitors compared with B-2 cells, have been controversial. However, a B-1 progenitor that appears distinct from a B-lineage progenitor that develops primarily into the B-2 population has been identified in murine fetal marrow, and to a lesser degree in adult marrow. B-1a cells and their natural antibody products provide innate protection against bacterial infections in naive hosts, while B-1b cells function independently as the primary source of long-term adaptive antibody responses to polysaccharides and other T cell–independent type 2 antigens during infection. The function and potential subpopulation status of human B-1 cells is less understood. MZ B cells are a unique population of murine splenic B cells with attributes of naive and memory B cells, and constitute a first line of defense against blood-borne encapsulated bacteria. Uncertainty regarding the identity of human MZ B cells partially reflects the fact that the microscopic anatomy of the human splenic MZ differs from rodents. Likewise, the microscopic anatomy of human follicular mantle zones is not recapitulated in mouse spleen and lymph nodes.

The B1, MZ, and GC B cell subsets all contribute to the circulating natural antibody pool, thymic-independent IgM antibody responses, and adaptive immunity by terminal differentiation into plasma cells, the effector cells of humoral immunity. Antigen activation of mature B cells leads initially to GC development, the transient generation of plasmablasts that secrete antibody while still dividing, and short-lived extrafollicular plasma cells that secrete antigen-specific germ line–encoded antibodies. GC-derived memory B cells generated during the second week of primary antibody responses express mutated BCRs with enhanced affinities, the product of SHM. Memory B cells persist after antigen challenge, rapidly expand during secondary responses, and can terminally differentiate into antibody-secreting plasma cells. In a manner similar to the early stages of B cell development in fetal liver and adult marrow, plasma cell development is tightly regulated by panoply of transcription factors, most notably Bcl-6 and BLIMP-1.

Persistent antigen-specific antibody titers derive primarily from long-lived plasma cells. Primary and secondary immune responses generate separate pools of long-lived plasma cells in the spleen, which migrate to the marrow where they occupy essential survival niches and can persist for the life of the animal without the need for self-replenishment or turnover. The marrow plasma cell pool does not require ongoing contributions from the memory B cell pool for its maintenance, but when depleted, plasma cells are replenished from the pool of memory B cells. Thereby, persisting antigen, cytokines, or Toll-like receptor signals may drive the memory B cell pool to chronically differentiate into long-lived plasma cells for long-lived antibody production.

B Cell Functions in addition to Antibody Production

In addition to their essential role in humoral immunity, B cells also mediate/regulate many other functions essential for immune homeostasis. Of major importance, B cells are required for the initiation of T cell immune responses, as first demonstrated in mice depleted of B cells at birth using anti-IgM antiserum. However, this has not been without controversy as an absence of B cells impairs CD4 T cell priming in some studies, but not others. Nonetheless, antigen-specific interactions between B and T cells may require the antigen to be first internalized by the BCR, processed, and then presented in an MHC-restricted manner to T cells. Recent studies depleting B cells from normal adult mice demonstrated that B cells are essential for optimal CD4 T cell activation during immune responses to low-dose foreign antigens and autoantigens, balancing this responsibility with DCs. The differential activation and expansion of CD4 T cells by B cells and/or DCs may impart characteristic features on immune responses, making this a critical area for future studies of host defense and autoimmunity.

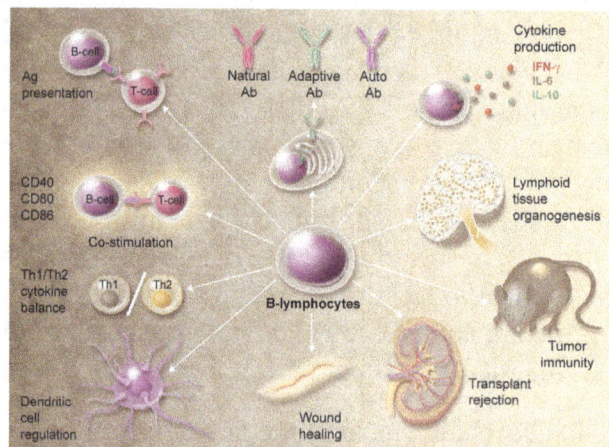

Multifunctional attributes of B cells. Selected examples of how B cells regulate immune homeostasis are shown; many of these functions are independent of Ig production.

The congenital absence of B cells during mouse development also leads to abnormalities within the immune system, including a profound decrease in thymocyte numbers and diversity, significant defects within spleen DC and T cell compartments, an absence of Peyer patch organogenesis and follicular DC networks, and an absence of MZ and metallophilic macrophages with decreased chemokine expression. While critical for normal immune system development, B cells are also important for its maintenance. For example, B cells can release immunomodulatory cytokines that can influence a variety of T cell, DC, and antigen-presenting cell functions, regulate lymphoid tissue organization and neogenesis, regulate wound healing and transplanted tissue rejection, and influence tumor development and tumor immunity. B cells can also function as polarized cytokine-producing effector cells that influence T cell differentiation. In addition, regulatory B cells have been described. One phenotypically distinct subset, designated B10 cells, has been shown to uniquely regulate T cell–mediated inflammatory responses through the production of IL-10. The further characterization of B cell subsets that carry out each of these functions and the molecular mediators for these diverse activities are exciting areas for future study.

Abnormalities in B Cell Development: Immunodeficiencies

The importance of genes encoding the pre-BCR and downstream signaling molecules has been demonstrated in gene-targeted mice and patients with primary immunodeficiencies. Perhaps the best studied is the Bruton tyrosine kinase *(BTK)* gene mutated in X-linked agammaglobulinemia (XLA). XLA was originally observed in a single male patient with recurrent bacterial sepsis and no detectable serum gammaglobulin. All XLA patients have a block at the pro-B to large pre-B cell transition in marrow, and a substantial reduction in the percentage of normal peripheral blood B cells. Btk plays a central role in signaling downstream of pre-BCR and BCR activation, primarily by promoting calcium flux. The BTKbase has cataloged more than 600 distinct mutations in 1100 patients, with many mutations leading to changes in Btk protein folding or stability. Although the perturbation in marrow B cell development is a universal characteristic of XLA patients, susceptibility to specific pathogens, age at diagnosis, number of circulating B cells, and level of serum Ig are more variable. Interestingly, the *Btk* mutations in the xid mouse and mice with a targeted disruption of Btk have a milder form of B cell immunodeficiency compared with most XLA patients. Future studies may reveal the contribution of individual genetic variation in either compensating for or exacerbating the phenotypic effect of a *BTK* mutation.

Two heterogeneous groups of immunodeficiencies impact primarily later stages of B cell development. Individuals with common variable immune deficiency (CVID) exhibit low serum Ig and an increased susceptibility to infection, accompanied by variable reductions in memory B cells, CSR, and B cell activation. Mutations in several genes have been identified in CVID patients, including the activated T cell stimulatory molecule ICOS, the B cell surface receptor CD19, and the TNF receptor superfamily member TACI. However, it is estimated that mutations in these 3 genes occur in only 10% to 15% of CVID patients. The age at diagnosis ranges from 3 to 78 years and is probably influenced by a host of genetic and environmental factors. A second group includes individuals with so-called hyper-IgM syndrome. These patients have recurrent infections, elevated serum IgM, a relative paucity of other serum Ig isotypes, and a general failure of B cells to undergo CSR and SHM. Mutations in several genes have been identified, the most common being a mutation in CD154 (CD40 ligand) expressed on activated T cells, which is inherited as an X-linked mutation. Rare patients with mutations in CD40, IKK-gamma/NEMO, and uracil-DNA glycosylase have also been reported. The critical function of AID in development of a functional Ig repertoire is underscored by the fact that patients with an autosomal recessive form of the hyper-IgM syndrome harbor a deficiency of this enzyme.

Abnormalities in B Cell Regulation: Autoimmunity

A series of checkpoints normally controls B cell selection, both centrally in the marrow and in the peripheral lymphoid tissues; in the latter a second screening process for reactivity with peripheral self-antigens results in apoptosis, receptor editing, or anergy. The outcome is the production of a diverse population of B cells capable of producing high-affinity effector antibodies that have been purged of pathological autoreactivity. However, disruption of the delicate balance between activating and inhibitory signals that regulate normal B cell activation and longevity can predispose to pathogenic autoantibody production and autoimmunity.

Autoantibodies represent important hallmarks for adaptive immune responses that are inappropriately directed against self-tissues. Autoantibody and rheumatoid factor identification during the 1950s to 1970s triggered a paradigm shift that some "connective tissue diseases" such as rheumatoid arthritis were actually autoimmune diseases. The identification of autoantibodies in glomerulonephritis patients in 1949 provided the first clinical and experimental evidence that disease is due to a continuous organ-specific antigen-antibody reaction. Equally remarkable is that rheumatoid factor was identified and biochemically characterized in 1957, prior to the identification of IgM and IgG. Although a close correlation between autoantibody production and systemic autoimmune disease is universally acknowledged, the precise contributions of autoantibodies and their autoantigen targets to disease pathogenesis remain to be elucidated in many human syndromes. Furthermore, B cells may contribute to autoimmune pathogenesis by presentation of autoantigen to T cells, or through production of proinflammatory cytokines.

A striking example of how dysregulated apoptotic regulatory genes can lead to autoimmunity is in *Bcl-2* transgenic mice. Enforced Bcl-2 expression allows the inappropriate survival of autoreactive B cell clones that normally are lost through negative selection and apoptosis. Bcl-2 transgenic mice develop antinuclear antibodies, immune complex deposition, and glomerulonephritis. MRL mice homozygous for mutations in *Fas* or *FasL* (frequently referred to as the *lpr* and *gld* phenotypes, respectively) spontaneously develop an autoimmune disease resembling human systemic lupus erythematosus (SLE). Subtle alterations in signaling pathways that influence BCR responses to autoantigen are also sufficient to predispose mice and possibly humans to autoantibody production and autoimmunity. For example, mice with lymphoproliferation phenotypes share similarities with Canale-Smith syndrome, a childhood disorder characterized by lymphadenopathy and autoimmunity due to novel *FAS* mutations. In most cases of human autoimmune disease, however, the combination of environmental factors and polygenic effects collectively dysregulate normal B cell function and thereby confer disease susceptibility.

As it has become more obvious that B cells contribute substantially to multiple human autoimmune diseases, highly targeted less toxic therapies focused on restoring normal B cell function and eliminating pathogenic autoantibodies are beginning to reduce the reliance on immunosuppressive drugs. Rituximab (CD20 mAb) effectively reduces B cell numbers without significant toxicity, and has become a standard therapy for rheumatoid arthritis and increasingly for other autoimmune diseases as well. Studies in the mouse have shown that rituximab leads to B cell elimination by monocyte-mediated Ab-dependent cellular cytotoxicity, but likely inhibits autoimmune disease initiation by regulating CD4$^+$ T cell expansion, thereby delaying the subsequent inflammatory phase of disease that leads to tissue pathology.

The BAFF/BlyS cytokine produced by DCs and monocyte/macrophages is particularly important in B cell survival and differentiation. BAFF binds 3 receptors—BCMA, TACI, and BAFF-R—and induces immature B cell survival and mature B cell proliferation within peripheral lymphoid tissues when coupled with BCR ligation. BAFF transgenic mice have SLE-like disease, and elevated BAFF levels are found in a significant number of SLE patients. Such findings suggest that antagonizing BAFF function may disrupt B cell survival. Disrupting CD22 ligand binding also disrupts B cell survival and may thereby provide an additional therapeutic strategy for patients with autoimmune disease.

B Cell Abnormalities: Leukemia and Lymphomas

Studies at the interface of hematology and immunology are exemplified by interchangeable lessons learned from parallel evaluation of B cell ontogeny and hematologic malignancies. Broadly speaking, the normal B cell developmental stages shown in figure have malignant counterparts that reflect the expansion of a dominant subclone leading to development of leukemia and lymphoma. Figures and show some specific subtypes of human leukemia/lymphoma and their approximate stage of B cell development, and selected morphologic images. The application of mAbs in multiparameter flow cytometry, detection of Ig gene rearrangements, detection of cytogenetic/molecular genetic abnormalities, and gene expression profiling have revealed an incredibly detailed portrait of gene expression and gene product function in normal and malignant B-lineage cells. For example, the marriage of Ig gene rearrangement detection and mAb phenotyping resulted in the so-called (at the time) "non-T, non-B" ALL being reclassified as a malignancy of B cell precursors. The antiapoptotic *Bcl-2* gene was discovered as the translocation partner with the IgH locus in the t(14;18)(q32;q21); frequently occurring in follicular lymphoma. Not only are the biologic and clinical consequences of Bcl-2 overexpression in follicular lymphoma profound, but the concept that increased expression of a single protein could promote cell survival has had an impact in areas of biology that go far beyond this lymphoma. The discovery that a substantial number of cases of diffuse large B cell lymphoma exhibit dysregulated expression of the transcriptional repressor Bcl-6 has led to new insight into the normal developmental program of antigen-activated B cells and the transformation events that underlie this lymphoma. The developmental origin of the Hodgkin/Reed-Sternberg cell in Hodgkin lymphoma, a controversy that was unsettled for many years, was resolved by single-cell analyses indicating a B-lymphocyte origin based on the demonstration of clonal Ig gene rearrangements.

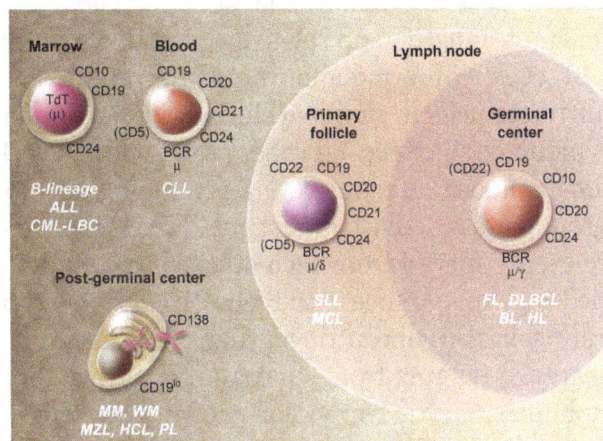

Human B cell malignancies.

In figure, selected cell surface, cytoplasmic, and nuclear markers expressed during normal B cell development that are generally expressed in malignancies. Molecules within parentheses are variable in their expression at the indicated stage of development. ALL indicates acute lymphoblastic leukemia; BL, Burkitt lymphoma; CLL, chronic lymphocytic leukemia; CML-LBC, chronic myelocytic leukemia–lymphoid blast crisis; DLBCL, diffuse large B cell lymphoma; FL, follicular lymphoma; HCL, hairy cell leukemia; HL, Hodgkin lymphoma; MCL, mantle cell lymphoma; MM, multiple myeloma; MZL, marginal zone lymphoma; PL, plasmablastic lymphoma; SLL, small lymphocytic lymphoma; and WM, Waldenström macroglobulinemia.

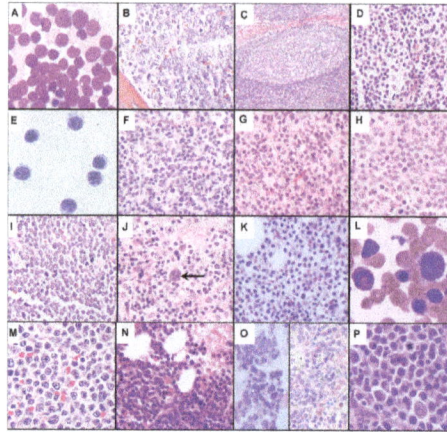

A histopathological montage of normal and malignant human B-lineage cells.

In figure, (A) Bone marrow aspirate of ALL cells exhibiting a high nuclear to cytoplasmic ratio, finely dispersed chromatin, indistinct nucleoli, and blue-gray cytoplasm. (B) Bone marrow biopsy showing effacement of the marrow architecture by a monotonous population of ALL lymphoblasts. (C) Representative normal lymph node follicle showing a reactive GC surrounded by mantle zone. (D) MCL cells display a heterogeneous morphology ranging from small round (true mantle zone/ CLL-like) cells to those showing irregular cleaved nuclei (FL-like). (E) A peripheral blood sample of CLL cells exhibiting closely condensed chromatin, indistinct nucleoli, and scant basophilic cytoplasm with a regular outline. (F) Normal GC centrocytes with vesicular chromatin and irregular nuclear outlines, along with larger round centroblasts showing a similar open chromatin. (G) FL with predominance of small cleaved centrocyte-like cells demonstrating significant nuclear irregularity. (H) DLBCL with classic post-GC immunoblastic morphology exhibiting a large nucleus, eosinophilic nucleoli, vesicular chromatin, and relatively abundant cytoplasm. (I) Biopsy from an abdominal mass showing BL cells with a monomorphic infiltrate of small to intermediate-sized cells with round nuclei, indistinct nucleoli, clumped chromatin, a basophilic cytoplasm, and a high apoptotic cell index. (J) A characteristic Reed-Sternberg cell (arrow) in HL. The cells are large and binucleated, with mirror image nuclei, demonstrating prominent eosinophilic nucleoli. Many of the other cells in the background are reactive lymphocytes. (K) Bone marrow biopsy showing hairy cell leukemia. The cells are evenly spaced from each other with round nuclei and clear abundant cytoplasm, imparting a "fried egg" appearance to the cells. (L) Peripheral blood smears of hairy cell leukemia (HCL) demonstrating classic concentric hairlike cytoplasmic projections. (M) MZL cells with a heterogeneous appearance ranging from small round cells to those manifesting a cleaved morphology. (N) WM/lymphoplasmacytic lymphoma showing considerable morphologic overlap with MZL. The cells demonstrate significant plasmacytoid features with pseudointranuclear inclusions (ie, Dutcher bodies). Many of the plasmacytoid cells contain globular collections of paraprotein in the cytoplasm, imparting a mulberry-like appearance to the cell. (O) Two cases of MM within the marrow. The cells show typical plasma cell features including the eccentrically disposed nucleus and abundant Ig-containing cytoplasm. (P) PL comprising enlarged plasmacytoid cells with enhanced atypia; mitoses are easily identifiable.

B Cell Activation

B cells are activated when their B cell receptor (BCR) binds to either soluble or membrane bound antigen. This activates the BCR to form microclusters and trigger downstream signalling cascades. The microcluster eventually undergoes a contraction phase and forms an immunological synapse; this allows for a stable interaction between B and T cells to provide bidirectional activation signals.

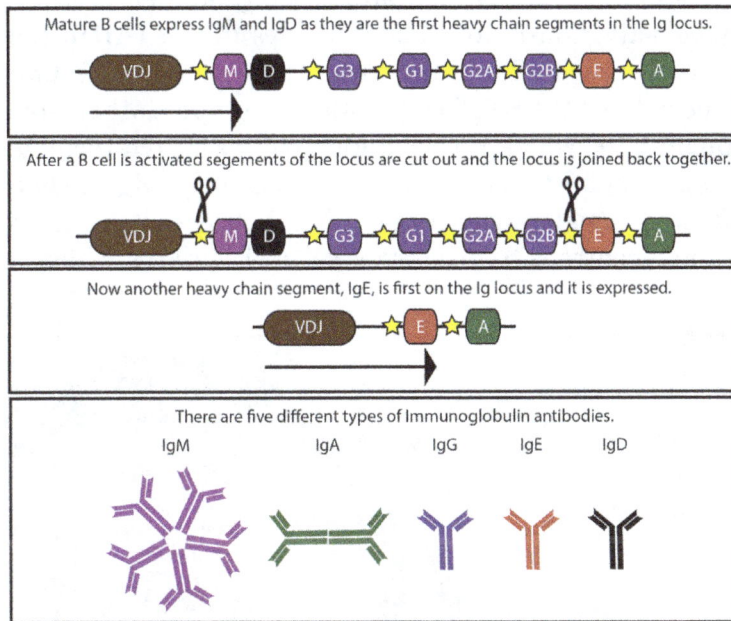

Class switch recombination.

Once activated B cells may undergo class switch recombination. In their inactivated state B cells express IgM/IgD but once activated they may express IgA, IgE, IgG or retain IgM expression. They do this by excision of the unwanted isotypes Cytokines produced by T cells and other cells are important in determining what isotype the B cells express.

In figure, after VDJ recombination class switch recombination may occur. In this process unwanted Immunoglobulin (Ig) genes are excised so that the desired gene can be expressed. In this depiction excision occurs and IgE is expressed. There are five isotypes which can be found in difference circumstances. For example, IgE is common in allergic responses such as asthma.

The Germinal Centre

B cells have two main types of immune responses. In a T-Independent immune response B cells can respond directly to the antigen. In a T-dependent immune response the B cells need assistance from T cells in order to respond.

In this situation activated B cells move to the border of the T cell zone to interact with T cells. CD40 ligand is found on these T helper cells and interacts with CD40 on the B cells to form a stable attraction. Cytokines secreted by T cells encourage proliferation and isotype switching and maintain germinal centre size and longevity. Without these signals the germinal centre response will quickly collapse.

B cells that have encountered antigen and begun proliferating may exit the follicle and differentiate into short-lived plasma cells called plasmablasts. They secrete antibody as an early attempt to neutralize the foreign antigen. They do not survive more than three days but the antibody produced can provide important assistance to stop fast-dividing pathogens such as viruses.

The germinal centre has a light zone and a dark zone. The germinal centre response begins in the dark zone where the B cells rapidly proliferate and undergo somatic hypermutation. During somatic hypermutation, random mutations are generated in the variable domains of the BCR by the enzyme activation-induced cytidine deaminase (AID). B cells then enter the light zone and compete with each other for antigen. If the mutation resulted in a BCR with an improved affinity to the antigen the B cell clone can out-compete other clones and survive. The light zone is also thought to be where B cells undergo class switch recombination, although a germinal centre is not crucial for this process. The B cells may migrate between both zones to undergo several rounds of somatic hypermutation and class switch recombination. The ultimate goal of the germinal centre is to produce B cells with a BCR which has high affinity for the initial antigen.

The migration of B cells in an immune response.

In figure, wWhen B cells (B) first encounter antigen (★) they migrate to the T-B border to receive survival signals from T cells (T). If they receive survival signals they will begin to proliferate and either become plasmablasts (Bl) or form a germinal centre (Blue). B cells can migrate between the light zone and dark zone of the germinal centre to undergo somatic hypermutation and class switch recombination. Eventually they may leave the GC as high-affinity memory cells (M) or plasma cells (P).

Plasma and Memory Cells

B cells leave the germinal centre response as high-affinity plasma cells and memory B cells. Plasma cells secrete antigen-binding antibodies for weeks after activation. They migrate to the bone marrow soon after formation where they can reside indefinitely, ready to encounter the antigen again and respond. Memory B cells circulate throughout the body on the lookout for antigen with a high-affinity for their BCR and then quickly respond to the antigen, stopping infection. This is how vaccination works. As your body has been previously exposed to the antigen the immune cells can quickly respond to remove the antigen if it is encountered again, stopping you getting sick.

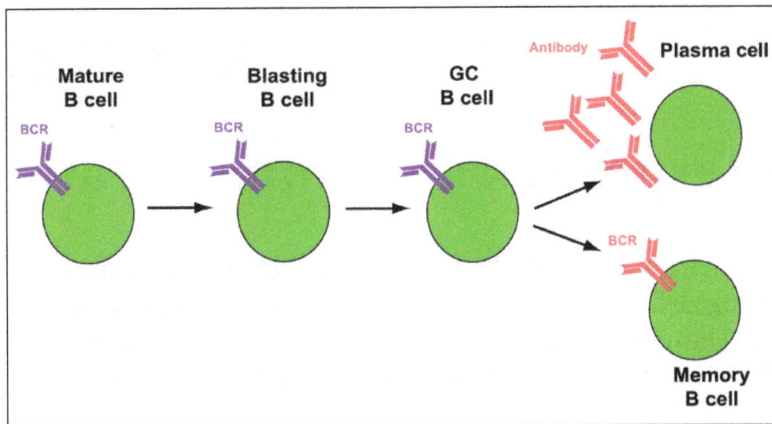

B cell differentiation after activation.

In figure, when a mature B cell encounters antigen that binds to its B cell receptor it becomes activated. It then proliferates and becomes a blasting B cell. These B cells form germinal centres. The germinal centre B cells undergo somatic hypermutation and class switch recombination. Plasma cells and memory B cells with a high-affinity for the original antigen stimuli are produced. These cells are long lived and plasma cells may secrete antibody for weeks after the initial infection.

References

- T-cells: leafscience.org, Retrieved 8 August, 2019

- T-cell-receptor: bio-rad-antibodies.com, Retrieved 17 March, 2019

- B-cells, cells: immunology.org, Retrieved 21 January, 2019

- B-cell-activation-and-the-germinal: immunology.org, Retrieved 18 July, 2019

Chapter 4

Immune Responses and Immunization

The body's response when antigens activate the immune system is known as the immune response. The process of fortifying an individual's immune system with respect to a particular agent is termed as the immunization. This chapter has been carefully written to provide an easy understanding of the varied facets of immune responses and immunization as well as the immunology of vaccination.

Immune Response to Infections

Immune response plays a vital role in protecting against infectious agents. It is the main impediment against the occurrence of disseminated infections that are usually associated with a high death rate. It is a well-known fact that for virtually all infectious diseases, the number of individuals exposed to infection is much higher than those actually presenting with a disease. This indicates that most persons are able to destroy these microorganisms and thus prevent the progression of an infection. By contrast immune deficiencies, whether of innate immunity (phagocytic cell dysfunction or complement deficiency) or adaptive immunity (antibody production deficiency or T-cell function deficiency), are strongly associated with increased susceptibility to infections.

Although immune response is fundamental for protecting against most infectious agents, evidence has been accumulating over the years as to how in many infectious diseases the main pathological aspects are not related to the direct action of an aggressor agent, but instead to abnormal immune response. In several such situations, there exists a hypersensitivity reaction with exaggerated and non-modulated immune response, the result of which is tissue damage. In other cases, infectious agents, whether by mimicking the antigens themselves, by inducing a proliferation of self-reactive cells or by increasing the expression of MHC and co-stimulatory molecules in infected cells can precipitate autoimmune diseases.

That different types of microbes are combated by different immune response components has been known since the beginning of the 1950s, when the importance of antibodies on the destruction of extracellular bacteria was first documented. Although antibodies on their own and in isolation are not able to destroy bacteria, they may neutralize microorganisms by preventing them from binding to the host tissue. Furthermore, in association with the complement, antibodies may lyse bacteria and function as opsonins, thereby facilitating phagocytosis. Neutrophils, eosinophils and macrophages exert their microbicid action most broadly against various types of agents and are extremely important cells for protecting the host. Documentation on how phagocytic cells express their receptor membranes like the toll-like receptor (TLR), which binds specifically with existing molecular patterns in various infectious agents, makes it inaccurate to name innate immune response non-specific. Neutrophils play a fundamental microbicid role against bacteria; macrophages are important cells for defending against intracellular agents (protozoan and intracellular bacteria). Eosinophils are essential not so much due to phagocytic activity as to cytotoxic activity against helminthes. T-cell mediated response is highly effective for the protection mechanism against intracellular agents, like viruses, protozoans, funguses and intracellular bacteria. T-cells may exercise their function through cytotoxicity mediated by CD8+ cells or through the secretion of cytokines, which activate macrophages to destroy intracellular agents. Other elements that may participate in the process of protecting against infectious agents included keratinocyte and Langerhans cell, since the skin is often invaded by various microorganisms. Keratinocytes are able to secrete innumerable cytokines, thereby activating and recruiting inflammatory cells and lymphocytes for the skin. The Langerhans cell in turn exercises a fundamental role of watching over the cutaneous territory, and phagocyting everything from particular inanimate proteins up to and including viruses, bacteria or other microorganism invaders. After phagocytosis the Langerhans cell migrates to the regional lymph node to carry out the antigenic presentation of the lymphocytes, which begins the development of specific protector immunity, tolerance or hypersensitivity.

The cells and mediators involved in protecting humans are well known. Yet the fact that TCD4+ (T helper) are heterogeneous and made up of two subpopulations, namely Th1 and Th2 cells, has only recently been documented. This observation has contributed a lot to understanding the immunopathogenesis of the most infectious diseases. Figure shows the dichotomy of the TCD4+ cells and mediators produced by them.

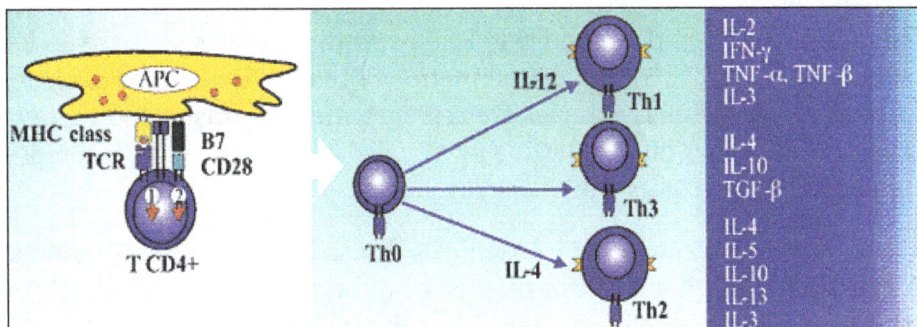

T CD4+ cell subpopulations and the main cytokines produced.

It is vital to understand that both Th1 and Th2 responses are important in the task of protecting the host against infection. Th1 response is related to protecting against protozoans, intracellular bacteria and viruses, while Th2 response is more effective against helminthes and extracellular bacteria. These responses are also antagonistic, insofar as the IFN-gamma negatively modulates Th2 response, and IL-4 and IL-10 negatively modulate Th1 response. This enables homeostasis in the immune system and a balanced immune response. In addition, the regulatory cells of immune response which express molecules CD4 and CD25 (Tr) and produce IL-10 and/or TGF-beta (Tr1 or Th3) are involved in modulating immune response. They prevent or reduce the consequences of hypersensitivity reactions and auto-immune diseases.

Immune Response against Bacteria

Bacteria are the microorganisms that most frequently cause infections in humans. The natural barriers against infection agents as well as innate and adaptive immunity participate in the protection mechanism against bacteria.

Intracellular Bacteria

The main characteristic is the ability to survive within the macrophages, for example *M. tuberculosis*, *M. leprae* and *L. monocitogenesis*. Penetration into the macrophage also constitutes the parasite's escape mechanism. Although paradoxical, the latter is benign for the host insofar as the lack of cellular penetration by the bacteria may induce a strong inflammatory response and excessive damage for the host. Within the macrophages these bacteria may stimulate either TCD4+ cells by an expression of the antigen associated to MHC class II or TCD8+ cells by an expression of the antigens associated with molecules of MHC class I. Activation of TCD4+ cells lead to the secretion of IFN-gamma, which activates the macrophages and leads to increased production of nitrous oxide (NO) and destruction of bacteria. TCD8+ cells participate in the protection mechanism through cytotoxicity, thereby destroying the infected macrophages. In the case of M. tuberculosis, despite having immune protection preventing its multiplication, there is no complete elimination of the bacillus. For this reason, individuals using corticosteroids and HIV-positive patients develop clinical signs of tuberculosis, despite having been infected much earlier and after remaining completely asymptomatic. The role of cellular immune response in controlling infections caused by mycobacteria is well demonstrated in how these infections have spread with the advent of AIDS.

Regarding infections caused by *M. leprae*, the clinical spectrum of the disease is intimately linked to immune response. In patients having a tuberculoid form, there is a strong response to Th1. Also, the disease is characterized by destruction of the nervous fibers in specific areas leading to the appearance of localized and well-delimited skin lesions, with a loss of sensitivity to heat and pain. When Th1 response is lacking, there is a dissemination of the bacillus, which leads to Virchowian Hanseniasis. In this event, the macrophages are replete with the parasite and there is a thickness of lymphocytes found on the lesion. Borderline forms, also known as dimorphic, represent a clinical and immunological pattern of intermediary response.

The importance of immune response in Hanseniasis disease is not limited to the determination of its clinical spectrum. With the onset of disease or often after treatment is started, some patients may show acute secondary clinical signs after the release of antigens and hypersensitivity reactions. These manifestations—also called reactions—are represented by erythema nodosum leprosum (ENL) and reverse reaction (RR). ENL is a systemic inflammatory response associated with high concentrations of tumor necrosis factor alpha (TNF-alpha) and the deposition of immunocomplexes with an infiltration of neutrophils and the activation of a complement, involving various organs. The immunopathogenesis of ENL is quite complex. High levels of circulating IL-1 and TNF-alpha, have been found in patients' feces, whereas a tissue increase in the expression of messenger RNA by IL-6, IL-8 and IL-10 indicates Th2 response. Moreover, the presence of the inductible nitrous oxide synthase enzyme (iNOS) has been documented as potentially being induced in the neutrophils and TNF-alpha and TGF-beta in the macrophages of the lesions. ENL may be accompanied by systemic toxicity, which is often treated with corticosteroids or TNF-alpha inhibitory drugs, like thalidomide. On the other hand, RR develops in the wake of the abrupt emergence of a delayed hypersensitivity mechanism against antigenic fractions of *M. leprae*, involving the active participation of T lymphocytes with tissue production of Th1 cytokines (IL-2, IFN-gamma) and inflammatory cytokines, like TNF-alpha. The lesions appear to be infiltrated by CD4+ lymphocytes, with increased expression of HLA-DR and of the receptor IL-2 in cells of the infiltrate, just as with those in the keratinocytes.

Extracellular Bacteria

Infections caused by extracellular bacteria are the most frequent of all. In these cases, the protection mechanisms are mainly related to the host's natural barriers, innate immune response and antibody production.

The importance of natural barriers in the fight against extracellular bacterial infections is well known. The integrity of skin and mucosas prevent adherence and penetration of bacteria; mucociliar movement eliminates bacteria from the respiratory tract; the stomach's acidic pH destroys bacteria penetrating by the upper digestive tract; and in the saliva and prostatic secretions there exist substances with antimicrobial activity. Chart provides details of the main protection mechanisms against extracellular bacteria.

Chart: Protection mechanisms against extracellular bacteria.

I. Natural barriers against infection
II. Innate immunity
1.   Ertracellular molecules (C reactive protein, complement)
2.   NR cells, nearophils, macrophages
3.   Chemokines. cytokines
III. Aquired immunity
1.   Antibodies
2.   Cytokines produced by T cells

The participation of innate immunity occurs through phagocyte cells, the activation of a complement system through an alternative path and by production of chemokines and cytokines. In addition, C-reactive protein (CRP), an acute phase protein produced mainly by hepatic cells in bacterial infections, exerts a diversified range of action against the bacteria. When binding to phospholipids of the membrane of some bacteria (for example, pneumoccocus) CRP works like opsonin, facilitating the phagocytosis by neutrophils. CRP also has the capacity to activate the complementary system and stimulates the synthesis of TNF-alpha, which induces the synthesis of NO and consequently the destruction of various microorganisms.

The complement performs its protection role by activating the attack complex at membrane (C5-C9) and facilitates opsonization through the C3b component, which binds to the bacteria and interacts at a second stage with the specific receptor existing in phagocytic cells. The deficiencies of the complementary system have been associated with serious infections by *Neisseria meningitides* and infections disseminated by Neisseria gonorheae.

All innate immunity cells participate in protecting against bacteria, though it is the role of neutrophils and monocytes/macrophages that are mainly emphasized by the phagocytic capacity of these cells. The basophiles and mastocytes activated by factors of the complement system, as in C5a, C3a and C4a for example, release mediators which, when combined with the aforementioned complement proteins, attract leukocytes to the site of aggression and contribute to the passage of these cells from the vessels to the tissues, namely the site at which the aggression against the host occurs. Apart from its phagocytic activity, eosinophils may destroy microorganisms by means of releasing proteins with microbicid activity, such as the main basic protein and eosinophil cationic protein. Neutrophils and macrophages play a key role in protecting against these agents provided that bacteria are susceptible to substances produced by these cells, for example NO and hydrogen peroxide. Within these cells, enzymes like myeloperoxidase and other substances like azurocidin having microbicid properties also exist. Although neutrophils as well as macrophages are phagocytic cells, they have much different characteristics. Whereas neutrophils have a short lifespan in either the blood or tissues, macrophages survive over extended periods of time. Neutrophils are only found in inflamed tissues, while macrophages are concentrated either in inflamed or healthy tissues. During the inflammatory reaction, neutrophils produce purulent secretion, whereas the macrophages form granuloma. Neutrophils mainly protect against extracellular bacteria, whereas macrophages are vital to eliminate the intracellular agents that house them.

Immune response cells are also the main sources of cytokines and chemokines at the onset of the infection. They exert inhibitory action either on the innate or adaptive phase. Due to their role of attracting cells to the lesion site, chemokines are very important in the process of protecting the host.

Among the various cytokines that participate in protecting against bacteria, the pro-inflammatory cytokines, like TNF-alpha, IL-1 and IL-6, are noteworthy. These cytokines are produced in the initial phases of the infection. By means of their action on the hypothalamus, they are responsible for the appearance of a fever that inhibits bacterial multiplication. They increase the expression of adhesion molecules (Seletine P and ICAM), thereby easing the passage of cells from the vessel to the infection site. They also stimulate neutrophils and macrophages to produce NO and destroy bacteria. Other cytokines produced in the initial infection phases interfere with the adaptive immune response. Produced by macrophages, IL-12 has an important role in the differentiation of Th0 cells into Th1 cells. By contrast, IL-4, produced by basophiles, mastocytes and macrophages, stimulates a differentiation of Th0 cells into Th2 cells, which end up collaborating with lymphocyte B in the production of antibodies, but especially of IgE.

Adaptive immunity, mainly by means of antibodies, performs an important role against these extracellular bacteria. The antibodies may perform their inhibitory action in three ways: 1) opsonization, 2) activating the complement system, 3) promoting the neutralization of bacteria or its products.

Extracellular bacteria are susceptible to destruction when phagocyted. They develop substances like the evasive mechanism that have antiphagocytic activity. Antibodies aimed against these substances not only impede upon their action, but facilitate phagocytosis, insofar as the neutrophils and macrophages have receptors for the FC portion of the immunoglobulin (opsonization). Antibodies also co-assist in destroying bacteria by the complement, and activate this system by a classic pathway. By means of the neutralization mechanism, the antibodies, primarily IgA, may bind with the bacteria and accordingly prevent the latter from establishing themselves in the mucosas, intestinal tract and respiratory tract. Antibodies often bind to bacteria-produced toxins, like tetanic and diphtheric toxins, and neutralize the action of these products.

Despite the protective importance of immune response, the difficulty in controlling the inflammatory response that develops may provoke tissue damage, which is nonetheless most often limited and without greater consequences for the host. However, infections caused by gram-negative germs may eventually result in septicemia and septic shock—very serious situations usually associated with a high mortality rate. Septic shock is triggered by lipopolyssacharides (LPS) present in the bacterial wall, which stimulate an exacerbated production of pro-inflammatory cytokines in the neutrophils, macrophages, endothelial cells and muscles (TNF-alpha, IL-1, IL-6, IL-8) and NO. Muscle tone and heart beat are reduced as a result, which leads to hypotension and poor tissue perfusion, and finally cellular death. By contrast, modulation of this exacerbated response may be obtained. As such, in an experimental model, the concomitant combination of IL-10 and LPS protects mice from death during septic shock by inhibiting the production of IL-12 and synthesis of IFN-gamma and TNF-alpha.

Immune Response in Viral Infections

Despite the manifold mechanisms of protecting against viruses, viral diseases are not only common, but in fact represent one of the most important infectious diseases today associated with mortality in the general population. Figure shows how viruses are destroyed by means of innate immune response. In the initial phase of viral infections, controlling the infections is done with interferons type I (IFN-alpha and IFN-beta), macrophages and NK cells.

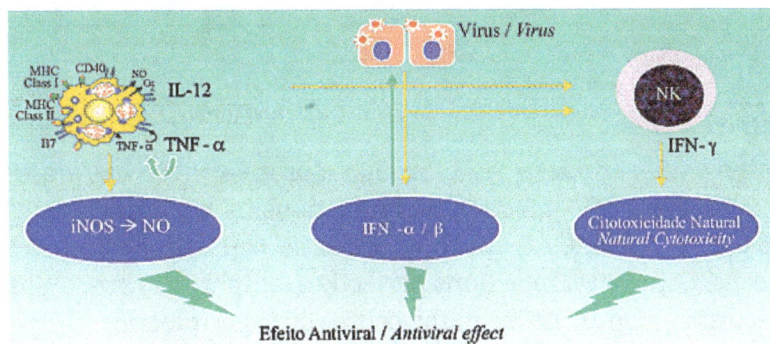

Diverse mechanisms of antiviral activity in innate immunity.

Type I interferons are produced by virus-infected cells. By interacting with a non-infected cell, their feature is to protect them against infection in addition to collaborating with adaptive immune response. IFN-gamma also acts against virus infections by means of activating the macrophages to destroy the virus as well as the NK cells (natural cytotoxic cells) to release granzyme and perforin and destroy infected cells. In addition, IL-12 plays an important part in the initial phase. It is produced by macrophages and other antigen-presenting cells. It stimulates NK to exert cytotoxicity and produce more IFN-gamma, which in turn increases the microbicid potential of macrophages.

Adaptive immunity against viral antigens occurs with the activation of TCD8+ cells that exert cytotoxicity when recognizing viral antigens via MHC class I in the target cells, with a result of releasing granzyme and perforins with the lysing of the infected cells and virus. During adaptive immune response TCD4+ cells are also activated, which then go on to collaborate with B cells to produce antibodies. In spite of viruses being intracellular agents, antibodies play an important role in fighting against viral infections insofar as the viruses break open these cells and remain free until penetrating into another cell. In this extracellular phase, antibodies may bind to the virus, and by means of the neutralization of the mechanism, prevent others from penetrating a non-infected cell. By contrast, antibodies may assist in the cellular cytotoxicity mechanism that depends on them, by binding to the infected cells and thereby allowing NK cell action. In various diseases, as in the examples of poliomyelitis, measles, hepatitis B and varicella, the antibody has a fundamental role in protecting against infection when it is a previously sensitized host, whether by a prior infection or immunization. This is because, in already sensitized individuals, the presence of antibodies can intercept the virus and thus prevent it from binding to the host cell.

In virtue of several protective mechanisms against viruses, a large part of viral infections are asymptomatic or have a subclinical presentation with nonspecific manifestations, like fever and cutaneous rash. Nonetheless, various viral infections do progress and important tissue damage can occur. The pathology associated with viral infection may be related to the virus' cytopathic effect, hypersensitivity reaction and auto-immune phenomena.

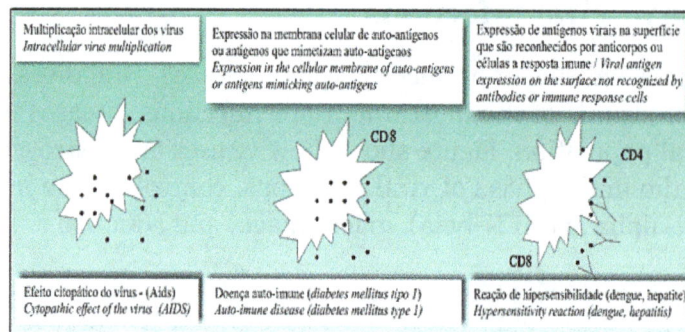

Pathology associated with viral infections.

In many viral infections, cells are destroyed through a process involving more than one of these mechanisms. For example, in HIV-infection and infections by hepatitis viruses B and C, the destruction of infected cells is mediated as much by the virus' cytopathic effect as through cytotoxicity by NK and CD8 cells. Some viral infections perfectly exemplify the broad dimension of aggression mechanisms occurring against tissue in the course of these infections.

Human Immunodeficiency Virus (HIV)

HIV infects TCD4+ cells predominantly. The destruction of these cells may occur by the virus' cytopathic effect. In addition, there exists increased apoptosis in these cells. Due to expressing viral antigens at the level of the membrane, the cells may also be destroyed by cytotoxicity mediated by the TCD8+ cell, a phenomenon also contributing to the reduction of CD4+ cells. As the CD4+ cell is one of the most important for obtaining the cooperation of immune response, the numerical reduction and alteration of its function leads to the suppression of immune response. This suppression is associated predominantly with a reduction of IL-2, IFN-gamma and TNF-alpha. This is why in AIDS patients, the main opportunistic infections are related to intracellular agents such as: *M. tuberculosis, P. carinii, cytomegalovirus, C. albicans* and *criptosporidium*. As in HIV infection, memory B lymphocytes keep functioning, antibodies are produced and the protection mechanism against extracellular agents does not experience large scale damage. However, this lack of greater susceptibility to extracellular bacterial infections observed in AIDS patients is observed in adults in whom the repertory of B-cell produced antibodies depending on T-cells had already formed prior to HIV infection. In infected children, as the alteration of TCD4+ cell functioning is premature, cellular cooperation is damaged with abnormalities also occurring in the synthesis of antibodies. This is why infections by extracellular bacteria are common in HIV-infected children.

Human T Cell Lymphocytotropic Virus (HTLV-1)

Infection by the HTLV-1 induces activation and intense cellular proliferation of infected T lymphocytes. This phenomenon is related mainly to the function of the virus' Tax gene, whose property is to transactivate IL-2 and IL-2-receptor genes. These T-cell proliferation anomalies may lead to the appearance of leukemia in adult T cells. Indiscriminate cell proliferation may also provoke an expansion of self-reactive T cells and accentuated secretion of pro-inflammatory cytokines like TNF-alpha. These abnormalities may associate with cutaneous and neurological tissue lesions.

Owing to the strong Th1 cell activation in HTLV-1 infection, there is reduced production of IL-4 and IL-5, and a drop in IgE synthesis, in mastocytes and in eosinophil activation. Both these components are features of the protective response against helminthes. Accordingly, there exists a higher prevalence of schistosomiasis and strongyloidiases in patients infected by HTLV-1. There may also be a dissemination of S. stercoralis with severe forms of strongyloidiasis.

Human Papilloma Virus (HPV)

HPV is a DNA virus that, apart from causing verruca vulgaris and condylomata acuminata, is strongly associated with the development of cervical neoplasia and skin cancer, mainly in immunosuppressed individuals. HPV involvement with skin cancer was also shown in patients with epidermodysplasia verruciform in which viral DNA was detected in macular lesions.

Immune response against HPV in general is mediated by cellular immune response, regardless of whether class IgG and IgA antibodies against antigenic fractions are found in the cervical mucus of patients with cervical neoplasia. Inflammatory infiltrate consisting of macrophages and CD4+ cells is observed in spontaneously regressing condylomata. The lymphoproliferative response of antigen-specific T CD4+ cells to E2 proved to be associated with the elimination of HPV. On the other hand, specific CD8+ cells for antigens E6 and E7 are found in patients with large lesions or a cervical tumor. Furthermore, type 1 response reduction with a low production of IL-2, IFN-gamma and TNF-alpha is observed in patients with a high-grade intraepithelial lesion.

Immune Response in Infections Caused by Protozoans

The main diseases caused by protozoans in human beings are leishmaniases, Chagas disease, malaria, toxoplasmosis and amebiasis. Protozoans are infectious intracellular agents that usually infect the host for long periods of time, owing to mechanisms that allow them to evade from aggressions mediated by the immune system. In addition, infections by protozoans usually only cause disease in some infected patients. This indicates that in most cases the immune system does not allow large scale multiplication of protozoans or the infection to spread, though it is unable to foster sterilization. Accordingly, these agents may remain in the host for its entire lifespan even without causing disease, unless this balance is lost by immune depression or by precipitation of an exacerbated immunitary response with tissue inflammation.

Various immune response components participate in the protection mechanism against protozoans, but these microorganisms manage to evade this protection mechanism. Whereas *in vitro* the

Leishmania promastigotes are highly sensitive to the complement, infectant forms resist their action. *Tripanosoma cruzi*, for instance, has a feature of preventing the complement's activation insofar it covers itself with the host's molecules as the degradation accelerator factor (DAF). Leishmania are also susceptible to the action of neutrophils, cells having a large potential to produce hydrogen peroxide and NO. But when penetrating the host, they infect the macrophages and make them vulnerable to a neutrophil attack. The adaptive response against protozoans occurs after the presentation of antigens by macrophages and dendritic cells, via MHC class II to the T cells. As other cells may be infected, and macrophages and dendritic cells also express MHC class I molecules, TCD8+ cells are also activated in protozoan infections. Chart shows the immune protection mechanisms against some clinically important protozoans.

Chart: Main protection mechanisms against protozoans.

Protozoans	Predominantly infected cells	Protection Mechanism
Leishmania	Macrophages	Prodution of IFN - γ, NO and cytotoxicity by CD8 cell.
Ameba	Neutrophil, macrophage	Production of IFN - γ and NO.
T. Cruzi	Cardiomiocytes	Cytotoxity by CD8 cells activation of macrophage by CD4 cells and NO production.
Toxoplasma gondii	SNC cells, eyes muscles, others	NO production by macrophages activated by TCD4+ and TCD8+ cells.
Plasmodium	Hepatocytes	Cytotoxicity by TCB8 + cells and production of IFN - alpha TNF – alpha and NO.

With the exception of Giardia lamblia, which may cause severe infection in patients who have an antibody production deficiency, immune cellular response is fundamental in protecting against infections caused by protozoans.

Whereas with infections caused by intracellular agents' immune response deviated by the Th2 pole could incur damages, due notably to the fact that susceptibility to infection increases and this in turn allows the multiplication and dissemination of the parasite, the concept of whether a potent Th1 response is protective must be addressed with some skepticism. In various protozoan-caused diseases, there is evidence that an exacerbated immune response is involved in tissue damage: in amebiasis, it depends on neutrophil action; in Chagas disease it is mediated by CD4+ and CD8+ cells; a massive production of TNF-alpha and NO, documented in the pathogens of cerebral malaria. These facts indicate that a balanced performance of the immune system is very important in order to contain the parasite without incurring any tissue destruction, so that despite remaining in the host, the infecting agent does not cause disease to the human being.

The pathogenesis of diverse clinical forms of leishmaniasis exemplifies well the importance of Th1 response in the control and genesis of tissue lesions. The most common clinical forms of leishmaniasis are tegumentary leishmaniasis (cutaneous leishmaniasis, mucous leishmaniasis and diffuse cutaneous leishmaniasis) and visceral leishmaniasis. Chart shows the association between diverse clinical forms of leishmaniasis, the Leishmaniasis species and immune response.

Chart: Immune response (production of IFN-gamma) and clinical forms of tbe infections caused by different species of Leisbmania.

Clinical Form	Specie	Production of IFN-gamma (pg/mI)
Visceral	L. chagasi	8 ± 5
Diffuse	L. amoznensis	4 ± 6
Cutaneous	L. braziliensis	1146 ± 382
Mucus	L. braziliensis	4284 ± 671

After inoculation of Leishmaniasis in the skin and the macrophage invasion, in individuals unable to produce IFN-gamma and activate macrophages, Leishmaniasis disseminates. Depending on the species, the latter causes visceral leishmaniasis (L. chagasi), or diffuse cutaneous leishmaniasis (L. amazonensis). In these patients, it is easy to understand the development of the disease, which occurs through IFN-gamma deficiency and high production of IL-10. Restoration of immune response *in vitro* in visceral leishmaniasis may be observed by neutralizing IL-10 or adding IL-12 to peripheral blood mononuclear cell cultures (PBMNCC).

More atypical is what occurs to cutaneous leishmaniasis and mucous leishmaniasis, situations in which a strong Th1 deviation exists. Even though the number of parasites in the skin is thick or even absent, the lesion tends to develop. PBMNCC of individuals with cutaneous leishmaniasis and mucous leishmaniasis stimulated with the Leishmania antigen produces large amounts of IFN-gamma, IL-2 and only slight amounts of IL-10. As the immune system does not usually manage to completely destroy leishmania, this strong Th1 response prompts the occurrence of a very intense inflammatory reaction and damage to the tissues themselves. This results in the appearance of ulcers on the skin and mucosa. This damaged tissue also participates considerably on the accentuated production of TNF-alpha and NO. The evidence that cellular immune response participates in the pathogenesis of cutaneous leishmaniasis and mucous leishmaniasis includes: 1) premature treatment of the infection does not prevent the appearance of the lesion; 2) the existence of a strong inflammatory reaction in the tissue with an increased expression of TNF-alpha, IFN-gamma and a few parasites on the lesion; 3) association of an antimonial with an inhibitor TNF-alpha drug cures patients with mucous leishmaniasis, which are otherwise refractory to antimonial treatment.

Immune Response to Fungus

The main protection mechanism against funguses is developed by phagocytes, which destroy them by producing NO and other components developed by these cells. In addition, there is participation of IFN-gamma. This enhances the function of neutrophils and macrophages, though there is no evidence of cytotoxic activity by T CD8+ cells. However, patients presenting with neutropenia (less than 500 neutrophils/mm^3) or that have frequent cellular immune deficiency present with recurrent mycoses and occasionally develop severe and deep forms.

Whereas a large number of fungus species may cause diseases in humans, the majority of them cause limited disease without greater clinical repercussions. Among the funguses associated with morbidity in Brazil, we can highlight *Candida albicans, Criptococcus neoformas* and Paraoccidiodis brasiliensis. In spite of the fact that infection by *C. albicans* regularly causes light infections with no greater consequences, HIV-positive patients not only present with a high prevalence of *C. albicans* infection, but esophagus, stomach, and intestine involvement are among the most recurrent infections. In children presenting alterations in cellular immune response and multiple endocrinal disturbances, a rare picture of chronic mucocutaneous candidiasis is described. In these children, one observes a reduction in Th1 response and severe cutaneous, mucous and ungual lesions.

Despite the fact that vaginal candidiasis is extremely frequent but with no greater repercussions, roughly 5% of women at reproductive age do present with a condition of recurrent vaginal candidiasis due to the absence of or low levels of IFN-gamma, which may be restored *in vitro* by neutralizing IL-10. Although there is no documentation of Th2 response against *C. albicans* antigens, the high rate of atopia in these patients suggest that an immediate hypersensitivity reaction to diverse antigens may participate in the disease pathogenesis. Moreover, some cases may bring benefits to immunotherapy.

Criptococcus neoformans may cause lung diseases and compromise the central nervous system in immunosuppressed patients. *P. braziliensis* is the causal agent of south-American blastomycosis. South-American blastomycosis is characterized by involvement of the ganglia, bucal mucosa and respiratory apparatus. In most infected patients, the agent is controlled and the individual remains completely asymptomatic. When there is no development of Th1, there is dissemination of the fungus with involvement of the organs of the reticuloendothelial and pulmonary system; in this context, the role of IL-4 seems important, given that in an experimental model the absence of this cytokine protects against severe pulmonary disease.

Immunological Response in Helminth Infections

The immune response mechanisms in helminth infections are manifold owing to the size and metabolic diversity of the parasites, which are antigenically complex. An additional problem is that the parasites may survive in the host for several years. As a result mechanisms are evaded, an example of which occurs with *S. mansoni* which ends up being covered by host antigens, and are no longer foreign for the immunological system.

Although the complement and other factors of natural immune response might contribute to protecting against the helminth infections, specific immune response with the production of antibodies and cytokines is important. The T CD4+ or TCD8+ type 2 cells are producers of cytokines like IL-4, IL-5 and IL-13 which, among their other functions, induce IgE production by B cells and activate the fundamental components in protecting against helminths, namely eosinophils, mastocytes and basophiles, respectively. Class IgE antibodies bind to circulating basophiles or tissue mastocytes. This induces the release of histamine and other reaction mediators of immediate hypersensitivity leading to the destruction of helminths. The IgE produced in high levels in type Th2 immunological response has been related to protecting against reinfection by *S. mansoni*. Eosinophils also have the capacity to destroy schistosomula and strongyloides through the cytotoxicity cellular mechanism that depends on the antibody. Th2 type cells are associated with a resistance to infection not only by *S. mansoni*, but by intestinal helminths, for example *S. stercoralis* and *A. lumbricoides*. IL-4 stimulates IgE production and, in combination with IL-13, mastocytes. This results in increased secretion of inflammation mediators, secretion of mucus and enhanced contractility of intestinal musculature, which facilitates the expulsion of adult worms.

In the acute phase of schistosomiasis, the clinical manifestations of fever, asthenia, weight loss, abdominal pain, diarrhea and coughing, in addition to complications such as pleuritis and peri-carditis, result from the presence of TNF-alpha, IL-1 and IL-6, and also the deposition of immune complexes. Improvement of symptomatology coincides with the production of IL-10 induced by egg antigens in the chronic phase. This phase also features secretion of IL-4, IL-5 and IL-13, that experimental models participate in the formation of granuloma and hepatic fibrosis, and yet in the pathogenesis of schistosomiasis.

Immunization

Immunization describes the process whereby people are protected against illness caused by infection with micro-organisms (formally called pathogens). The term vaccine refers to the material used for Immunization, while vaccination refers to the act of giving a vaccine to a person.

Immunity describes the state of protection that occurs when a person has been vaccinated or has had an infection and recovered.

Vaccination, like infection, confers immunity by interaction with the immune system. The term micro-organism refers to infectious agents that can only been seen under the microscope and here covers bacteria, viruses, fungi and protozoa.

Antigens are the components/fragments from pathogens or their toxins. The purpose of Immunization is to prevent people from acquiring infections and to protect them against the shortand longer-term complications of those infections, which can include chronic illnesses, such as cancer, and death.

Vaccines work by stimulating the body's defence mechanisms against infection. These defence mechanisms are collectively referred to as the immune system. Vaccines mimic and sometimes improve on the protective response normally mounted by the immune system after an actual infection. The great advantage of Immunization over natural infections is that Immunization has a much lower risk of adverse outcomes.

Immunization Harnesses the Body's own Defence Mechanisms

To understand how Immunization protects against the diseases produced by pathogens such as viruses and bacteria, we first need to understand how the immune system works.

The immune system consists of trillions of specialised blood cells, known as white blood cells, and their products, such as antibodies. These cells are located throughout the body, not only in the bloodstream, but also in lymph glands, the spleen, the skin, lungs and intestine.

The skin and the lining of the lungs and intestine are the first line of defence against infection. These tissues and the white blood cells located at these sites form the innate immune system. The white blood cells of the innate immune system (or guardian white blood cells) detect the presence of infection using sensors on their surfaces that recognise parts of pathogens or the toxins released by them. These fragments from pathogens or toxins are collectively known as antigens.

When guardian white blood cells detect the presence of pathogens, a second set of white blood cells (called lymphocytes) is activated. Lymphocytes are categorised into two types: B-cells and T-cells.

T-cells respond to infections by releasing chemicals called cytokines, which trigger protective inflammation. Furthermore, T-cells can help combat pathogens by killing cells that harbour a pathogen hidden inside them. B-cells, sometimes with help from T-cells, make antibodies, which are complex proteins that attach in a 'lock-and-key' fashion either to pathogens or to the toxins released by them. When antibodies attach to a pathogen, they flag it for destruction, and when they attach to a toxin, they neutralise its ability to cause damage.

In most cases, the outcome of these immune responses is termination of the infection followed by repair of any associated damage to the body's tissues. However, some infections outstrip the immune system's capacity to respond, leading to disease and sometimes death. By giving a vaccine before exposure to the infection, such serious outcomes can be avoided through generation of protective immunity in advance.

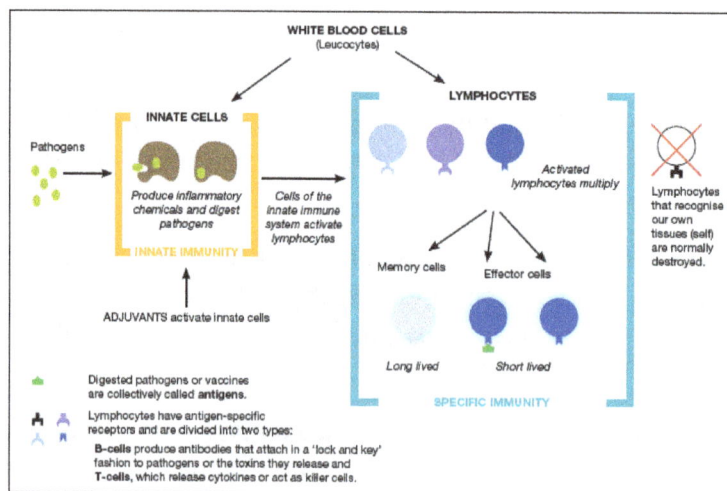

All blood cells originally come from the bone marrow. There are three main cell types in our blood: red blood cells, which carry oxygen to our tissues; platelets, which help the blood clot; and white blood cells (leucocytes), which are the main component of the human immune system. There are two main types of leucocytes: guardian cells responsible for innate immunity and lymphocytes responsible for specific immunity. The guardian cells of the innate immune system form the first line of defence against infection and can digest pathogens or vaccine particles and use these to activate lymphocytes. In addition they produce chemicals capable of causing inflammation and amplifying specific immunity. These cells are the target of adjuvants in vaccines. Lymphocytes have receptors for one antigen; that is, they are antigen specific. After infection or vaccination, specific lymphocytes recognise their target antigens, multiply and turn into short-lived effector cells or long-lived memory cells. Lymphocytes (T- and B-cells) have receptors on their surface for one particular antigen; that is, they are antigen specific.

Immunization is Disease-specific

A healthy immune system has the capacity to generate hundreds of millions of T- and B-cells, each of which targets one particular antigen. Consequently, healthy people have the capacity to mount a protective response to essentially every infection they could possibly encounter during their lifetimes.

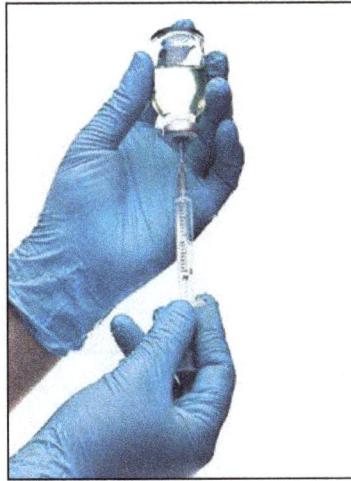

However, pathogens have evolved to overcome this defence and can sometimes overwhelm the immune response. Vaccines give the immune system a head start, providing valuable early protection against aggressive pathogens.

The specificity of these immune responses is the reason we need to have a separate vaccine for each disease. The capacity of the immune system to respond independently to each micro-organism in the environment also explains why the system cannot be 'overloaded' or damaged by giving the full range of currently available vaccines or by having multiple antigens in one vaccine preparation.

Vaccines Harness the Immune System's Capacity for Memory

When a pathogen is recognised by the immune system, individual lymphocytes not only make antibodies and cytokines against the infection, but also multiply quickly. As a result, the number of lymphocytes (T- and B-cells) specific for that infection increases greatly, enabling the body to fight the infection more efficiently. Most of the cells involved in immune responses live for only a few days as effector cells, but a small number of lymphocytes survive for months or years after the infection has been cleared and retain a 'memory' of the invading pathogen. In the case of measles, for example, that memory has been shown to last for more than 60 years.

The immune system's memory of infections it has been exposed to previously is one of its most valuable assets. This memory means the immune system is ready to mount a much quicker, larger and more sustained response if it encounters the same pathogen again.

That response can control subsequent infection more efficiently, without leading to the unwanted and serious complications that can be associated with infection in non-immune people.

A successful vaccine, like the corresponding infection, can harness the immune system's memory capability by generating a population of long-lived lymphocytes (T- and B-cells) that are specific for the targeted pathogen. Again, the result is long-term protection against subsequent exposures to that pathogen and avoidance of the complications associated with a natural infection.

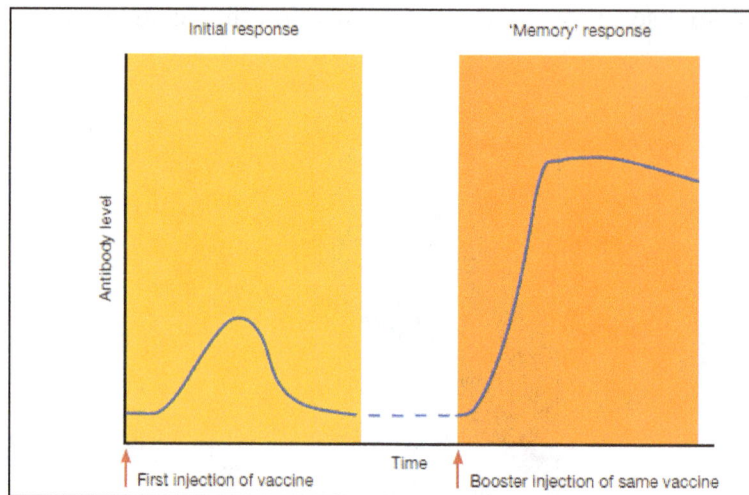

Figure shows effect of giving booster doses of vaccines: After first Immunization of a non-immune person, a small and brief response occurs. When second (booster) doses are given, memory lymphocytes created during the initial response are switched on to generate a much more rapid and longer lasting protective response. This figure shows the levels of antibodies from B-cells after first and booster vaccinations. A similar, more effective memory response is also a property of T-cells.

Infant Vaccines Work with the Newborn Immune System

The body's immune system begins developing before birth 26. In the period during and soon after birth, when the functions of the immune system are still maturing, newborns are protected against many, but not all, serious infections by antibodies from their mothers (maternal antibodies). This protection usually lasts for about four months.

These maternal antibodies cross the placenta into the baby's circulation before birth and are present in the mother's breast milk. If the mother has been vaccinated recently or has recovered from infection during pregnancy, the amount of antibody transmitted to the baby can be sufficient to ensure complete protection. On the other hand, if the mother's infection (particularly with the pathogen that causes whooping cough) or Immunization occurred a long time ago, the antibody levels may be lower and protection suboptimal.

The current Immunization programs are designed to balance the capacity of the baby's immune system to respond to the vaccine, against the risk of infection.

In the case of hepatitis B, for example, exposure to the virus at birth can result in the infant becoming a chronic carrier for life; hence the policy of starting vaccination within two weeks of birth.

The situation is different for other infections, which have a lower risk of infection at birth. Thus, administration of the Haemophilus influenzae type b (Hib) and pneumococcal vaccines is delayed until 6–8 weeks of age, when the infant's immune system can respond better. Moreover, the measles-containing MMR (measles, mumps and rubella) vaccine is not given until 12 months of age, when maternal antibodies against measles, which can interfere with vaccine responses, have essentially disappeared.

Passive Immunization Provides Immediate Protection

Most vaccines work by actively switching on the recipient's own immune system to make the antibodies and memory cells needed to provide long-term protection against infection. Such 'active immunity' is the primary goal of all Immunization programs.

However, this kind of active immune response takes 7–21 days to develop fully. Consequently, in the case of overwhelming infections, there is sometimes a role for 'passive' Immunization, which involves giving pre-formed antibodies obtained from healthy blood donors, as these can act much more quickly.

Vaccine

Vaccines Contain Antigens and Adjuvants

Vaccines generally have two major types of ingredients, antigens and adjuvants. Antigens are designed to cause the immune system to produce antibodies and/or T-cells against a specific pathogen or its toxin. Adjuvants amplify immune responses more generally.

Disease-specific Vaccine Ingredients are Called Antigens

Pathogens (such as viruses and bacteria) are assembled from building blocks—proteins, sugars, nucleic acids (such as DNA) and fats. Each pathogen has a unique set of these building blocks. Some can be recognised by the body's immune system and are termed antigens. The antigens used in a vaccine are designed to trigger a specific protective response by the immune system to a particular pathogen. Therefore, each vaccine contains a different set of antigens.

Several Types of Antigen are used in Vaccines

Some vaccines comprise the killed whole pathogen that the vaccine is designed to protect against. The virus or bacterium is grown in the laboratory and killed by heat and/or chemicals to render it non-infectious. The injectable poliomyelitis (polio) vaccine and inactivated hepatitis A vaccine are examples of this type of vaccine.

Other vaccines contain only components of the pathogen as their antigens. These components can be prepared by purifying them from the whole bacterium or virus, or by genetically engineering them. Engineered vaccines include the hepatitis B virus vaccine and the human papillomavirus vaccine, which protects against cervical cancer.

In some vaccines, sugar components of the pathogen are joined with proteins to create an antigen that can generate a stronger response—this allows even 6-week-old babies to make significant amounts of antibody, which they otherwise could not do until they are older. These vaccines are called conjugate vaccines, and include those against meningococcal and pneumococcal disease.

Another group of vaccines is based on the toxin produced by the pathogen that causes the disease symptoms. The toxin is chemically treated to make it into a harmless toxoid. The antibodies produced against this toxoid are still able to neutralise the toxin, and to prevent disease symptoms from developing. Examples of this type include the tetanus and diphtheria vaccines.

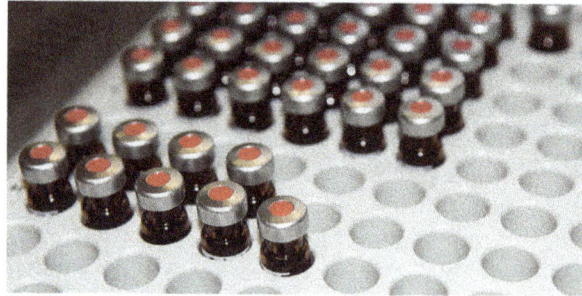

Some Vaccines Contain Live Organisms

Some vaccines contain an infectious microorganism. These are called live vaccines. The micro-organism may be derived from the pathogen (bacterium or virus) that the vaccine aims to protect against. This is usually achieved by growth of the pathogen in the laboratory under conditions designed to weaken or 'attenuate' it. This attenuation process permanently alters the pathogen so that it is still infectious, but is unable to cause the disease. Examples include the injectable MMR vaccine, the oral polio vaccine, and the chickenpox vaccine.

Alternatively, a live vaccine may consist of a naturally occurring organism that is closely related to the pathogen, but does not cause disease in healthy humans with intact immune systems. An example is the BCG vaccine against tuberculosis and leprosy.

Vaccines containing live pathogens are not recommended for people whose immune systems are impaired due to use of immunosuppressive drugs, serious illness or genetic abnormalities of the immune system because of the risk of causing disease. Similarly, live vaccines are not recommended during pregnancy as a precautionary measure, in case the pathogens they contain cross the placenta. This is because a baby's immune system is not completely developed until after birth. Vaccines without live micro-organisms ('killed' vaccines), in contrast, are not harmful in pregnancy.

Adjuvants Amplify the Immune System's Response

Adjuvants are substances that promote a more vigorous immune response to vaccine antigens. They can also help target the body's response. In doing so, they may cause mild local reactions (soreness, redness and swelling) at the injection site. These reactions are a healthy indicator of the strength of the underlying immune response.

Most killed vaccines incorporate adjuvants, to make the body's defences think a significant infection is present. They stimulate stronger, longer-lasting immune responses to the vaccine antigens, leading to better protection against subsequent infection. Adjuvants are not needed in vaccines based on live organisms, as these naturally produce inflammation and amplify protective immunity.

In most human vaccines that contain adjuvants, the adjuvant is an aluminium salt (known as alum), which has a track record of safety dating back to the 1950s. Some newer vaccines incorporate more active adjuvants, derived from naturally occurring oil in water emulsions, fats from bacterial cell walls, or sugars. These can produce more vigorous and better targeted immune responses against the infectious agent.

Vaccine Quality is Carefully Monitored

In addition to adjuvants and antigens, vaccines can contain minute quantities of materials from the manufacturing process. These can include trace amounts of detergents, nutrients from the laboratory cultures, chemicals used to kill the pathogens, stabilisers like gelatin or small amounts of DNA and parts of dead organisms.

Vaccine developers are required by regulatory authorities to test for the presence of these extra materials during the manufacturing process to ensure they do not exceed levels known to be safe.

Occasionally, individuals can be allergic to an ingredient of a vaccine, although such reactions are rare. Fewer than one in 100,000 vaccine doses delivered cause a significant allergic reaction.

Beneficiaries of Vaccines

Individuals Benefit in the Short and Long Term

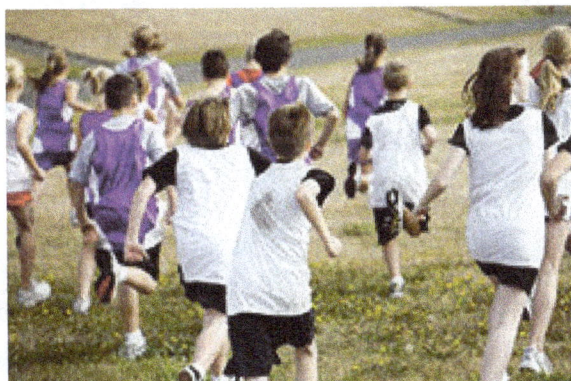

An effective vaccine protects an individual against a specific infectious disease and its various complications. In the short term, the efficacy of a vaccine is measured by its capacity to reduce the overall frequency of new infections, and to reduce major complications, such as serious tissue damage and death.

All vaccines currently in use in Australia confer high levels of protection that are sufficient to prevent disease in the great majority of vaccinated individuals, and in the wider community. In other countries where the use of vaccination is widespread, there has been a dramatic reduction in the number of people who become ill and die from formerly common and severe infections. For example, the whooping cough vaccine prevents disease in 85% of recipients, while the measles vaccine prevents disease in 95% of recipients. The remaining individuals may not be fully protected and remain at least partially susceptible to infection. This may be due to genetic factors, or to the presence of other medical conditions that impair the capacity of the vaccine recipient to mount a protective immune response.

Booster doses of some vaccines are required to maintain protection. Examples include the whooping cough, tetanus, and polio vaccines, as well as the more recently introduced conjugate pneumococcal and meningococcal vaccines. In contrast, a single course of others, such as the hepatitis B vaccine, appears to be sufficient to provide lifelong protection.

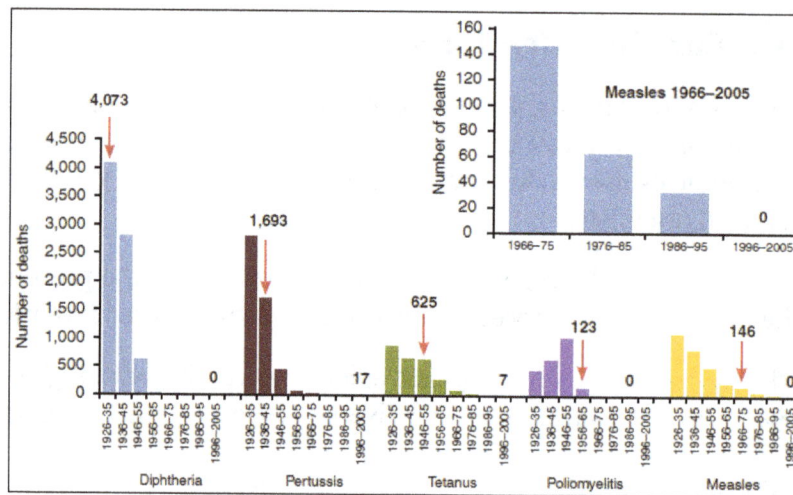

Number of deaths in Australia from diseases now vaccinated against, by decade (1926–2005).
Red arrow indicates when vaccine was introduced.

Vaccines can Protect against Long-term Complications of Infections

The efficacy of vaccines is most often thought of in terms of their capacity to protect against the immediate consequences of serious diseases such as meningitis, pneumonia, hepatitis, chickenpox and measles. By preventing infection, vaccines can also prevent long-term complications associated with chronic infections, where the pathogen persists in the body after the initial infection has passed.

Certain viruses can cause dormant infections. Such persistent infections can eventually lead to chronic damage of infected organs (e.g. encephalitis induced by measles, called SSPE, or cirrhosis of the liver, caused by hepatitis B or hepatitis C virus infection).

Persistent viral infections can also lead to late complications, including cancer and shingles. Viruses known to cause cancer and for which vaccines are available include hepatitis B and the human papillomavirus (HPV). Hepatitis B can lead to liver cancer and liver damage, whereas HPV can cause cervical and anal cancers. At present there is no protective vaccine available against hepatitis C infection; however, drug treatment is now effective in curing the disease in around 95% of cases at the two-year mark.

On the other hand, currently available vaccines are generally not capable of eliminating a virus infection once it has been acquired. This is why hepatitis B vaccine is administered from birth, and why HPV vaccine is delivered in late childhood or very early adolescence, before the individual is at risk of being exposed to the virus through sexual encounters.

An exception to the rule of vaccines being unable to control established viral infections is seen with the chickenpox vaccine. This vaccine protects against the development of a long-term complication of the infection, shingles (also known as herpes zoster). Shingles is a debilitating condition characterised by the appearance of painful blisters on parts of the skin above nerves where the chickenpox virus has lain dormant since infection in childhood. Adults who had chickenpox in childhood can be given a high-dose chickenpox vaccine to boost immunity, resulting in a substantial reduction in their subsequent risk of developing shingles.

Community at Large Benefits

An important feature of Immunization is that it brings benefits not only for the individual who receives the vaccine, but also for the entire population through a phenomenon called herd immunity.

Herd immunity occurs when a significant proportion of individuals within a population are protected against a disease through Immunization. This situation offers indirect protection for people who are still susceptible to the disease, by making it less likely that they will come into contact with someone who is carrying the pathogen.

In addition to protecting unvaccinated individuals, herd immunity benefits the small proportion of people who fail to respond adequately to vaccination. In the case of a highly infectious disease such as measles, more than 95% of the population must be vaccinated to achieve sufficient herd immunity to prevent transmission if the disease recurs.

For other childhood infections, the proportion of the population that need to be vaccinated is lower, because the diseases are less infectious—for instance, until very recently no cases of diphtheria had occurred in Australia since the 1970s, despite Immunization coverage of much less than 95% of the population.

The effectiveness of herd immunity is well illustrated by reference to the introduction of a new form of the pneumococcal vaccine, which protects against disease caused by the bacterium *Streptococcus pneumoniae*. In addition to protecting susceptible infants and young children from the disease, this vaccine also reduces circulation in the community of the bacteria present in the vaccine. Consequently, older people are also protected, even though they have not been vaccinated against this organism.

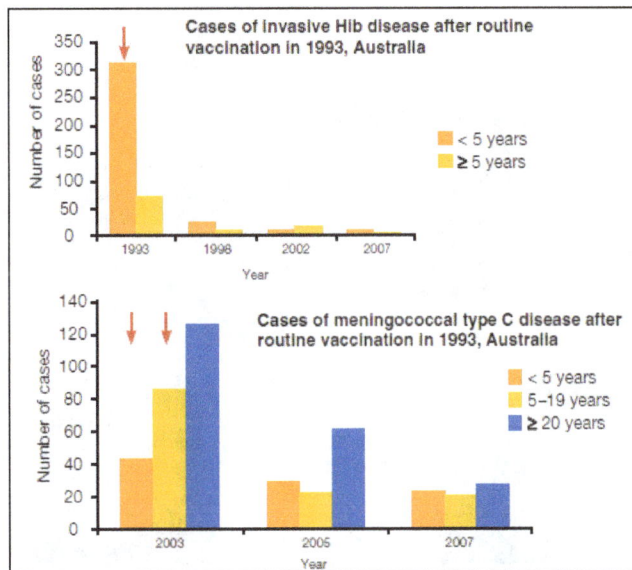

Cases of Haemophilus influenzae (Hib) and meningococcal type C disease since the introduction of routine vaccination. Red arrows indicate when vaccine was introduced and for what age group(s). Note the reduction in both the vaccinated children and unvaccinated children.

Vaccines can Control, Eliminate and Eradicate Diseases

When a large proportion of a community is immunised, it can lead to a situation where there are very low levels of the disease in that population. This is referred to as control of the disease.

Even more effective and prolonged vaccination programs can result in interruption of transmission in the population for long enough to ensure that there is no residual disease— elimination of disease. However, even when high levels of community coverage with a vaccine are achieved, infection may be reintroduced, for example by unvaccinated travellers or, for some pathogens, an animal that is a carrier. In Australia, isolated outbreaks of infectious diseases such as measles have been attributed to transmission from unvaccinated carriers.

Once a high degree of control is achieved worldwide, it is theoretically possible to eradicate an organism and the associated risk of infection, provided there is no other animal that can carry the infection and transmit it back to humans. This was achieved with smallpox in the 1970s and there is hope that such a goal may also be achievable for polio and measles, for which, as for smallpox, humans are the only host. Compared with 350,000 cases in 1988, only 650 polio cases were reported worldwide in 2011, a figure that now stands at less than 150 for 2015. The only countries in which transmission of polio has never been interrupted are Nigeria, Pakistan and Afghanistan.

Vaccination brings Economic Benefits

Cost-effectiveness of community Immunization programs is determined by measuring the benefits—in terms of cost and quality of life—that result from preventing illness, disability and death, and comparing them with the costs of vaccine production and delivery to the population. A striking example is the benefits of polio vaccination. In the first six years after introduction of the vaccine, it was calculated that more than 150,000 cases of paralytic polio and 12,500 deaths were prevented worldwide. This represented a saving of more than US$30 billion annually in 1999 dollars.

Safety of Vaccines

Benefits of Vaccines outweight the Risks

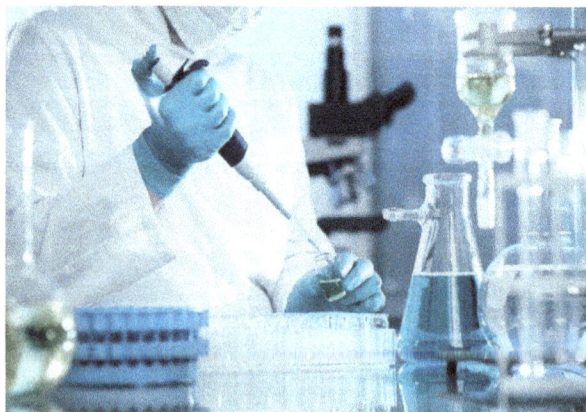

Vaccines, like other medicines, can have side effects. However, all vaccines in use in Australia provide benefits that greatly outweigh their risks.

Most Reactions from Vaccination are Minor

The great majority of side effects that follow vaccination are minor and short-lived. The most common side effects for all vaccine types are 'local' reactions at the injection site, such as redness or swelling, which occur within hours and are clearly caused by the vaccine. More general or 'systemic' reactions, such as fever or tiredness, can also occur after vaccination, but careful studies have shown that they are much less common than local reactions.

Local reactions are outward signs that the vaccine is interacting with the immune system to generate a protective response. The nature of these reactions varies, depending on the type of vaccine given.

For example, if a person develops a fever due to an inactivated vaccine, they almost always do so within 24 to 48 hours—the time when the immune system is making an immediate response to the components of the vaccine. In contrast, the onset of fever caused by a live attenuated vaccine, such as the MMR vaccine, is delayed for seven to 12 days because this is the time needed for the attenuated virus in the vaccine to multiply sufficiently to induce a protective response from the immune system.

Some Adverse Events Coincide with but are not Caused by Vaccination

Symptoms such as fever, rashes, irritability and nasal snuffles are common, especially among children. Consequently, it can be difficult to determine how many of these reactions are caused by a vaccine when the 'background rate' (how often it occurs anyway) in the same age group is unknown.

In some cases, these kinds of reactions may be caused by the vaccine. But in other situations, the symptoms may be unrelated, occurring by chance at the same time as the vaccination. For this reason, scientists refer to these kinds of symptoms as adverse events following Immunization to indicate that events that follow vaccination may not be caused by the vaccine.

One unique study from Finland addressed this issue. Researchers analysed common symptoms in 581 pairs of twins after one twin received the MMR vaccine and the other was given a dummy vaccine (a placebo). Between one and six days after the injection, the number of adverse events in the twin who received the MMR vaccine was almost identical to those in the twin who received placebo. Between seven and 12 days after the injection, the vaccinated group had a measurable increase in symptoms that are known to be associated with administration of the attenuated measles vaccine, such as fever, irritability and rash. On the other hand, no difference between the two groups could be detected over that period in the frequency of cough and cold-like symptoms—which occur commonly with or without vaccination. Moreover, even some of the symptoms known to occur after MMR vaccine were also seen in the group who received placebo, but at a lower rate.

In summary, this valuable study showed that many common symptoms that occur after a vaccine is given are not caused by the vaccine, but occur by chance at that time.

However, safety surveillance systems in countries like Australia require health care providers to report adverse events that occur following vaccination regardless of the cause. The reports are compared with historical trends to identify any changes that require special investigation and to assess whether adverse events are vaccine-related. For example, new vaccines are often reported more often than old vaccines, and reported events decrease as health carers gain familiarity with the vaccine. It can be misleading to rely on the reported raw numbers of adverse events, as a number of factors must be taken into account to determine if an event is coincidental or caused by the vaccine. The vast majority of adverse events are coincidental.

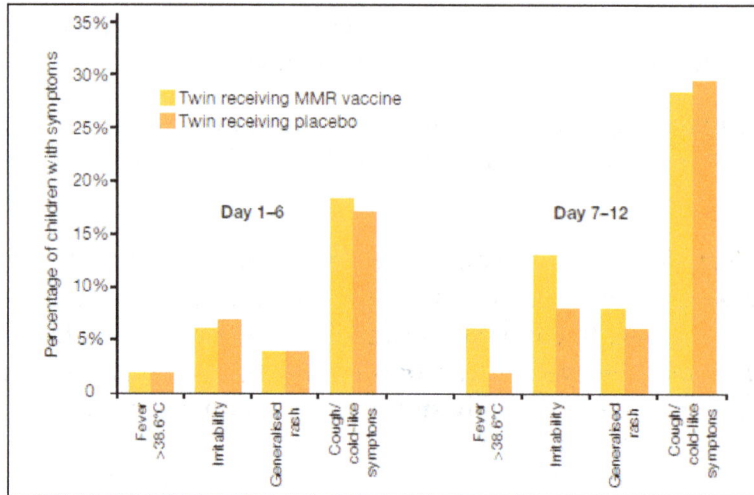

Comparison of common symptoms in a paired twin study, where one twin received an MMR vaccine and the other received a placebo.

Serious Side Effects from Vaccines are Extremely Rare

Potentially serious side effects, such as transient febrile seizures, have been reported after vaccination. However, such severe side effects occur much less often with the vaccine than they would if a person caught the disease itself.

This is well illustrated in young children by comparing the frequency of adverse events from the MMR vaccine with the frequency of adverse events with measles itself. Severe complications due to MMR vaccine and measles among 1 million children aged less than 5 years.

MMR vaccine	Measles
Uncommon complications	
300 children have seizures	10,000 children have seizures or convulsions induced by fever.
Rare complications	
26 children have a temporary tendency to bruise or bleed more easily (thrombocytopenia)	330 children develop thrombocytopenia.
Very rare complications	
Up to four children get a severe allergic reaction (anaphylaxis). This is readily treated with complete recovery	No anaphylaxis cases.
No children will get subacute sclerosing panencephalitis (SSPE). SSPE causes progressive brain damage and death	10 children get SSPE several years later.
Uncertain; a maximum of one child may develop inflammation of the brain (encephalitis). Encephalitis from any reason may result in permanent brain damage or death	2000 children may develop encephalitis.

About three in every 10,000 children who receive the MMR vaccine develop a fever high enough to cause short-lived seizures. In contrast, the risk of such a fever is more than 30 times greater among children who develop the disease—affecting about 100 in 10,000 children. Importantly, worldwide measles vaccination was estimated to prevent 9.6 million deaths from the infection during 2000. Similarly, around one in 10 young children develop a fever after receiving influenza vaccine 3, whereas around nine in 10 children develop a fever after a proven influenza infection.

The frequency of side effects associated with some earlier vaccine preparations (no longer in use in developed countries such as Australia) was higher than with the current generation of vaccines. Lastly, some alleged links between administration of certain vaccines and onset of diseases, particularly when the causes are unknown, have proven to be unfounded.

Vaccine Safety Testing

Safety Testing is an Integral Component of Vaccine Development and use

Careful testing of safety is an essential part not only of vaccine development and manufacture, but also of ongoing surveillance programs after vaccines have been introduced into the community.

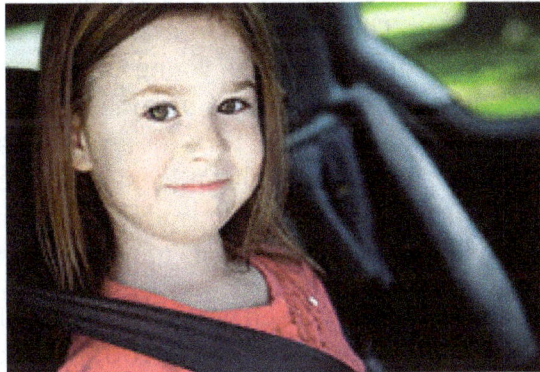

The importance of strict routine testing is illustrated by an incident that occurred in 1955, before such testing was introduced, when a batch of polio vaccine had not been fully inactivated and still contained live virus. As a result, some recipients and their close family members developed polio infections, leading to paralysis and some deaths. No such events have been reported since.

Vaccine Safety is always Assessed before Licensing for use

During vaccine development, initial safety testing procedures occur in two stages. The first stage involves preclinical assessment in the laboratory. If a vaccine fails these safety tests, it cannot progress into clinical trials. Vaccines are then evaluated in three phases of clinical trials. In phase I clinical trials, the vaccine candidate is given to small numbers (25–50) of healthy adults with the primary goal of assessing safety.

Phase II trials involve hundreds of participants and are designed to demonstrate how effective a vaccine is in mounting an immune response, and to determine the optimal dose regimen. Phase III clinical trials aim to demonstrate protection against the target disease and safety, and this usually requires administration of the vaccine to many thousands of potentially susceptible people. Only after the vaccine has passed each of these safety and efficacy hurdles is it approved for widespread community use.

Safety Assessments Continue once a Vaccine is Licensed for use

Some side effects of vaccines are so uncommon; they are not detected during the extensive safety testing before vaccine licensure. To ensure that authorities can detect such unanticipated side effects, careful surveillance continues even after a vaccine candidate has proven to be effective and has passed all safety checks in thousands of people. The formal term for this systematic collection of data and analysis of reports of any suspected adverse events is post-licensure assessment.

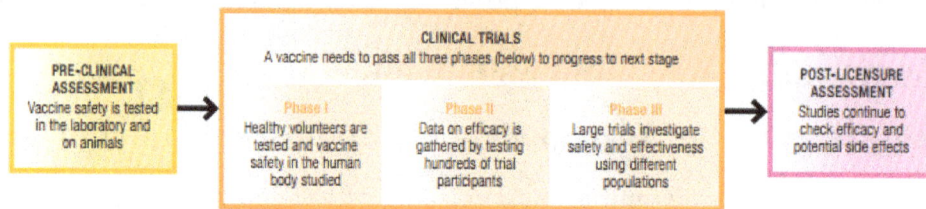

The phases of vaccine safety testing.

The value of ongoing safety testing of licensed vaccines is demonstrated by the successful identification of potential clinical problems. The most recent example is the detection of an increased risk of febrile seizures that unexpectedly occurred in young children given a particular influenza vaccine in Australia in 2010. When the problem first became apparent, the use of all influenza vaccines in young children was suspended to allow time for authorities to identify the one type of vaccine preparation causing the problem. Meanwhile, influenza vaccines shown not to be associated with unacceptable rates of febrile seizures were reintroduced to ensure that protection against influenza remained available for children at high risk of complications from the disease.

Likewise, in adults, long-term surveillance has been used to determine the risk of developing Guillain – Barré syndrome (GBS), a rare (one to two cases per 100,000 people) but serious condition characterised by temporary paralysis which has occasionally been reported to occur after influenza vaccination. The conclusion of these long-term studies was that, at most, one additional case of GBS occurs for every million people vaccinated against influenza. On the other hand, the risk of developing GBS after influenza infection is much greater.

The Benefits of Vaccination Worldwide will Continue

Vaccination represents the most successful form of disease prevention available today. In the past 20 years, vaccine technology has improved, resulting in production of vaccines against a broad range of infectious diseases.

Nevertheless, the burden of infectious diseases worldwide remains high, particularly in developing countries. According to the World Health Organization, infections still account for about 40% of all recorded deaths worldwide.

Future strategies to meet this challenge include extending the use of existing vaccines, new technologies to deliver vaccines and generating new vaccines. Priority targets for future vaccines include viruses, bacteria and parasites.

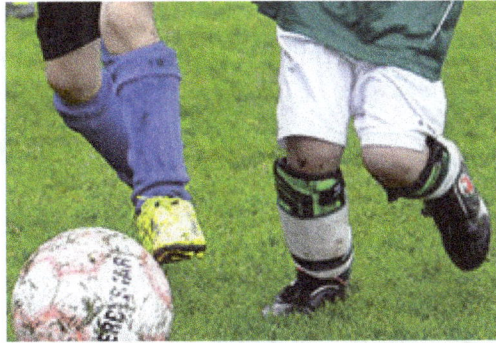

Existing Vaccines will be used in New ways

Using existing vaccines in different ways shows promise. One example is administration of a killed vaccine, normally given during childhood, to a pregnant woman. This Immunization boosts antibody levels in the mother, allowing the extra antibodies to reach her baby by crossing the placenta, and via the mother's breast milk. Doing this protects her newborn baby while the baby's immune system is still maturing. In the future, giving a malaria vaccine in this way could be beneficial to protect newborns from becoming chronically infected from birth. Another way of applying existing vaccines more effectively is to target them to elderly people, who make up a growing proportion of the population. For instance, elderly people in hospitals are more prone to infections with vaccine-preventable diseases such as *Streptococcus pneumoniae*, influenza virus and shingles-causing varicella.

New Technologies will Change Vaccine Delivery

Many technologies under development will improve the simplicity and effectiveness of vaccine delivery.

To make a vaccine that only needs to be given once, it must either be very powerful, or be packaged in such a way that its contents are released intermittently once it has been administered. Under development are multilayer particle technologies and alternative adjuvants, which have the potential to remove the need for multiple shots.

Needle-free administration is already possible for some vaccines, such as live vaccines given orally (polio vaccine) or via a nasal spray (influenza vaccines). Currently, many vaccines need to be injected, but researchers are working on edible (plant-based) vaccine materials, needle free skin patches and microneedle injection technologies to get the vaccine through the skin without discomfort.

Technologies for delivering multiple vaccines in one injection are improving— many different killed vaccines can already be given in one injection without impairing the immune response to any of them, and some live virus vaccines can also be given together.

Novel Vaccines

Most successful vaccines protect against acute infections largely through production of antibodies. Vaccines for chronic infections, in particular malaria, HIV and tuberculosis remain a problem.

One of the major reasons for this is the viruses, bacteria and parasites that cause these infections 'hide' from the immune system in the person's own cells. To overcome this, an immune response mediated by T-cells is required, instead of, or in addition to, an antibody response.

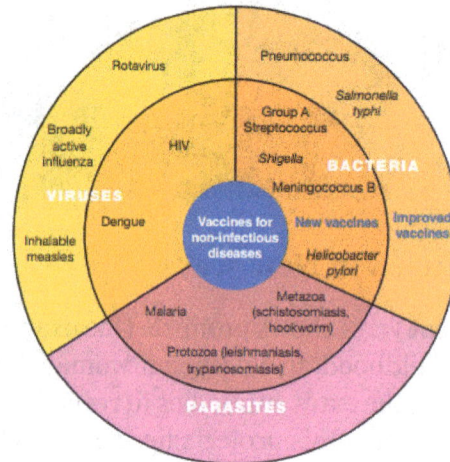

Current research is aiming for entirely new vaccines and improved versions of existing vaccines.

There are effective vaccines to target infections that predispose people to long-term complications, such as cancer. Examples include vaccines to the human papillomavirus (HPV), hepatitis B and the shingles-causing varicella virus. On the other hand, there are still no vaccines for other infections associated with many serious long-term complications. For instance, infection with the bacterium *Helicobacter pylori* predisposes patients to stomach cancer, group A streptococcus infection is responsible for rheumatic fever-still a major cause of death and disability in developing countries, and chlamydia infection can lead to infertility and blindness.

Vaccines have the potential to be used to treat rather than prevent infectious and non-infectious diseases. Such therapeutic vaccines are being targeted at persistent infections, such as shingles, and also at non-infectious conditions, including autoimmune disorders, allergies and cancers not related to infections. In the case of tumours, the vaccine can either be directed against the tumour itself or be designed to amplify the anti-tumour immune response. By contrast, for autoimmune or allergic disorders, the vaccines are being designed to switch off unwanted immune responses, so-called negative vaccination—rather than switching on the useful immune response needed for infections and cancer.

Immunology of Vaccination

It is easy to define the properties of an ideal vaccine. Most of these are obvious, but few vaccines approach the ideal. In addition, vaccines do not yet exist for many organisms and it is worth considering why this is so. First it is notable that most successful vaccines are against relatively small organisms. There are excellent vaccines against several viruses and some against bacteria, although several of these do not protect against infection but rather the toxic effects of infection. As yet there are no satisfactory vaccines against parasites. Generally, therefore, successful vaccines are against organisms with smaller genomes although there are of course exceptions to this general rule, for example so far we do not have an effective vaccine against HIV or hepatitis C.

Properties of an ideal vaccine:

- Should give life-long immunity.

- Should be broadly protective against all variants of an organism.

- Should prevent disease transmission, e.g. by preventing shedding.

- Should induce effective immunity rapidly.

- Should be effective in all vaccinated subjects, including infants and the elderly.

- Should transmit maternal protection to the fetus.

- Requires few (ideally one) immunisations to induce protection.

- Would not need to be administered by injection.

- Should be cheap, stable (no requirement for cold chain), and safe.

Without prior Immunization, most organisms gain a foothold in their host but from very early on in the infectious process must deploy mechanisms to interfere with the host immune response. Even those organisms that rely on rapid multiplication and spread to new hosts must combat innate (non-specific) immune mechanisms. Organisms with a life-style involving co-existence with their host over long periods have also to combat the adaptive (specific) immune response. Thus all micro-organisms have evolved complex defence mechanisms that interfere with every stage of the immune response. Organisms with large genomes have sufficient genetic capacity to carry multiple genes capable of affecting immune response. The sheer magnitude of the enterprise involved in working out all these mechanisms means that there is more complete information available for smaller organisms. A number of viruses have been well studied. Numerous viral gene products that interfere in immune function have been described. These include a large variety of molecules that mimic important regulatory molecules of the immune system, such as interferons, interleukins and chemokines and their receptors. Interference with antigen processing is common and viruses may also prevent apoptosis. Genes dedicated to viral escape may represents at least 10% of viral genomes, indicating the potential magnitude of the task involved in understanding how a complex organism such as a bacterium avoids elimination by the immune system since 10% of a bacterial genome might be 200–400 genes.

Smaller organisms do not have the luxury of devoting tens or hundreds of genes to combating the immune system and must adopt other strategies, one of which is rapid change. Many viruses use this method including influenza, HIV and hepatitis C. Larger organisms also employ this strategy including malaria. Most often, the variation takes place after infection of the host. Of course if the organism has a secondary host, change may take place during infection of this species as is thought to occur in the case of influenza virus. Pre-existing immunity can prevent the opportunity for multiplication and development of escape variants such as have been well described for HIV. Thus Immunization against an epidemic strain of influenza virus can provide very effective preventive immunity against spread of that strain but not against future variants.

The ability of micro-organisms to deploy escape mechanisms even early in immune responses suggests that, for organisms so far insusceptible to vaccines, we need to decide what the vaccine is intended to do. Do we wish to prevent infection completely, or simply suppress replication of the organisms to an extent compatible with a normal life-span? Is prevention of transmission to other and perhaps more susceptible individuals (for example infants) the objective, or is the aim not the prevention of infection but pathology? Recent understanding of the complex interactions of micro-organisms with their hosts suggests that if we are to make progress in containing many infectious diseases caused by complex organisms, we should better define our objective and tailor our vaccine strategies accordingly. Better understanding of the crucial events in immune responses will help in doing this and may lead to development of new vaccines capable of combating infections in very different ways.

Initiation of Immune Responses

Danger Signals

A key stage of any immune response is the phase of initiation. Antigens must be recognised as foreign for an immune response to occur. Micro-organisms are usually recognised because they carry 'danger' signals that signal the immune system through conserved pattern recognition receptors. Tissue damage also leads to the expression of self-molecules that can also activate cells of the innate immune system. The receptors for external and internal 'danger' signals are diverse. They include low affinity IgM, serum mannan binding protein, pentraxins and cellular receptors such as complement receptors, mannose and other lectin-like receptors for carbohydrates, the phosphatidylserine receptor, heat shock proteins and the recently described family of IL-1R-Toll-like molecules. The latter may function as homodimers, but they frequently form heterodimers with other Toll-like receptors or may work in concert with other cell surface or soluble molecules such as CD14. They recognise molecules that are often abundant, contain repeating subunits and are not produced by vertebrates. These include bacterial polysaccharides and lipopolysaccharides, complex fungal polysaccharides, flagellin and bacterial DNA or viral RNA.

Table: Pattern recognition receptors.

Receptor	Ligands
TLR2 + (TLR6 or TLRx)	Bacterial lipoproteins, peptidoglycan
	Zymosan, GPI anchor (T. cruzi)
	LPS (Leptospira interrogans)
	LPS (P. gingivalis)
	Lipoarabinomannan (M. tuberculosis)
	Phosphatidylinositol dimannoside (M. tuberculosis)
TLR3	dsRNA
TLR4	LPS, Taxol, HSP60 (human and chlamydial)
	Fibronectin, F protein (respiratory syncytial virus)
TLR5	Flagellin
TLR9	CpG DNA
FcγRs	Pentraxin-opsonised zymosan, serum amyloid P, C-reactive protein
CR1 (CD35)	Complement opsonised bacteria and fungi
CR3 (CD11b-CD18)	Complement opsonised bacteria and fungi
CR4 (CD11b-CD18)	M. tuberculosis

CD43 leukosialin	M. tuberculosis
CD48	Enterobacteria
Mannose receptor	Mannosyl/fucosyl residues, P. carinii, Candida albicans
Scavenger receptor	Apoptotic cells, Gram +ve cocci, leipoteichoic acid
MARCO	E. coli
MER	Apoptotic thymocytes
PSR	Apoptotic cells
CD36	Apoptotic PMN
CD14	P. aeruginosa

Initial recognition of micro-organisms as foreign is likely to take place in non-lymphoid tissues and the most important cells in this process are tissue resident macrophages and dendritic cells (DCs). Activation of dendritic cells is crucial as these cells have been shown to be uniquely capable of initiating a primary immune response. DCs are also actively pinocytic and take up soluble antigens as well as those bound by their surface receptors. Uptake of antigen and ligation of one or more DC receptors, initiates three key processes: antigen processing, migration to lymph nodes, and maturation of the DCs.

Antigen Processing

Antigens entering cells by endocytosis are broken down in lysosomal vesicles and peptides from them encounter major histocompatiblity class II antigens (MHC II) in a specialised intracellular loading compartment where the peptides are loaded onto MHC II molecules for transport to the cell surface (exogenous antigen processing). Antigens synthesised in the cell, as is the case for viruses and other intracellular pathogens, are broken down to peptides by the proteasomes and the resulting peptides are transported into the rough endoplasmic reticulum for loading onto MHC class I molecules (endogenous antigen processing). Loaded MHC molecules are then transported to the cell surface.

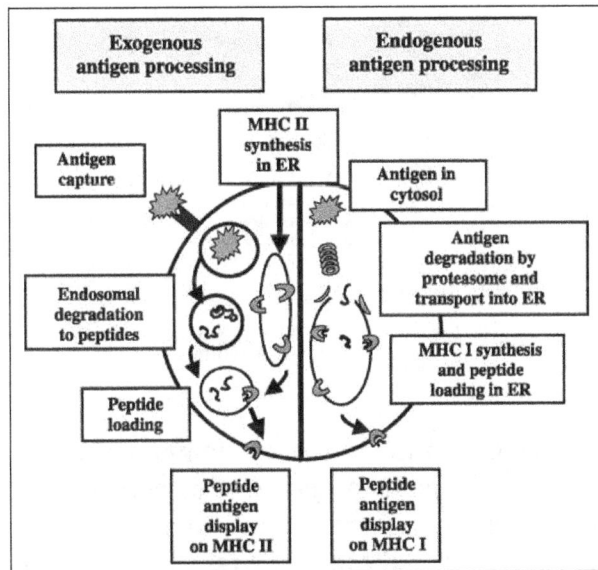

The figure shows the two modes of antigen processing. In the exogenous modes, antigens are captured from the extracellular space, degraded to peptides in endosomes and the peptides displayed on MHC II molecules. Endogenous processing of intracellular antigens is carried out by the pro-teasomes and the resulting peptides are loaded on to MHC class I molecules in the endoplasmic reticulum.

Tissue resident DCs are active antigen processing cells. Following activation by 'danger' signals, surface expression of MHC increases greatly and subsequently antigen processing decreases.

Migration and Maturation

At the same time, the cells migrate from the tissues to the draining lymph nodes, a process con-trolled by chemokines and their receptors. Thus in the tissues, DCs express CCR1, CCR5 and CCR6 – the receptors for chemokines produced by tissue cells. Down-regulation of these receptors and up-regulation of CXCR4 and CCR7 are induced by 'danger' signals and signals from inflammato-ry cytokines such as tumour necrosis factor-α (TNF-α) and interleukin-1 (IL-1). This allows the DCs to receive chemotactic signals from the lymph node chemokines, secondary lymphoid tissue chemokine (SLC) and EBV-induced-receptor ligand chemokine. During migration and entry of DCs into the T-cell areas of nodes, the DCs show considerable changes in phenotype (maturation) in addition to the up-regulation of MHC already described. The most important is the up-regu-lation of surface molecules that are important for interaction of DCs with T-cells. CD40, CD80 and CD86 (B7.1 and B7.2) deliver crucial co-stimulatory signals for T-cell activation, while several members of the TNF–TNFR (tumour necrosis factor receptor) family of molecules are up-regu-lated. These include CD40, Ox40 and 4-1BB and they appear to play important roles in differenti-ation of different types of effector T-cells. In concert with this, the DCs up-regulate production of many different cytokines that affect T-cell differentiation and function.

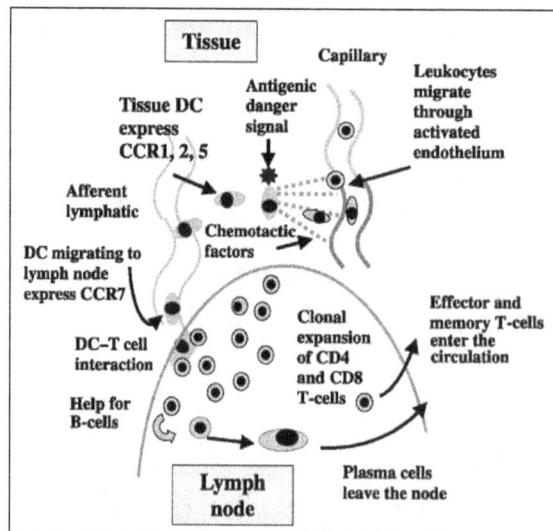

The figure illustrates key events in the initiation of an immune response. Introduction of antigen and an accompanying danger signal, leads to release of cytokines and chemokines and influx of inflammatory cells. Dendritic cells take up antigen and migrate to draining nodes where they in-teract with T- and B-cells to generate specific immune responses. Effector cells leave the node and some of these homes to the inflammatory site.

Two aspects of this complex series of processes are particularly crucial from the point of view of vaccines. The first is the need for 'danger' signals to initiate responses. While whole micro-organisms, even if killed, may well deliver appropriate signals, subunit vaccines may be poorly immunogenic so that adjuvants are needed. In humans, the most commonly used is alum. Alum has been shown to favour Th2 responses in mice, inducing strong antibody responses. This observation leads to the second crucial point, that the nature of the 'danger' signal has an important bearing on the type of immune response generated. Clearly for vaccines where a Th1 type of response is required, alum may not be an appropriate adjuvant and, furthermore, the danger signals carried by the vaccine itself or a live vector must also be taken into account. So far, few alternative adjuvants are available for routine use in humans. However, better understanding of the mechanisms of action of adjuvants and the signals that control differentiation of DCs and, therefore, T-cells will eventually allow design of vaccine-adjuvant preparations tailored to induce appropriate protective responses for particular infections.

Immunological Memory

Irrespective of the type of immune response required for protection, for almost all vaccines long-lasting protection (memory) is a desirable objective. However, while it is easy to state this, it is less certain how it should be achieved, although a great deal has been learnt about immunological memory over the last two decades. During a primary immune response, lymphocytes proliferate and change their phenotype. Memory populations of cells are, therefore, both quantitatively and qualitatively different from those that have not yet encountered antigen. Thus memory consists of expanded clones of lymphocytes with altered function. Among thymus-derived (T) lymphocytes, this is reflected in rapid production of effector cytokines such as IFN-γ or interleukins. Primed cells express higher levels of several adhesion molecules, such as ICAM-1 and integrins, as well as homing molecules such as CD44, CD62L and the cutaneous lymphocyte antigen (CLA). Among B-cells, the hallmark of immunological memory is the production of isotype switched, somatically mutated, high affinity immunoglobulin. It is also clear that memory is a dynamic state. In both man and experimental animals, phenotypically defined memory cells have been shown to divide more rapidly than naive cells. This appears to be an inherent property of memory cells since division continues in the absence of antigen.

Constraints on the duration of Memory

In vitro at least, human T lymphocyte clones can only undergo a finite number of cell divisions and, as they approach senescence, no longer express the co-stimulatory molecule CD28, can no longer up-regulate telomerase on activation, and show progressive shortening of telomeres. These mechanisms may limit the duration of memory in the absence of re-exposure to antigen, which would recruit new clones. In addition to these constraints on survival of individual clones, there is also the constraint of space in the memory pool. Although during an acute infection lymphocyte numbers may increase greatly, in the longer term numbers of cells with naive and memory phenotypes change only slowly. Thus every time a new antigen is encountered and a new set of clones undergoes expansion and enters the memory pool, other cells must die to provide space. What factors favour one cell or clone over another in this competition for survival are not known. However, experimental evidence suggests that memory persists longer if the initial clonal expansion is large.

Alternatively, persistence of antigen may favour clonal survival as occurs in chronic infections such as EBV or CMV. It is now clear that there is considerable heterogeneity among antigen-specific T-cell populations detected by binding to MHC-peptide tetramers and it is thought that some memory cells may revert to a more slowly dividing state. This suggests two alternative strategies for ensuring persistence of memory. Either vaccine should be designed to ensure maximal clonal expansion by providing an optimal dose of antigen and appropriate adjuvant, or vectors should be chosen to ensure long persistence of antigen.

Appropriate Immune Responses

Heterogeneity of Immune Responses

One of the major discoveries of the modern era of immunology is that not all immune responses are the same. In truth, this is not a new discovery since it has been long been known that there are many types of immune response and these may be both beneficial, for example the development of neutralising antibody to viruses, or pathological, for example the production of IgE antibody leading to anaphylaxis. What is new is the greatly increased, though not complete, understanding of how different types of response are generated.

Immune responses are influenced by many factors, but key cells that control the functions of other immune cells are the T helper cells (Th cells). These cells, which express the CD4 surface antigen and recognise antigenic peptides displayed by MHC II molecules, influence the function of important effector cells such as CD8 cytotoxic cells, antibody producing B lymphocytes and macrophages, both by cell–cell contact and production of soluble cytokines. Two major types of Th cells (and analogous CD8 subsets) have been described. Th1 effectors produce IL-2, IFN-γ, and lymphotoxin and mediate 'cellular' immunity. The dominant cytokine is IFN-γ, immune CD4 and CD8 cells are both readily demonstrable, and antibody is not a prominent feature of the response.

In contrast, in Th2 cell responses, the dominant cytokines produced are IL-4, IL-5, IL-10, and IL–13. CD8 cytotoxic cells are not prominent and high titres of antibody may be produced, with a bias toward IgG as well as IgA and IgE. In general, Th1 cell responses are adapted to deal with intracellular parasites through direct and indirect mechanisms – cell killing or production of cytokines (particularly IFN-γ) that activate cellular protective mechanisms. Th2 cell responses are particularly effective at coping with extracellular parasites through antibody-dependent mechanisms. It should be emphasised that, although some response are almost exclusively Th1 or Th2 and very biased responses are associated with some disease states, in most immune responses both Th1 and Th2 components can be detected. Furthermore, many cytokines including TNF-α, IL-3, IL-6 and GM-CSF are produced by both Th1 and Th2 cells.

Control of T-cell Responses

It is important to understand what controls the development of a Th1 or Th2 biased response. In experimental animals, the genetic background of the host has been shown to be important. Thus Balb/c mice mount a Th2 response to the parasite *Leishmania major*, while other strains of mice make a Th1 response. The former strain is susceptible to infection while others are resistant, demonstrating the important of making the 'right' type of response. This model illustrates another important aspect of the Th1/Th2 balance – that manipulation of the balance of cytokines can have profound effects. Treatment of susceptible Balb/c mice with antibody to the Th2 cytokine IL-4 or administration of the Th1-inducing cytokine IL-12 makes them resistant. Apart from the genetic background of the host, it has been shown that the route, dose and form of the antigen and whether an adjuvant is given can have profound effects on the type of immune response generated.

More recent experiments show that treatment of DCs with products of micro-organisms such as lipopolysaccharide (LPS) or the filarial worm antigen ES62, can bias their ability to stimulate Th1 and Th2 responses to a protein antigen. Thus it appears that micro-organisms signal DCs, probably through binding to Toll-like, lectin-like and other surface receptors, to differentiate along different pathways that have been termed DC-1 and DC-2. These DC subtypes show different patterns of cytokine production, which in turn influence Th1 cell generation. IL-12 produced by DCs has been shown to be a key cytokine for induction of Th1 cells while IL-4 and IL-10 are important for generation of Th2 cells.

The observations discussed above indicate why particular adjuvants may induce Th-biased responses. Although the exact mechanisms of action of alum are not well understood, it induces strong Th2 responses in mice and humoral responses in man, presumably by inducing DCs to produce Th2-inducing cytokines. In contrast, the experimental adjuvant, Freund's complete adjuvant, which contains BCG in mineral oil, generates a strongly Th1-biased response. Since the mechanism underlying Th bias is a cytokine milieu, it is perhaps not surprising that strong cytokine inducers can bias not only on-going immune responses but appear to be able to bias other subsequent responses. Thus BCG vaccination (a Th1 response) has been shown to protect against subsequent development of allergy (a Th2 response). This has led to attempts to use the strong Th1 inducer, *Mycobacterium vaccae*, as an immunomodulating agent for treatment of a number of diseases. Similarly, it has led to the suggestion that early exposure to micro-organisms capable of biasing the immune response may have a life-long effect on subsequent immune responses (the hygiene hypothesis).

In conclusion, a key issue in vaccine development today is what type of immune response is needed to best protect against the 'difficult' organisms for which there are currently no effective vaccines. Most of the present generation of successful vaccines depend principally on generating high titres of antibody and many are given with the Th2-biasing adjuvant alum. However, natural protection against many organisms, particularly intracellular parasites, is mainly Th1 in nature. Furthermore, for organisms that vary rapidly (*e.g.* HIV, malaria) even if neutralising antibody could be induced, escape variants would rapidly make this ineffective, as is the case with influenza virus. For these difficult organisms, it remains unclear whether a strong cellular response, induced by a vaccine, could either prevent infection becoming established or suppress it to a subclinical level compatible with normal life, although it is clear that the cellular immune response does contribute to protection against HIV.

Nevertheless, in the absence of concrete evidence that cellular immunity can be protective, many new vaccines are being designed to induce strong Th1 and CD8 cytotoxic T lymphocyte (CTL) responses. To induce CTLs, presentation of antigen via MHC I is required and, as yet, the most effective way of doing this is through the use of live vectors that infect cells and thereby introduce antigens into the cytosol, although particulate antigens and some adjuvants can also induce CTLs. DNA has the advantage that, like live vectors, it can generate antigens inside cells, and the additional advantage that the DNA may also code for genes such as cytokines that have adjuvant effects and can bias responses in a desired direction.

There is an additional problem for vaccines that induce cellular immunity. Clearly, for cells to have a protective effect and prevent establishment of detectable infection, they must be able to enter tissues that are the site of entry for micro-organisms, particularly the respiratory, gastrointestinal and genito-urinary tracts. It is clear that among CD4 and CD8 memory cells, not all cells can do this. Among CD4 cells, central and effector memory has been defined. Central memory cells express the chemokine receptor CCR7 which enables them to re-circulate through lymphoid tissues, while effector memory cells express CCR3 and CCR5 and can enter non-lymphoid tissues. CD8 memory cells have similarly been further divided into subsets with differing expression of chemokine receptors and other surface molecules. While as yet it is not clear how to influence the proportions of these re-circulating or tissue homing memory cells, it has been shown experimentally that recent activation by antigen provides memory that is optimally protective against tissue infection. This may indicate that means of ensuring persistence of antigen over long periods of time will be essential if protective cellular immunity is to be maintained and be useful. Novel adjuvants and vectors will be needed to achieve this.

Chapter 5

Immunodeficiency, Immunosuppression and Autoimmunity

The state where the ability of the immune system to fight infectious diseases or cancer is reduced or completely absent is called immunodeficiency. Immunosuppression refers to the reduction of the activation of the immune system. The network of immune responses of an organism against its own healthy tissues and cells is termed as autoimmunity. The diverse aspects of immunodeficiency, immunosuppression and autoimmunity have been thoroughly discussed in this chapter.

Immunodeficiency

In healthy individuals the immune response comprises two phases. The first line of defence is the innate system, made up of specialised cells that provide a rapid response that is not tailored to the specific microbe that has infiltrated the body. Sometimes this can clear the infection alone but usually the innate response will contain the infection long enough for the adaptive immune system to activate. The adaptive response is the second line of defence and takes several days to assemble. The response is specific to the microbe and leaves a lasting immune memory, which makes the response to future reinfection more efficient. In a person with an immunodeficiency disorder, one or more components of either the adaptive or innate immune response is impaired, resulting in the body being unable to effectively resolve infections or disease. This leaves immunodeficient individuals at high risk of recurrent infection, and vulnerable to conditions that would not usually be of concern to otherwise healthy individuals. There are two types of immunodeficiency disorder:

- Primary immunodeficiency (PID): Inherited immune disorders resulting from genetic mutations, usually present at birth and diagnosed in childhood.

- Secondary immunodeficiency (SID): Acquired immunodeficiency as a result of disease or environmental factors, such as HIV, malnutrition, or medical treatment (e.g. chemotherapy).

Primary Immunodeficiency (PID)

PID disorders are inherited conditions sometimes caused by single-gene mutations, or more often by an unknown genetic susceptibility combined with environmental factors. Although some PIDs are diagnosed during infancy or childhood, many are diagnosed later in life. PIDs are categorised based on the part of the immune system that is disrupted.

Examples of Primary Immunodeficiency Disorders

- B cell immunodeficiencies (adaptive): B cells are one of two key cell types of the adaptive immune system. Their main role is to produce antibodies, which are proteins that attach to microbes, making it easier for other immune cells to detect and kill them. Mutations in the genes that control B cells can result in the loss of antibody production. These patients are at risk of severe recurrent bacterial infections.

- T cell immunodeficiencies (adaptive): T cells are the second of two key cell types of the adaptive immune system. One role of the T cell is to activate the B cell and pass on details of the microbe's identity, so that the B cell can produce the correct antibodies. Some T cells are also directly involved in microbe killing. T cells also provide signals that activate other cells of the immune system. Mutations in the genes that control T cells can result in fewer T cells or ones that do not function properly. This can lead to their killing ability being disrupted, and can often cause problems with B cell function too. Therefore, T cell immunodeficiencies can often lead to combined immunodeficiencies (CIDs), where both T and B cell function is defective. Some forms of CIDs are more severe than others.

- Severe combined immune deficiencies (SCID) (adaptive): SCID disorders are very rare but extremely serious. In SCID patients there is often a complete lack of T cells and variable numbers of B cells, resulting in little-to-no immune function, so even a minor infection can be deadly. SCID patients are usually diagnosed in the first year of life with symptoms such as recurrent infections and failure to thrive.

- Phagocyte disorders (innate): Phagocytes include many white blood cells of the innate immune system, and these cells patrol the body eating any pathogens they come across. Mutations typically affect the ability of certain phagocytes to eat and destroy pathogens effectively. These patients have largely functional immune systems but certain bacterial and fungal infections can cause very serious harm or death.

- Complement defects (innate): Complement defects are some of the rarest of all the PIDs, and account for less than 1% of diagnosed cases. Complement is the name given to specific proteins in the blood that help immune cells clear infection. Some deficiencies in the complement system can result in the development of autoimmune conditions such as systemic lupus erythematosus and rheumatoid arthritis. Patients who lack certain complement proteins are highly susceptible to meningitis.

Treatments and Outcomes

The prognosis of patients with PIDs is extremely variable and depends on the condition. Most SCID patients will die before the age of 1 without prompt treatment, although 95% of those that receive a bone marrow transplant (BMT) before 3 months of age will survive. Forty-three states in the USA now screen for SCID disorders at birth, but this is not yet routinely available in the UK. A famous SCID disorder patient was David Vetter, known as "the boy in the bubble", who from birth was isolated into a sterile environment while his family searched for a suitable bone marrow match. He died at the age of 12 from Burkitt's lymphoma probably triggered by the Epstein - Barr virus, which lay dormant and undetected in the transplanted bone marrow he received. BMT is the preferred long-term treatment option for CIDs/SCIDs and some phagocyte disorders, although some SCIDs are now routinely treated with gene therapy. Supportive therapy for all PID conditions involves routine preventative use of antibiotics and antifungals. B cell disorders can also be managed with immunoglobulin (antibody) replacement therapy, where immunoglobulin G is purified from the blood plasma of healthy donors and infused into the patient.

Key vaccines are recommended for patients with innate deficiencies, but live vaccines (such as MMR) must be avoided for CID/SCID patients. It is therefore crucial that there is enough vaccine coverage in their local communities to generate "herd immunity", where vaccine rates are at 95% or above ensuring resistance to disease transmission exists across the whole community, even for the few patients who cannot be vaccinated.

Secondary Immunodeficiency (SID)

SIDs is more common than PIDs and is the result of a primary illness, such as HIV, or other external factor such as malnutrition or some drug regimens. Most SIDs can be resolved by treating the primary condition.

Examples of secondary immunodeficiency disorders:

- Malnutrition: Protein-calorie malnutrition is the biggest global cause of SIDs which can affect up to 50% of the population in some communities in the developing world. T cell numbers and function decrease in proportion to levels of protein deficiency, which leaves the patient particularly susceptible to diarrhoea and respiratory tract infections. This form of immunodeficiency will usually resolve if the malnutrition is treated.

- Drug regimens: There are several types of medication that can result in secondary immunodeficiencies, but these drugs also perform critical roles in certain areas of healthcare. Immunosuppression is a common side-effect of most chemotherapy used in cancer treatment. The immune system usually recovers once the chemotherapy treatment has finished. Another common use for immunosuppressive drugs is the prevention of transplant rejection, where medication is required to suppress the transplant recipient's immune system and prevent it from targeting the transplanted tissue. These drugs can have significant side-effects and often suppress more areas of the immune system than are required, leading to susceptibility to opportunistic infections. Uses of a new generation of medicines called biologics are becoming more widespread in treating transplant rejection. These drugs are derived from biological sources like cells, rather than chemical structures. Monoclonal antibodies are one such class of biologics and these drugs are made by farming antibodies from B cells that will act against a specific part of the disease process. These agents are more specific in their action than traditional drugs and have fewer side effects on non-target immune cells.

- Chronic infections: There are a number of chronic infections which can lead to SID disorders, the most common of which is acquired immune deficiency syndrome (AIDS), resulting from HIV infection. The virus attacks CD4+ T cells, a type of white blood cell that plays a critical role in preventing infection, and gradually depletes their numbers. Once the T cell count is less than 200 cells per ml of blood, symptoms of AIDS begin to manifest and the patient is at high risk of recurrent infections that will eventually lead to death. Anti-viral therapies, such as the HAART regimen (Highly Active Antiretroviral Therapy), allow the T cell population a chance to recover and resume normal function. These drugs have had a huge impact on increasing the life expectancy for HIV/AIDS patients and improving their quality of life. Prior to the introduction of HAART, patients with HIV diagnosed at age 20 had an average of 10 years before developing AIDS. Nowadays on average, patients diagnosed at age 20 can expect to live well into their 60s. However; these drugs must be taken every day for life as they are not curative, and are only available to patients and healthcare systems that can afford them.

Treatments and Outcomes

For many SID disorders treatment of the primary condition will lead to resolution of the immunodeficiency. This is of limited use in chronic conditions such as organ transplantation or HIV where the emphasis is on managing the condition to minimise immunodeficiency. With advances in medical science the prognosis for these patients is now much improved. There is evidence to suggest that more patients with HIV now die from toxicity associated with the anti-retroviral therapy than the disease itself, and that managing this is the next big challenge. Comorbidities, such as secondary infections, are a major cause for concern and account for a high proportion of deaths in SID patients. As with PIDs, high community vaccine rates and herd immunity are vital to prevent transmission of common diseases to immunocompromised individuals, who cannot be vaccinated.

How many People are affected by Immunodeficiency?

No figures exist for the total number of people affected by all individual PID and SID disorders but some estimates are as follows:

- Around 6 million people live with a PID worldwide but between 70-90% are undiagnosed.
- Around 5,000 individuals in the UK are thought to have a PID disorder.
- According to the NHS there were 39,000 PID-related hospital admissions in England in 2014-2015.
- Up to 50% of the poorest communities in the developing world are affected by malnutrition-related SID disorders.
- There were around 100,000 patients with HIV in the UK in 2015, of which 96% are on treatment.
- Around 600 UK deaths were attributed to HIV/AIDS in 2015.
- According to the NHS there were 15,000 HIV-related hospital admissions in England in 2014-2015.

Although the numbers of people affected by these illnesses are relatively small, the specialist nature of their care and the risk of severe complications add up to a significant cost-burden for their treatment. For example, delayed diagnosis of SCID in infants can result in treatment costs of well over $1million (USD) per patient. Diagnosis before 3.5 months of age could reduce costs to $50,000 (USD) per child, as recurrent infections are prevented. Estimates of transplant patient numbers are not available but over 4 million prescriptions for immunosuppressant drugs were dispensed in England during 2015 at a cost of £220 million.

Importance of Supporting Immunodeficiency Research

Primary immunodeficiencies are rare but can be extremely serious, and a PID diagnosis is life-changing for both the young child affected and their families. Current therapies provide some management of the condition but patients may remain susceptible to severe, recurrent infections. Novel therapies such as gene therapy represent an opportunity to fix the faulty gene responsible and allow these children the chance to have a normal life. Gene therapy is currently offered for a small number of immunodeficiency conditions, but with further research it is hoped that the therapy can be offered to more patients in the coming years. The technique involves replacing a mutated copy of the gene with a healthy copy in stem cells isolated from the patient, which are then transfused back into the body – a process known as autologous stem cell transplantation. Results from a recent trial of this technique in a SCID disorder show 100% survival rates at 7 years post-treatment, compared with 85% survival in patients receiving a stem cell transplant from a healthy sibling. However, a major limitation of this technique is that the vector carrying the healthy copy of the gene is inserted randomly, sometimes close to genes that have the potential to cause cancer. Therefore, in some cases the process of inserting the healthy gene can increase the activity of cancer-linked genes, leading to tumour formation.

Use of gene therapy in conjunction with a new genome-editing technology, CRISPR/Cas9, would allow the specific insertion of the healthy gene into sites in the genome that are known to be located far away from cancer-linked genes, reducing the risk of tumour formation. The first UK license for CRISPR/Cas9 use in editing genes in human embryos was granted in 2016, and CRISPR-edited cells to treat lung cancer were administered in the world's first human trials for the technique by a Chinese group in late 2016. This technology is still in the early stages of development and continued research is vital in order to translate the technology into the clinic for PID gene therapy as soon as possible.

Secondary immunodeficiencies are more common and some of the primary causes of them are global health issues. While immunological research will not solve SID issues related to malnutrition, further research into HIV/AIDS prevention and treatment is essential to reducing the impact of this devastating disorder, particularly in the developing world. Anti-retroviral therapy has been very successful in reducing mortality from HIV/AIDS but relies on the patient taking an oral dose every day. There are myriad reasons why access to reliable supplies of anti-retroviral therapy may not be possible in the developing world, and HIV patients in the developed world are not immune from forgetting to take their daily dose. Non-compliance in teenagers and young adults is particularly high, with around 40-50% of adolescents and young adults not adhering to the therapy regimen in Europe and the USA. Research into long-acting anti-retroviral therapy represents an exciting opportunity to tackle these issues and reduce the global burden of HIV related secondary immunodeficiency.

Immunosuppression

Immunosuppression means that your immune system is not functioning as it should. This can be caused by disease, but it is more often induced by medications such as chemotherapy and immunosuppressant. Some procedures can cause immunosuppression too.

The immune system is the collection of all the cells, tissues, and organs that help the body stave off infection. Without an intact immune system, infections can become very aggressive, and may even be fatal. Immunosuppression also increases the risk of cancer, because the immune system helps protect the body from cancer.

Common Causes

There are a number of medications that reduce inflammation or suppress the immune system. Immunosuppressant are used for treating a variety of inflammatory and autoimmune diseases, such as lupus and arthritis. Human immunodeficiency virus (HIV) can cause AIDS, another cause of immunosuppression.

Corticosteroids

Because steroids reduce inflammation, they are prescribed for a variety of autoimmune, allergic, and inflammatory conditions, such as rheumatoid arthritis, inflammatory bowel disease, asthma, and atopy. Taking a high dose of steroids makes you susceptible to infections from a variety of organisms, such as Pneumocystis jirovecii, which causes deadly Pneumocystis pneumonia, and well as Strongyloides, a potentially deadly roundworm infection. Corticosteroids can also increase the risk of reactivation of tuberculosis or other latent infections.

Chemotherapeutic Agents

Chemotherapy is used to shrink cancer cells. There are a number of different chemotherapeutic medications. Sometimes, treatment of cancer requires a combination of several different chemotherapeutic agents. Cancer cells rapidly reproduce, and chemotherapeutic agents work by targeting cells that rapidly reproduce. Hair and skin cells rapidly reproduce, and this is why hair loss is such a common (and visible) side effect of chemotherapy.

Unlike skin cells, immune cells are hidden inside the body. They tend to be substantially reduced during treatment with chemotherapy, resulting in a high risk of infection.

Monoclonal Antibodies

These medications target disease-causing cells in the body. Rituximab is an example of a monoclonal antibody used to treat non-Hodgkin lymphoma, rheumatoid arthritis, and chronic lymphocytic leukemia. It is linked to rare illnesses such as progressive multifocal leukoencephalopathy (PML), which is caused by JC virus, and pure red cell aplasia, which is associated with parvovirus infection. Furthermore, immunosuppression secondary to rituximab administration can lead to reactivation of hepatitis B infection.

Tumor Necrosis Factor-alpha (TNF-α) Inhibitors

These medications are cytokines; cytokines are usually produced by immune cells. TNF-α inhibitors include drugs like infliximab and certolizumab pegol and are used to treat autoimmune conditions like rheumatoid arthritis and Crohn's disease. Of note, immunosuppression resulting from the administration of these drugs opens the door to infection with Listeria monocytogenes, a foodborne pathogen that can cause fetal death in pregnant women.

Human Immunodeficiency Virus (HIV)

HIV is a virus that can be transmitted by sexual contact, intravenous (IV) drug use with contaminated needles, or from a pregnant mother to her infant. The virus may destroy a large number of immune cells called helper T cells, which are necessary to mount an immune response.

The progression of HIV to AIDS is marked by severe immunocompromise. Once the infection advances to the AIDS stage, a person can develop opportunistic infections, including:

- Candidiasis
- Coccidioidomycosis
- Cryptococcosis
- Cytomegalovirus disease
- Encephalopathy, HIV-related
- Herpes simplex
- Histoplasmosis
- Kaposi's sarcoma (a type of cancer)
- Tuberculosis
- Pneumocystis carinii pneumonia
- Toxoplasmosis of brain

Medical and Surgical Procedures

There are several procedures that result in immunosuppression, either directly or indirectly. Removal of the spleen, bone marrow ablation, and organ transplant are all associated with immunosuppression.

Asplenia

Asplenia, the loss of splenic function, can occur due to conditions like sickle cell anemia, which can damage the spleen. Surgical removal of the spleen, called splenectomy, may be necessary for treatment of cancer, trauma, or blood disorders (like refractory idiopathic thrombotic purpura).

People with asplenia are at increased risk of infection with encapsulated organisms, such as Streptococcus pneumoniae, Haemophilus influenzae, and some forms of Neisseria meningitides. These infections are more likely to occur within the first few years of developing asplenia or of having a splenectomy.

Post Organ Transplant

After receiving a solid organ transplant, such as a kidney, liver, heart, or pancreas, lifelong treatment with immunosuppressant medications is needed to decrease the risk of rejecting the organ.

During the first few months after an organ transplant, infections related to the surgery itself can develop. Common infections during this period include urinary tract infections, skin infections, and wound infections, as well as reactivation of herpes virus or other latent infections.

Six months after transplant and beyond, recipients are most susceptible to community-acquired infections like those caused by encapsulated organisms such as Streptococcus pneumoniae and Haemophilus influenzae.

Bone Marrow Ablation

Prior to a stem cell transplant, a bone marrow transplant, or treatment for leukemia or lymphoma, the suppression of the cells in the bone marrow involves the use of radiation or powerful medications. The immune system becomes very weak during this time, and there is a high risk of infection.

Radiation Therapy

Radiation can be used as a treatment for cancer, or as preparation for certain procedures, such as bone marrow transplant. Radiation therapy can be targeted to certain areas of the body, so it does not always result in immunosuppression. However, radiation targeted to the bone marrow results in immunosuppression.

Genetics

Inherited immune diseases, called primary immunodeficiencies, are rare. These conditions, such as severe combined immunodeficiency and chronic granulomatous disease, are diagnosed at an early age. Common variable immunodeficiency (CVID) and immunoglobulin A deficiency may begin to cause infections during adolescence and young adulthood, with a later diagnosis.

With CVID, the immune cells fail to produce immunoglobulins necessary to mount an immune response. Consequently, people with CVID are more likely to suffer from respiratory infections as well as infections of the gastrointestinal system like Giardia lamblia.

The treatment of CVID is complicated and requires specialist care in part because people with this condition don't respond to immunization and instead require an infusion of immunoglobulin in a hospital setting.

Advice

Chemotherapy, HIV, and bone marrow ablation are examples of severe immunosuppression that can make a person susceptible to fatal infections. If you have any of these types of immunosuppression, you need to avoid contact with people who could carry contagious illnesses, such as schoolchildren and toddlers. You may need to avoid public places or wear a mask when out in public to protect yourself from common community infections.

There are several other causes of milder immunosuppression, such as malnutrition, cytomegalovirus (CMV) infection, alcoholism, diabetes, and kidney failure. Having a suppressed immune system can expose you to more frequent infections which may take longer than usual to recover from.

Autoimmunity

Autoimmune disorders result from a breakdown of immunologic tolerance leading to an immune response against self-molecules. In most instances the events that initiate the immune response to self-molecules are unknown, but a number of studies suggest associations with environmental and genetic factors and certain types of infections. Approximately 3% of the populations in Europe and North America currently suffer from autoimmune diseases, many with symptoms of multiple disorders. This may be an underestimate, as epidemiologic studies are not available for some of the less common diseases. In addition, there are suggestions that a number of common health problems such as atherosclerosis and inflammatory bowel disease may have an autoimmune component. Women have a significantly higher risk of developing an autoimmune disease than men, as > 75% of those suffering from autoimmune diseases is female. Young, postpubescent women have been shown to be approximately 10 times more susceptible than men to developing autoimmune disease. Although the underlying mechanisms for this predisposition are currently being investigated, it is known that females and castrated males produce much higher levels of estrogen and reduced levels of testosterone, and it is well documented that estrogen and estrogenlike chemicals may alter the immune response. Much of the evidence supporting a role for estrogen in the development of autoimmune diseases comes from animal models rather than human studies. In autoimmune prone mice, estrogen administration greatly enhances mortality in both males and females. Testosterone is found in much higher levels in sexually functionally males. Recent studies have found that testosterone given to lupus-prone autoimmune mice exerts a powerful suppressive effect on this disorder in both adult and prenatally treated animals, and male autoimmune MRL/Ipr mice exhibit abnormally low testosterone levels.

Autoimmune Diseases

Autoimmune disorders are a spectrum of diseases ranging from organ specific, in which antibodies and T cells react to self-antigens localized in a specific tissue, to systemic, which are characterized by reactivity against a specific antigen or antigens spread throughout various tissues in the body. In general, ThI cytokines such as IL-2 and IFN-y predominate in organ-specific diseases, and the effector responses tend to occur via cell-mediated immune responses such as killing by cytotoxic T cells through the release of cytokines or through IgG and IgM antibodies directed toward cell-surface antigens, triggering Fc receptor-mediated killing. Systemic autoimmune disorders are characterized by elevated levels of Th2 cytokines such as IL-4, IL-5, and IL-10, the widespread circulation of autoantibodies and immune complex deposition, opsonization with antibody, and cell damage via complement-mediated lysis. Some autoimmune syndromes such as multiple sclerosis are not easily classified, as they demonstrate both organ-specific and systemic components. The most common targets for organ-specific autoimmune disease are the thyroid (Hashimoto thyroiditis, thyrotoxicosis), stomach (pernicious anemia, autoimmune atrophic gastritis), adrenal glands (Addison disease), and pancreas (type I or insulindependent diabetes mellitus [IDDM]). Systemic autoimmune disorders commonly involve the skin (scleroderma), the joints (rheumatoid arthritis), and the muscle tissue (idiopathic inflammatory myopathies [IIM]). In many instances multiple autoimmune diseases may occur in the same patient, and certain diseases are sometimes associated, such as IIM and vasculitis or rheumatoid arthritis and systemic lupus erythematosus (SLE).

Table: Spectrum of autoimmune diseases and putative autoantigens.

	Disease	Autoantigen
Organ specific	Hashimoto thyroiditis	Thyroglobulin
	Thyrotoxicosis	Thyroid-stimulating hormone
	Pernicious anemia	H'/K' -ATPase
	Autoimmune atropic gastritis	Intrinsic factor
	Addison disease	21-Hydroxylase
	Insulin-dependent diabetes mellitus	Glutamic acid decarboxylase 65
	Goodpasture syndrome	Type IV collagen
	Myasthenia gravis	Acetylcholine receptor
	Male infertility(few cases)	Epididymal glycoprotein FA-1
	Sympathetic opthalmia	Interphotoreceptor retinol binding protein
	Multiple sclerosis	Myelin basic protein
	Autoimmune hemolytic anemia	X antigen, glycophorin
	Ulcerative colitis	Catalase, α-enolase
	Rheumatoid arthritis	Rheumatoid factor
	Scleroderma	Topoisomerase 1, laminins
Non-organ specific	Systemic lupus erythematosus	DNA nucleotides and histones. Sm-RNP

In recent years it has been recognized that many other diseases in a variety of target organs/tissues may have an autoimmune component. In general, the etiology of these diseases is not well understood, and multiple factors such as genetics, infectious agents, and lifestyle may contribute in some fashion to disease induction and progression. There is significant evidence that an immune response to self-antigens is involved in atherosclerosis. Increased levels of autoantibodies to heat shock protein 65/60, gangliosides, and oxidized low-density lipoproteins have been demonstrated in atherosclerotic lesions. The role of heat shock protein 65/60 as a candidate autoantigen is supported by animal studies in which immunization with this antigen led to the development of atheroslcerotic lesions in rabbit aorta. In addition, elevated levels of MHC class II expression and increased production of growth-promoting and chemotactic cytokines have been shown in atherosclerotic plaques. There is also evidence for an autoimmune pathology in schizophrenia, with immunologic abnormalities, such as increased prevalence of antinuclear and platelet-associated antibodies, altered cytokine production, and increased levels of soluble cytokine receptors being reported. Abnormal antibody production and autoimmunity have also been implicated in both male and female infertility and are associated with recurrent spontaneous abortion, endometriosis, premature ovarian failure, and abnormal sperm maturation.

Mechanisms of Autoimmune Disease

A small number of autoreactive B and T cells constitute a normal part of the immune cell pool, as the production of autoantibodies is frequently observed in normal healthy individuals. Tolerance is normally maintained by the regulatory interactions of a variety of cell types and soluble mediators. However, under certain conditions, tolerance can be broken and an autoimmune pathology may result. It is apparent that development of autoimmune disease is highly dependent on a permissive genetic background but that other triggering factors such as viral, bacterial, or chemical insult lead to altered self-reactivity. This section is meant to introduce the reader to several of the hypotheses regarding the role that genetics and environmental factors may play in breaking down the barrier to reactivity with self-antigens.

Release of Isolated Autoantigens

T cells reactive to self-antigens not present in the thymus during the early stages of T-cell development may escape thymic deletion. These antigens (cryptic or hidden antigens) generally have relatively low circulating levels or are anatomically sequestered in specific tissues (e.g., myelin basic protein or thyroglobulin) where vascular and cellular basement membranes constitute an effective barrier that prevents access by autoreactive cells. Induction of organ-specific autoimmune disease following tissue trauma has been frequently reported and likely occurs via tissue damage that results in the availability of previously isolated antigens, as is the case in ophthalmia following eye injury or orchiditis following vasectomy. Infection with tissue-tropic pathogens such as viruses may induce similar autoimmune phenomenon, and these infections also provide the additional stimulus of the production of soluble mediators and costimulatory molecules important in the perpetuation of the immune response. This may be best exemplified in rodents and humans who develop diabetes after infection with Coxsackie B viruses.

Chemical Alteration of Self-peptides

T lymphocytes that bind with low affinity to self-proteins in the thymus may not be deleted. However, these T cells are normally functionally anergized in the periphery. Responses to and presentation of these cryptic self-peptides can be enhanced under certain conditions. In a murine model of IDDM, viral infection stimulates the secretion of IFN-y, which in turn upregulates levels of antigen-presenting MHC molecules and enhances presentation of low-affinity selfpeptides. Some metals induce autoimmune disease via the creation of new high-affinity binding sites for MHC molecules on chemical-bound self-peptides, allowing activation of previously anergized T cells. Expression of altered nucleolar proteins appears to be an important step in the development of mercuric chloride ($HgCl_2$) - induced autoimmunity in a rodent model of SLE. In addition, many drugs induce autoimmunity via formation of hapteninduced autoantibodies. Compounds such as penicillin and halothane induce reactions in which hapten-specific T cells provide help to antibody-producing B cells that recognize the modified hapten but not the native form of the self-protein.

Molecular Mimicry

Many peptide fragments of infectious agents are homologous with host proteins and induce organ-specific autoimmune responses. A membrane protein on the P-hemolytic streptococcus bacterium has a high degree of homology with cardiac myosin, and antibodies that target the bacterium also cross-react with cardiac muscle and induces rheumatic fever. Yersinia enterocolitica, a bacterium normally associated with food poisoning outbreaks, has also been associated with various autoimmune diseases. Increased levels of antibodies to Yersinia have been demonstrated in patients with Graves' disease or autoimmune thyroiditis. These antibodies cross-react with a variety of thyroid antigens.

Polycoial Acivators

Microbial antigens have also been implicated in the precipitation and exacerbation of systemic autoimmune diseases. Exogenous polyclonal activators may mutually stimulate T cells that react with both MHC class IIbound superantigens (peptides that activate large numbers of Th cells, promoting cytokine overproduction) on B cells and the B cells them, leading to the production of polyclonal Ig, some of which may be autoreactive. Mycoplasma arthriditis superantigen stimulates cytokine production and upregulates MHC class II expression in human T cell lines and stimulates T lymphocytes with arthritis-associated TCR-P chains. In a rodent model, Mycoplasma arthriditis superantigen stimulated Th cells, resulting in polyclonal B-cell activation and differentiation of antigenspecific B cells.

Genetic Factors

Familial studies suggest a clear association between genetics and autoimmune diseases, particularly those with an organ-specific pathology. Further, although concordance rates between identical twins can be relatively low depending on the disease, this may be explained by nonidentity in immune repertoires because of TCR and Ig gene recombination, variations in receptor assembly, and somatic mutation of B-cell receptors. The most clearly established genetic association is with specific alleles within the MHC gene complex. Certain haplotypes (HLA-B8, DR2-DR5) tend to be associated with certain autoimmune diseases. However, a specific MHC haplotype is not sufficient for development of autoimmune disease, and autoimmunity-associated haplotypes are found in individuals with no clinical signs of disease.

Table: Experimental models for autoimmune diseases.

Autoimmune disease	Classification		
	Organic or chemical induction	Autoimmunization	Genetically pre-disposed strains
Autoimmune thyroiditis		Thyroglobulin – experimental autoimmune thyroiditis (m,r)	MRL (m)
			BB (r)
Insulin-dependent diabetes mellitus	Streptozotocin (m)		OS (ch)
			NOD (m)
			BB (r)
			DRBB (r)
			BN (r)
Myasthenia gravis	Penicillamine (m,r)	Acetylcholine receptor - experimental autoimmune myasthenia gravis (m,r)	
Multiple sclerosis		Myelin basic protein - experimental autoimmune encephalomyelitis (m,r,ch)	
Rheumatoid arthritis	Streptococcal cell wall (r)	CFA + type 11 collagen (m,r,mo) CFA + mycobacterium heat shock protein (m,r)	MRL/Ipr(m)
			SCID (m)
			HLA B27 (r)
Systemic lupus erythematosus	Mercury (m,r,mo)	CFA + anti-DNA antibodies (m,r)	MRL +/+ (m)
	Penicillamine (m,r)		MRL-mp-lpr/lpr (m)
	Procainamide (m,r)		NZW 2410 (m)
			NZB/NZW (m
			TSK (m)
Systemic sclerosis (scleroderma)			

There are also a number of non-MHC genes that may contribute to autoimmunity. Many studies have examined the possibility that predisposition for certain autoimmune diseases in the human population may lie in the germline genes for the TCR. The strongest evidence for TCR involvement comes from studies of sibling pairs with recurrent/relapsing multiple sclerosis. Siblings with multiple sclerosis shared specific TCR-j3 haplotypes at a frequency much higher than would be expected because of random segregation. TCR-ax gene polymorphisms have also been associated with disease susceptibility.

Animal Models of Autoimmune Disease

Three basic types of animal models may be employed to identify the potential of environmental agents to induce autoimmune responses: a) organic- or chemical-induced, b) autoimmunization, or c) genetically predisposed animals.

In models where autoimmunity is induced by exposure to chemical or biologicagents, foreign substances are used to initiate the autoimmune disease state. These may indude chemicals, drugs, or biologic substances such as bacterial or viral antigens. One of the more commonly employed models of this type is the Brown Norway rat model, in which the animals are injected with nontoxic amounts of $HgCl_2$. The chemical exposure produces no overt signs of toxicity, yet the rats develop an immunologically mediated disease characterized by T-cell-dependent polyclonal B-cell activation, autoantibodies to laminin, collagen IV and other components of the glomerular basement membrane, and nephrotic syndrome with proteinuria similar to that observed in humans with autoimmune glomerulonephritis.

Autoimmunization with purified selfantigens can elicit a specific autoimmune response, particularly when adjuvants are administered in conjunction with selfproteins. A frequently used model of this type-experimental autoimmune encephalomyelitis-is induced by immunization of rodents with myelin basic protein with Freund's complete adjuvant. The resulting pathology is a Th-cell-mediated autoimmune disease characterized by central nervous system perivascular lymphocyte infiltration and destruction of the myelin nerve sheath with resultant paralysis similar to that observed in patients with multiple sclerosis.

The genetically predisposed models, whether naturally occurring, transgenic, or knockout based, tend to be the most reliable and therefore have been more commonly employed in autoimmunity research. In these models, mild to severe syndromes spontaneously develop, usually because of specific MHC allele mutations encoding class II molecules and often inducing functional abnormalities of the Th cell.

In each type of model the development and severity of symptoms have multiple components in that the presence of the disease and its progression can be influenced by age, hormonal, and/or environmental factors. In addition, there is a tendency for more than one autoimmune disorder to occur in several of the individual models. Nevertheless, a number of syndromes similar to those clinically observed in humans can be mimicked in animal models.

Permissions

Index